Textbook of

Gastroenterology

SELF-ASSESSMENT REVIEW

Third Edition

Textbook of

Gastroenterology

SELF-ASSESSMENT REVIEW

Third Edition

Editor

TADATAKA YAMADA

Special Editor

WILLIAM D. CHEY

Associate Editors
DAVID H. ALPERS
LOREN LAINE
CHUNG OWYANG
DON W. POWELL

Section Editors
MICHELLE A. ANDERSON
JEFFREY L. BARNETT
LAUREL R. FISHER
JOHN M. INADOMI
HYE-RANG KIM
KENNETH S. LOWN
TIMOTHY T. NOSTRANT
ELLEN M. ZIMMERMANN

LIPPINCOTT WILLIAMS & WILKINS
A **Wolters Kluwer** Company
Philadelphia • Baltimore • New York • London
Buenos Aires • Hong Kong • Sydney • Tokyo

Acquisitions Editor: Beth Barry
Production Editor: John C. Vassiliou
Manufacturing Manager: Benjamin Rivera
Cover Designer: Christine Jenny
Compositor: Circle Graphics
Printer: Edwards Brothers

Library of Congress Cataloging-in-Publication Data

Textbook of gastroenterology : self-assessment review / editor, Tadataka Yamada ;
special editor, William D. Chey ; associate editors, David H. Alpers . . . [et al.] ; section
editors, Timothy T. Nostrant . . . [et al.].—3rd ed.
   p. ; cm.
   ISBN 0-7817-2056-7
   1. Gastroenterology—Examinations, questions, etc. I. Yamada, Tadataka.
   [DNLM: 1. Gastrointestinal Diseases—Examination Questions. WI 140 T3551 1999 Suppl.]
RC801.T48 1999 Suppl.
618.3′3′0076—dc21

                                                      00-042440

---

10 9 8 7 6 5 4 3 2 1

CONTENTS

CONTRIBUTING AUTHORS

EDITOR

Tadataka Yamada, M.D.
Adjunct Professor
Departments of Internal Medicine and Physiology
University of Michigan Health System
Ann Arbor, Michigan

SPECIAL EDITOR

William D. Chey, M.D.
Assistant Professor of Internal Medicine
Division of Gastroenterology
University of Michigan Health System
Ann Arbor, Michigan

ASSOCIATE EDITORS

David H. Alpers, M.D.
William B. Kountz Professor of Medicine
Washington University School of Medicine
St. Louis, Missouri

Loren Laine, M.D.
Professor of Medicine
University of Southern California School of
*   Medicine; and*
Chief, Gastroenterology Section
Los Angeles County and University of Southern
*   California Medical Center*
Los Angeles, California

Chung Owyang, M.D.
Professor of Internal Medicine
H. Marvin Pollard Collegiate Professor of
*   Gastroenterology; and*
Chief, Division of Gastroenterology
University of Michigan Health System
Ann Arbor, Michigan

Don W. Powell, M.D.
Edward Randall and Edward Randall Jr.
*   Distinguished Chairman and Professor of*
*   Internal Medicine*
Professor of Physiology and Biophysics
The University of Texas Medical Branch at
*   Galveston*
Galveston, Texas

SECTION EDITORS

Michelle A. Anderson, M.D.
Lecturer of Internal Medicine
Division of Gastroenterology
University of Michigan Health System
Ann Arbor, Michigan

Jeffrey L. Barnett, M.D.
Associate Professor of Internal Medicine
Division of Gastroenterology
University of Michigan Health System
Ann Arbor, Michigan

Laurel R. Fisher, M.D.
Clinical Instructor of Internal Medicine
Division of Gastroenterology
University of Michigan Health System
Ann Arbor, Michigan

John M. Inadomi, M.D.
Assistant Professor of Internal Medicine
Division of Gastroenterology
Ann Arbor Veterans Affairs Medical Center
University of Michigan Health System
Ann Arbor, Michigan

Hye-Rang Kim, M.D., Ph.D.
Research Fellow of Internal Medicine
Division of Gastroenterology
University of Michigan Health System
Ann Arbor, Michigan

Kenneth S. Lown, M.D.
Assistant Professor of Internal Medicine
Division of Gastroenterology
University of Michigan Health System
Ann Arbor, Michigan

Timothy T. Nostrant, M.D.
Professor of Internal Medicine
Division of Gastroenterology
University of Michigan Health System
Ann Arbor, Michigan

Ellen M. Zimmermann, M.D.
Assistant Professor of Internal Medicine
Division of Gastroenterology
University of Michigan Health System
Ann Arbor, Michigan

CONTRIBUTING AUTHORS
Division of Gastroenterology
Department of Internal Medicine
University of Michigan Health System
Ann Arbor, Michigan

Frederick K. Askari, M.D., Ph.D.
Ezra Burstein, M.D.
Manish M. Chokshi, M.D.
John Del Valle, M.D.
Matthew J. Dimagno, M.D.
William L. Hasler, M.D.
Keith S. Henley, M.D.
John Y. Kao, M.D.
Mark D. Marrilley, M.D.
Juanita L. Merchant, M.D., Ph.D.
Kimya-Anchina L. Nguyen, M.D.

Ernest Ofori-Darko, M.D.
Chung Owyang, M.D.
Leonard G. Quallich, M.D.
John C. Rabine, M.D.
Melissa Rich, M.D.
James M. Scheiman, M.D.
Thomas M. Shehab, M.D.
Mimi S. Takami, M.D.
Andrea Todisco, M.D.
D. Kim Turgeon, M.D.
John W. Wiley, M.D.

PREFACE

The *Textbook of Gastroenterology* is a comprehensive and encyclopedic review of the science, technology, and clinical practice of gastroenterology. Its purposes are to teach the scientific basis of gastroenterology, to provide practical approaches to common gastrointestinal problems, to serve as an encyclopedic reference for gastrointestinal diseases, and to indicate the current applications and future directions of the technology of gastroenterology. A useful adjunct to a textbook of this sort is a self-assessment study guide that will permit the reader to focus on specific questions that arise from the reading. Moreover, the demands of the current guidelines for credentialing in gastroenterology include not only examinations for specialty qualification, but also recertification examinations. Thus, we developed the first edition of the *Self-Assessment Review* to assist the student of gastroenterology in assimilating the details of the knowledge presented in the *Textbook of Gastroenterology*.

As we have advanced the knowledge base of the *Textbook of Gastroenterology* in its third edition, so we have had to revise the *Self-Assessment Review*. As in the first edition of the *Review*, the questions are presented in a variety of formats but organized by organ system. Every question presented in the second edition of the *Review* has been reevaluated, and over 40% of the questions in this third edition are new. Although most of the questions focus on clinically relevant issues, knowledge of the pathophysiology of disease in each organ system is required to answer the questions correctly. Each answer is followed by a short comment and a reference to a specific page in the third edition of the *Textbook of Gastroenterology* for further information. For this endeavor, we were greatly assisted by Dr. William D. Chey, who served as the overall editor of this volume, and his associates in the Gastroenterology Division of the Department of Internal Medicine in the University of Michigan Health System. We hope that this *Self-Assessment Review* proves to be a useful adjunct to the *Textbook of Gastroenterology*.

Tadataka Yamada, M.D.

1

Esophagus

MULTIPLE CHOICE

(one best answer)

1. Regarding preparing to swallow, which of the following statements is true?

   a. The bolus passively transfers to the soft palate, where the pharynx is the major propulsive force for bolus movement.
   b. Gravity is more important than peristalsis in the passage of liquids through the esophageal body.
   c. Pharyngeal contraction and upper esophageal sphincter (UES) relaxation occur simultaneously.
   d. UES pressures return to baseline immediately after the bolus passes.

2. Which of the following statements about oropharyngeal swallowing is true?

   a. The entire swallowing cycle takes 3 to 4 seconds to complete.
   b. Closure of the nasopharynx occurs just after the opening of the upper esophageal sphincter.
   c. The pharynx is most important in solid food clearance.
   d. The epiglottal ridge is the most sensitive trigger zone for swallowing.

3. Which of the following statements about the effect of esophageal acid reflux and distention on the upper esophageal sphincter (UES) is true?

   a. The highest increase in UES pressure is induced by distention of the mid esophagus.
   b. Acid induces a lower pressure increase than saline in healthy subjects.
   c. Bilateral blockade of the vagosympathetic trunks abolishes acid-induced increases in UES pressure.
   d. Air distention of the esophagus causes contraction of the UES.

4. Which of the following statements about esophageal peristalsis is true?

   a. It is almost entirely produced by cholinergic excitation.
   b. It is more important in liquid as opposed to solid food movement.
   c. It requires only intact esophageal neurocircuitry for normal function.
   d. It requires nitric oxide–induced relaxation prior to cholinergic excitation.

5. Relaxation of the lower esophageal sphincter (LES) is stimulated by all of the following except:

   a. cholinergic excitatory input
   b. vasoactive intestinal polypeptide (VIP)–induced neural inhibition
   c. central vagal input
   d. nitric oxide–induced LES relaxation increases with 5′-phosphate of guanosine (GMP)

6. Which of the following statements about lower esophageal sphincter (LES) function is true?

   a. Somatostatin increases LES contraction.
   b. Gastrin increases LES relaxation.
   c. Cholecystokinin induces LES relaxation.
   d. Vasoactive intestinal polypeptide (VIP) increases LES contraction.

7. Which of the following statements regarding transient lower esophageal sphincter relaxations (TLESRs) is false?

   a. TLESRs represent the major mechanism by which acid reflux occurs.
   b. TLESRs reduce or obliterate the resting pressure of the lower esophageal sphincter.
   c. Gastric distention increases the frequency of TLESRs.
   d. TLESRs cannot be induced by pharyngeal stimulation.

8. After a cerebrovascular accident (CVA), a 60-year-old man complains of oropharyngeal dysphagia, marked sputum production, and difficulty

swallowing his saliva. Which of the following statements is false?

a. Poor tongue movements and an impaired swallowing reflex are common after a CVA.
b. Cricopharyngeal achalasia is an unlikely possibility.
c. Upper esophageal sphincter relaxation is normal in most patients with this clinical presentation.
d. Esophageal manometry will be more useful than barium studies in this patient.

9. A 57-year-old man who recently received a diagnosis of bronchogenic carcinoma is admitted to the hospital with fever, cough, and pneumonia of the right lower lobe of the lung. The recent onset of oropharyngeal dysphagia suggests aspiration. What is the most likely explanation for his aspiration?

a. unilateral adductor paralysis of the vocal cords with impaired laryngeal closure
b. primary pharyngeal dysfunction resulting from tumor involvement of the recurrent laryngeal nerve
c. soft palate and pharyngeal constrictor dysfunction resulting from metastatic disease
d. metastasis to the medulla

10. A 60-year-old man complains of a 5-year history of cervical dysphagia after the ingestion of both solid and liquid food, regurgitation of undigested food, and halitosis. He shows a bulge in the left side of his neck during eating. Which of the following statements is false?

a. His upper esophageal sphincter probably exhibits reduced compliance.
b. He has at least a 5% chance of having or developing squamous cell carcinoma.
c. Surgery is the treatment of choice.
d. A barium swallow is the initial diagnostic procedure of choice.

11. Each of the following statements regarding a Zenker diverticulum are true except:

a. Zenker diverticula are typically located above the upper esophageal sphincter (UES).
b. Poor coordination between pharyngeal contraction and UES relaxation is believed to be an important predisposing factor.
c. Classic symptoms include cough, postprandial regurgitation, and aspiration.
d. A loss of UES elasticity may restrict the esophageal diameter in this disorder.

12. Which of the following clinical presentations could be most expected to respond well to cricopharyngeal myotomy?

a. poor tongue motion and absence of the swallowing reflex on cinefluoroscopy

b. normal tongue movement, pharyngeal stasis, and a cricopharyngeal bar on cinefluoroscopy
c. dysphagia, a Zenker diverticulum, and normal upper esophageal sphincter (UES) relaxation on barium swallow examination and esophageal manometry
d. globus sensation and normal UES pressures on esophageal manometry

13. A 50-year-old woman presents with a 6-month history of progressive cervical dysphagia. A barium swallow reveals weak contractions of the pharyngeal musculature. Possible physical findings could include all of the following except:

a. sclerodactyly
b. skin rash
c. proximal muscle weakness
d. heliotropic rash

14. A 31-year-old woman presents with a history of dysphagia that has been progressively worsening for years. She reports that initially she had problems only with solid foods, but more recently her ability to consume liquids has become affected as well. She notes frequent episodes of regurgitation of undigested food, a chronic cough, and two episodes of pneumonia over the past year. Which of the following studies will most likely establish the correct diagnosis?

a. upper endoscopy
b. esophageal manometry
c. ambulatory pH monitoring
d. esophageal scintigraphy
e. upper gastrointestinal radiographic series

15. Which of the following statements is true about the treatment of achalasia?

a. Medications decrease lower esophageal sphincter and esophageal body pressures.
b. Sublingual calcium channel blockers are more effective than oral calcium channel blockers.
c. Medications are most effective in healthy patients with a dilated esophagus.
d. Surgery is more cost-effective than pneumatic dilation.

16. Which of the following statements about pseudo-achalasia is correct?

a. Most patients older than 50 who experience the rapid onset of dysphagia and significant weight loss have pseudoachalasia, not primary achalasia.
b. It can be reliably diagnosed by esophageal manometry alone.
c. It is most commonly caused by carcinoma of the gastric antrum.

d. It may be associated with antibodies to enteric neurons.

17. A 20-year-old man presents with a 3-year history of dysphagia. There has been no weight loss, and the patient's nutrition is good. The findings of upper endoscopy and esophageal manometry are consistent with a diagnosis of achalasia. Which of the following statements is true?

a. The risk of esophageal perforation with pneumatic dilation is about 1 in 500.
b. Esophageal dilation must be repeated in fewer than 10% of patients.
c. Heller myotomy affords a good to excellent response in more than 80% of cases.
d. Acid reflux is more common after pneumatic dilation than after surgical myotomy.

18. Which of the following is the best predictor of a prolonged clinical response following pneumatic dilation for achalasia?

a. prompt clinical response in the first days following dilation
b. normal relaxation of the lower esophageal sphincter (LES) on manometry
c. mean LES pressure
d. normal esophageal peristalsis following dilation

19. Which of the following statements about Chagas disease is false?

a. Loss of ganglion cells occurs as a result of infection with the protozoan *Trypanosoma cruzi*.
b. The diagnosis can be confirmed with immune fixation assays.
c. Treatment with benzimidazole is effective, even after the symptoms have become chronic.
d. This diagnosis should be considered in the presence of megacolon or megaduodenum.

20. Which of the following statements regarding spastic motor disorders of the esophagus is true ?

a. Diffuse esophageal spasm is the most common motility disorder documented by manometry.
b. After achalasia is ruled out, nutcracker esophagus is the most common esophageal motor abnormality in patients with dysphagia.
c. A decrease in the amplitude of high-pressure contractions predicts the patient's response to medical treatment.
d. Esophageal motility disorders can improve spontaneously.
e. Many patients have coexistent acid reflux, but reflux rarely causes motility disturbances.

21. A 40-year-old man presents with intermittent and nonprogressive dysphagia to both solid and liquid food. Chest pain and abnormal findings on cardiac evaluation suggest diffuse esophageal spasm. Which of the following findings supports this diagnosis?

a. barium column segmentation is visible on an esophagram
b. simultaneous, nonperistaltic contractions on manometry
c. prolonged (>6 seconds) and high-amplitude (>180 mm Hg) contractions on manometry
d. all of the above

22. Which of the following statements about esophageal dysphagia is true?

a. Localization of esophageal dysphagia symptoms by the patient is often confirmed by endoscopic and radiologic findings.
b. Manometry is the best initial test.
c. Multiple dry swallows inhibit the passage of a bolus through the esophagus.
d. Heartburn in achalasia is produced by hydrochloric acid.
e. Esophageal dilation is helpful in patients with solid food dysphagia and normal findings on upper endoscopy.

23. The treatment of pain from spastic dysmotility syndromes should begin with which of the following substances?

a. nitrates
b. antireflux medications
c. calcium channel blockers
d. anxiolytics

24. A 50-year-old woman complains of solid food dysphagia, pain in her fingertips during cold weather, and difficulty opening her mouth. Which of the following statements is false?

a. Esophageal manometric abnormalities are likely to include body aperistalsis and increased lower esophageal sphincter pressure.
b. Gastroesophageal acid reflux is likely to be present.
c. A stricture of the esophagus must be ruled out.
d. Barrett esophagus with cancer has been reported in this setting.

25. Which of the following statements about food impaction is false?

a. It usually occurs in the setting of underlying esophageal disease.
b. An underlying esophageal stricture should be dilated immediately after disimpaction of the food bolus.
c. An overtube should be used in conjunction with endoscopy when disimpacting a food bolus.
d. A history of prior food impaction is common.

26. Which of the following statements concerning esophageal chest pain is true?

    a. The character of chest pain induced by acid is different from the character of chest pain induced by distention.
    b. The correlation between distinct acid reflux events and chest pain is poor in patients with esophageal chest pain.
    c. Esophageal symptoms are less common after exercise than are cardiac symptoms.
    d. Left arm pain is more common in cardiac-associated pain.

27. A 44-year-old man presents with substernal chest pressure. The discomfort is not exercise-induced and the patient has a completely normal gastrointestinal history. The findings from a cardiac evaluation which included stress echocardiography and cardiac catheterization are normal. Which of the following statements is true?

    a. The next best diagnostic test is upper endoscopy.
    b. This history is highly predictive of an abnormal finding on esophageal manometry.
    c. This condition is best diagnosed by observing the patient's response to an empiric trial of standard doses of H_2-receptor antagonists.
    d. This condition may be produced by a combination of a decreased pain threshold and an increased esophageal contractility.

28. Which of the following statements regarding the psychologic profiles of patients with noncardiac chest pain (NCCP) is false?

    a. Psychologic stress is associated with higher acid reflux scores in patients with NCCP.
    b. Patients with NCCP and patients with irritable bowel syndrome have similar levels of somatic anxiety on standardized testing.
    c. Patients with chest pain and nutcracker esophagus have higher levels of somatic anxiety than patients with esophageal rings and esophagitis.
    d. Anxiety disorders, panic attacks, and neuroticism are more common in patients with NCCP than in hospitalized patients without chest pain.

29. All of the following statements concerning provocation testing for chest pain are true except:

    a. The diagnostic yield is low even if all test types are used.
    b. A positive result from a Bernstein test predicts gastroesophageal reflux.
    c. Ambulatory testing during chest pain predicts the cause better than elective testing.
    d. Pain produced by balloon distention is severe in patients with acid sensitivity.

30. All of the following statements about intraesophageal balloon tests are true except:

    a. Commercial balloons are not available.
    b. Pain thresholds are higher in women than men.
    c. Pain occurs at lower levels of distention in patients with chest pain.
    d. Balloon distention reproduces pain in more patients with noncardiac chest pain than does acid infusion or edrophonium.

31. A 40-year-old man presents with episodic chest pressure. The findings of a cardiac evaluation that included cardiac catheterization are normal. The patient denies experiencing heartburn or regurgitation. Which of the following statements is true?

    a. Mortality rates from cardiac disease in this patient population are greater than in the general population.
    b. Normal findings on upper endoscopy rule out gastroesophageal reflux–induced pain.
    c. Esophageal dysmotility is an unlikely cause of the chest pain if baseline esophageal motility is normal.
    d. Ambulatory 24-hour pH monitoring of the esophagus is likely to be the most useful test in the diagnostic evaluation of this patient.
    e. Balloon distention– or acid infusion–induced pain define an esophageal source of the chest pain.

32. Risk factors for gastroesophageal reflux disease include all of the following except:

    a. *Helicobacter pylori* infection
    b. male
    c. obesity
    d. hiatal hernia

33. Symptoms often associated with gastroesophageal reflux disease include all of these except:

    a. water brash
    b. dysphagia involving solid food
    c. regurgitation during sleep
    d. odynophagia
    e. atypical chest pain

34. Which of the following diagnostic studies has the highest sensitivity and specificity for gastroesophageal reflux disease?

    a. upper endoscopy
    b. barium esophagram
    c. empiric trial of a proton pump inhibitor
    d. radionuclide scintiscanning

35. Which of the following statements concerning hiatal hernias and gastroesophageal reflux disease (GERD) is true?

a. Most patients with GERD have a hiatal hernia.

b. A hiatal hernia occurring together with erosive esophagitis is rare.

c. Poor acid clearance is a feature in patients with a hiatal hernia and GERD.

d. Hiatal hernias decrease the frequency of transient lower esophageal sphincter relaxations.

36. Which of the following statements about reflux laryngitis is true?

    a. It most commonly affects the anterior laryngeal surface.
    b. It occurs with distal acid reflux only.
    c. It can go undetected by current acid monitoring technologies.
    d. It is caused by poor acid clearance from the pharynx.

37. Esophageal bougienage of peptic strictures is least likely to induce perforation at which of the following sites?

    a. cervical esophagus
    b. thoracic esophagus above the stricture
    c. the stricture itself
    d. for midesophageal strictures, a site distal to the stricture

38. All of the following statements about Barrett esophagus are true except:

    a. It is the most common precursor lesion for esophageal adenocarcinoma.
    b. It is less common in patients who are infected with *Helicobacter pylori.*
    c. It is discovered more frequently at autopsy than at endoscopy.
    d. Effective treatment to completely remove Barrett epithelium will decrease mortality from esophageal adenocarcinoma.

39. Which of the following statements about Barrett esophagus is false?

    a. Barrett esophagus occurs more frequently in white males.
    b. Up to one-third of patients report no symptoms at the time of diagnosis of Barrett esophagus.
    c. The histologic subtype of Barrett esophagus with the highest risk for development of adenocarcinoma is gastric metaplasia.
    d. The estimated lifetime risk for the development of esophageal cancer in patients with Barrett esophagus is approximately 1%.

40. All of the following statements about Barrett esophagus are false except:

a. Barrett esophagus is a premalignant condition if columnar epithelium is present.

b. Alcohol and cigarette smoking are key risk factors in the development of Barrett epithelium

c. Barrett esophagus typically affects white women older than 55.

d. Barrett esophagus is no more common in *Helicobacter pylori*–infected persons than in persons not infected with *H pylori.*

41. The most important prognostic finding of endoscopic ultrasonography in managing esophageal cancer is:

    a. a T3 lesion
    b. malignant-appearing nodes at the tumor site
    c. a tumor abutting the aorta
    d. positive celiac axis lymph nodes

42. A benign stricture of the esophagus can be differentiated from carcinoma of the esophagus in the following way:

    a. Benign strictures produce intermittent dysphagia.
    b. Benign strictures rarely produce progressive symptoms.
    c. Benign strictures, unlike esophageal carcinoma, are typically associated with heartburn.
    d. The two diagnoses can be reliably differentiated by radiographic evaluation.
    e. none of the above

43. Endoscopic ultrasonography is more sensitive and specific for the staging of esophageal malignancy with respect to all of the following criteria except:

    a. depth of invasion into the esophageal wall
    b. local and celiac lymph node involvement
    c. invasion into surrounding vascular structures
    d. hepatic metastases

44. What is the correct esophageal stent length for treating malignant lesions?

    a. long enough to traverse the lower esophageal sphincter
    b. 1 to 2 cm longer than the tumor
    c. 3 to 4 cm longer than the tumor
    d. none of the above

45. A Maloney dilator may be blindly passed to dilate each of the following lesions except:

    a. lower esophageal rings
    b. esophageal webs
    c. short, 12-mm diameter peptic strictures
    d. long, 10-mm diameter peptic strictures

46. Risk factors for the development of squamous cell carcinoma include all of the following except:

    a. alcohol and tobacco
    b. celiac sprue

c. diet high in acidic fruit juices

d. Asian heritage

47. All of the following statements about tylosis are true except:

a. About 50% of patients with tylosis will develop esophageal cancer by age 45.

b. Tylosis is associated with oral leukoplakia.

c. It is an autosomal recessive disorder.

d. It is characterized by hyperkeratosis of the palms and soles.

e. Tylosis is linked to a locus on chromosome 17q.

48. All of the following statements about cancer of the gastroesophageal junction are true except:

a. Barrett esophagus is the most common preceding event.

b. *Helicobactor pylori* infection is less common in patients with cancer of the gastroesophageal junction than in controls.

c. Risk factors for gastroesophageal reflux disease are more common.

d. Women and men have an equal risk.

49. Which of the following statements about photo-dynamic therapy is not true?

a. Photodynamic therapy requires photoradiation to activate a previously administered photo-sensitizer.

b. It may be complicated by sunburn or eye damage for 48 to 72 hours after treatment.

c. It is contraindicated in patients with esophageal pulmonary fistulas secondary to tumor.

d. Photodynamic therapy may be used to palliate esophageal cancer.

50. Which of the following statements about radiation-induced esophageal injury is true?

a. Doses of 20 Gy consistently induce damage.

b. Radiation of esophageal cancer before stenting increases the risk of perforation after esophageal stenting.

c. Radiation-induced dysphagia typically presents in the first year after radiation of the esophagus.

d. Hemorrhage and perforation are early complications of radiation therapy.

51. Which of the following statements regarding radiation-induced esophagitis is not true?

a. Chemotherapy potentiates radiation injury.

b. Fibrosing esophagitis usually occurs at the time of radiation treatment.

c. The development of severe esophagitis usually requires radiation doses of at least 50 Gy.

d. The esophagus is one of the most radioresistant gastrointestinal organs.

52. Which statement about medication-induced esophagitis is most accurate?

a. Most affected patients have an underlying esophageal disorder.

b. Common medications that cause medication-induced esophagitis include cimetidine and prednisone.

c. Esophageal transit time is longer for oval tablets than for round tablets.

d. The onset of symptoms can be delayed for weeks after ingestion of the medication.

53. Which statement about medication-induced esophagitis is incorrect?

a. Direct mucosal contact is the mechanism of non-steroidal antiinflammatory drug–induced esophageal damage.

b. Underlying esophageal dysmotility disorders or strictures increase the risk for esophagitis.

c. Antibiotics are the most frequent cause of medication-induced esophagitis.

d. The best way to prevent medication-induced esophagitis is to swallow pills in the upright position and to consume at least 100 mL of fluid at the same time.

54. Which of the following is not a risk factor for hemorrhage from esophageal varices?

a. an elevation in portal vein pressure of 10 mm Hg

b. variceal size

c. the severity of the underlying cirrhosis (e.g., a Child classification)

d. red wale markings on the varix wall

55. Which statement regarding sclerotherapy for esophageal varices is true?

a. Sclerotherapy significantly improves the long-term survival of patients in Child classes B and C.

b. Patients with prior esophageal variceal bleeding who are enrolled in a sclerotherapy program are at significant risk of rebleeding before variceal obliteration is achieved.

c. Sclerotherapy is rarely successful for the control of active variceal bleeding.

d. It is more expensive than surgical shunt therapy for the prevention of rebleeding.

56. Which of the following therapies is contraindicated in the management of a caustic esophageal burn?

a. broad-spectrum antibiotics

b. oral corticosteroids
c. "late" esophageal dilation
d. oral sucralfate
e. neutralizing mild acids or alkalis

57. All of the following statements regarding Boerhaave syndrome are true except:

a. Ninety percent of spontaneous esophageal ruptures occur in the distal esophagus.
b. Acute massive esophageal rupture is characterized by hypotension, pneumothorax, and shock.
c. The Mackler triad of vomiting, chest pain, and subcutaneous emphysema occurs in most patients with spontaneous esophageal rupture.
d. Some patients lack a muscularis mucosae.

58. Which of the following statements regarding Mallory-Weiss tears is incorrect?

a. Up to 50% of patients present without antecedent retching or emesis.
b. Mallory-Weiss tears can occur in both the stomach and the esophagus.
c. Most lesions stop bleeding without invasive treatment.
d. Balloon tamponade is the treatment of choice if bleeding continues.
e. A hiatal hernia is often present.

TRUE/FALSE

The following statements pertain to achalasia:

59. _____ Botulinum toxin is a potent inhibitor of acetylcholine uptake by cholinergic neurons.

60. _____ Age older than 50, severe weight loss, and short duration of symptoms are highly predictive of pseudoachalasia.

61. _____ The primary endoscopic finding in esophagitis caused by the herpes simplex virus is diffuse ulcerative esophagitis.

Candida esophagitis in patients with AIDS

62. _____ is best treated with ketoconazole because it is cheaper than fluconazole and most patients have normal gastric acid secretion

63. _____ is characterized primarily by fever and chest pain

64. _____ should be diagnosed by endoscopy in the absence of oral thrush

Reflux esophagitis

65. _____ is the most common finding in patients with severe heartburn and regurgitation

66. _____ Healing is directly correlated with the percentage of time the gastric pH is greater than 4.

67. _____ is best diagnosed by an empiric trial of acid suppression

The following characteristics (68–71) pertain to gastroesophageal reflux during pregnancy:

68. _____ is most common in the first trimester

69. _____ is most commonly caused by increased intra-abdominal pressure

70. _____ is mediated by high estrogen levels

71. _____ should be initially treated with an H_2-receptor antagonist

72. _____ Upper esophageal sphincter recontraction precedes upper esophageal body contraction.

73. _____ Lower esophageal sphincter relaxation lasts less than 2 seconds after swallowing.

74. _____ Lower esophageal sphincter relaxation occurs simultaneously with upper esophageal sphincter relaxation.

75. _____ A lower esophageal sphincter pressure of zero represents an open sphincter

76. _____ The most important determinant of opening of the upper esophageal sphincter is hypopharyngeal intrabolus pressure.

Which of the following findings (77-79) are considered to be abnormal on esophageal manometry?

77. _____ failure of lower esophageal sphincter relaxation with 5% of all wet swallows in an 80-year-old man

78. _____ simultaneous esophageal body contractions with 20% of all dry swallows in a 60-year-old man

79. _____ a mean esophageal body contractile amplitude of 200 mm Hg in a 20-year-old man

80. _____ Activation of the muscles of swallowing is centrally mediated by the sequential activation of specific brain stem nuclei.

81. _____ Pain associated with gastroesophageal acid reflux occurs more commonly when the pH of the refluxate is less than 2 compared to when it is more than 2.

82. _____ Positive 24-hour pH monitoring of the esophagus has been shown to predict a satisfactory response to antireflux therapy, whereas a positive result from a Bernstein test has not.

83. _____ Among all patients who present with symptoms of heartburn, fewer than 10% will have endoscopic evidence of injury in the distal esophagus.

84. _____ Antidepressant medications can reduce chest pain in some patients who have an underlying esophageal motility disorder.

85. _____ Ingestion of an acidic agent usually causes more damage to the stomach than to the esophagus.

86. _____ Patients with esophageal strictures resulting from previous lye ingestion are at increased risk of developing esophageal carcinoma and should undergo periodic surveillance by upper endoscopy.

87. _____ Culturing of exudate or biopsy specimens is the most accurate means for the diagnosis of candidal infection of the esophagus.

88. _____ Patients with clinical evidence of chronic graft-versus-host disease of the esophagus usually show no other organ involvement.

89. _____ The depth of invasion of squamous cell carcinoma of the esophagus correlates best with the duration of survival.

90. _____ As with squamous cell cancer of the esophagus, endoscopically performed cytology and biopsy are both highly accurate in detecting the presence of adenocarcinoma in patients with Barrett esophagus.

Esophageal rings and webs:

91. _____ produce progressive dysphagia

92. _____ produce symptoms when the diameter of the esophageal lumen is less than 13 mm

93. _____ are best diagnosed by routine barium radiography studies

94. _____ can be asymptomatic

Pharyngeal dysphagia:

95. _____ can be produced by disease of the distal esophagus

96. _____ can be associated with gastroesophageal reflux

97. _____ produced by disease of the upper esophageal sphincter may be a manifestation of scleroderma

Features of the patient history that make it possible to distinguish between cardiac and esophageal sources of chest pain include:

98. _____ relief of pain with nitroglycerin

99. _____ precipitation of pain by exercise

100. _____ radiation of pain to the jaw or hand

101. _____ radiation of pain to the back and posterior neck

102. _____ gradual onset and gradual relief of chest pain

MATCHING

(match each question or statement with the correct answer)

Match the following diseases with the corresponding oral lesions:

103. _____ Familial adenomatous polyposis (Gardner syndrome)

a. trichilemmomas

104. _____ Cowden's disease

105. _____ Peutz-Jeghers syndrome

106. _____ Cronkhite-Canada syndrome

b. melanin spots

c. supernumerary teeth

d. hyperpigmentation

Match the following diseases with their corresponding orocutaneous manifestations:

107. _____ scleroderma

108. _____ graft-versus-host disease

109. _____ lead poisoning

110. _____ AIDS

a. gingival discoloration

b. telangiectasias

c. oral mucositis

d. white verrucous lesions on the tongue

Match the following disorders with their corresponding abnormalities:

111. _____ blue rubber bleb nevus syndrome

112. _____ pseudoxanthoma elasticum

113. _____ Osler-Weber-Rendu disease

114. _____ Ehler-Danlos syndrome

a. nasal bleeding

b. hamartomas

c. pseudotumors

d. angioid streaks

Match the following deficiencies with their corresponding abnormalities:

115. _____ vitamin B deficiency

116. _____ vitamin C deficiency

117. _____ vitamin A deficiency

118. _____ folate deficiency

a. cheilosis

b. gingival bleeding

c. lingual atrophy

d. dysgeusia

Match the following conditions of dysphagia with the appropriate symptom:

119. _____ solid or liquid food, intermittent dysphagia

120. _____ progressive heartburn with solid or liquid food dysphagia

121. _____ intermittent solid food dysphagia

122. _____ progressive solid food dysphagia with long-standing reflux

123. _____ progressive solid or liquid food dysphagia with prior aspiration events

124. _____ rapidly progressive solid food dysphagia and anorexia in an elderly man

125. _____ daily solid food dysphagia in a child

a. peptic stricture

b. carcinoma

c. diffuse esophageal spasm

d. achalasia

e. scleroderma

f. vascular ring

g. lower esophageal ring

Match the following clinical manifestations with viruses that can infect the esophagus:

126. _____ most likely to infect a normal host

127. _____ does not infect squamous epithelium

128. _____ necrotizing panesophagitis

129. _____ ulcers and cytoplasmic inclusions

130. _____ vesicles, ulcers, intranuclear inclusions

a. cytomegalovirus

b. varicella zoster virus

c. herpes simplex virus

Match the following esophageal motility disorders with their characteristic motor abnormalities:

131. _____ nutcracker esophagus

132. _____ hypertensive lower esophageal sphincter (LES)

133. _____ nonspecific esophageal dysmotility

134. _____ diffuse esophageal spasm

135. _____ achalasia

a. simultaneous contractions, preserved peristalsis

b. high LES pressures, normal LES relaxation

c. high esophageal body pressures, normal motility

d. isolated incomplete LES relaxation

e. aperistalsis, poor LES relaxation

Match the malignancy with a potential serologic marker:

136. _____ esophageal cancer

137. _____ colon cancer

138. _____ gastric cancer

139. _____ hepatocellular carcinoma

140. _____ pancreatic cancer

a. carcinoembryonic antigen (CEA)

b. CA19-9

c. α-fetoprotein (AFP)

d. no marker has been identified

e. CA72.4

2

Stomach

1. A 35-year-old nonsmoking man is referred to your office for the evaluation of recurrent peptic ulcer disease. A prior evaluation revealed multiple ulcers in the duodenal bulb despite an 8-week course of ranitidine (300 mg/day) and no evidence of *Helicobacter pylori* in antral biopsy specimens. Laboratory studies disclose the following values:

   fasting gastrin: 350 pg/mL (normal, 100 pg/mL)
   gastric acid analysis:
      basal acid output (BAO) = 12 mEq/h
      maximal acid output (MAO) = 23 mEq/h
   secretin stimulation: basal gastrin = 325 pg/mL
   peak gastrin level after secretin injection: 390 pg/mL

   Select the best choice regarding this patient:

   a. This patient has clear-cut evidence of Zollinger-Ellison syndrome and should be referred to the surgeon for exploratory laparotomy.
   b. The BAO:MAO ratio is less than 0.6 and therefore excludes Zollinger-Ellison syndrome.
   c. The clinical and biochemical picture is consistent with antral G-cell hyperplasia. A standard meal study will help in making a definitive diagnosis.
   d. The next step in the evaluation should be endoscopic ultrasonography.

2. Each of the following conditions can cause hypergastrinemia except:

   a. renal failure
   b. diabetes insipidus
   c. rheumatoid arthritis
   d. pheochromocytoma

3. All of the following statements regarding the pathogenesis of diarrhea in patients with Zollinger-Ellison syndrome are true except:

   a. Hypergastrinemia leads to colonic hypersecretion of fluid and electrolytes.

   b. Acid hypersecretion leads to extreme acidification of the duodenum, resulting in inactivation of pancreatic enzymes and concomitant steatorrhea.
   c. Extreme acidification of the small intestine can lead to mild disruption of enterocyte integrity, resulting in mild malabsorption.
   d. Gastric hypersecretion can lead to significant volume overload of the small intestine.

4. The following statements regarding the medical therapy for Zollinger-Ellison syndrome are true except:

   a. The somatostatin analog octreotide is the drug of choice for controlling the clinical manifestations of this syndrome.
   b. Chemotherapy and radiation therapy are of limited benefit in the treatment of metastatic gastrinoma.
   c. Strict control of gastric acid secretion leads to decreased morbidity in patients with gastrinoma.
   d. Tachyphylaxis in terms of acid inhibition is observed less often with omeprazole than with H_2-receptor antagonists.

5. The following statements regarding multiple endocrine neoplasia (MEN) type I syndrome are true except:

   a. Twenty-five percent of patients with gastrinoma have MEN I syndrome.
   b. Pancreatic tumors are the most common manifestation of this syndrome.
   c. MEN I is an autosomal dominant genetic disorder; there is a genetic defect in the long arm of chromosome 11.
   d. Patients with MEN I syndrome and gastrinoma may develop gastric carcinoid tumors.

6. All of the following are currently considered valid therapeutic options for the initial treatment of Zollinger-Ellison syndrome except:

   a. surgical resection of the gastrin-producing tumor
   b. H^+,K^+-ATPase inhibitors
   c. total gastrectomy
   d. combination chemotherapy with streptozocin, 5-fluorouracil, and doxorubicin

7. Each of the following are associated with a favorable outcome in patients with gastrinoma except:

    a. negative exploratory laparotomy revealing no abnormalities
    b. Cushing syndrome in sporadic gastrinoma
    c. isolated lymph node tumor
    d. primary duodenal wall tumor

8. A 42-year-old man seeks a second opinion from you after receiving a diagnosis of gastrinoma. Upon reviewing his history and biochemical studies, you concur with this diagnostic impression. He is concerned that his previous physician recommended surgery without further testing (i.e., structural studies of the abdomen). Which of the following options would you recommend to this patient?

    a. You agree with his physician and recommend exploratory laparotomy without further studies.
    b. You recommend endoscopic ultrasonography before surgery.
    c. The patient should proceed to computed tomography, magnetic resonance imaging, or somatostatin receptor scintigraphy (e.g., octreoscan) depending on the local expertise, before further studies and therapy.
    d. Selective arterial secretin injection (SASI) is the first study you would recommend before considering further evaluation and therapy.

9. Select the most accurate statement regarding the sensitivity and specificity of the imaging studies used to evaluate Zollinger-Ellison syndrome.

    a. Transcutaneous ultrasonography has a sensitivity exceeding 50% for detecting metastatic gastrinoma.
    b. Computed tomography of the abdomen provides a sensitivity of greater than 80% for detecting both primary and metastatic gastrinoma.
    c. Endoscopic ultrasonography can detect metastatic gastrinoma with a sensitivity of 80% to 100%.
    d. Somatostatin receptor scintigraphy can detect a primary gastrinoma with a sensitivity of greater than 65%.

10. Each of the following conditions can be associated with elevations in serum gastrin levels to greater than 1000 pg/mL (normal, 100 pg/mL) except:

    a. pernicious anemia
    b. retained gastric antral segment
    c. Zollinger-Ellison syndrome
    d. cirrhosis

11. The following statements regarding the management of foreign bodies in the stomach are true except:

    a. The clinician should consider removing objects that are more than 2 cm in diameter or more than 5 cm in length, because they are unlikely to pass through the duodenum.
    b. In the case of battery ingestion, levels of heavy metal in the blood and urine should be measured.
    c. Batteries that have passed through the esophagus to the stomach should always be removed.
    d. Between 80% to 90% of ingested foreign bodies that reach the stomach will pass without specific therapy.

12. All of the following are treatments for symptomatic bezoars except:

    a. cellulase
    b. acetylcysteine
    c. atropine
    d. mechanical fragmentation at the time of endoscopy

13. Acute gastric volvulus typically presents with all of the following signs and symptoms except:

    a. acute localized epigastric distention
    b. copious vomiting
    c. inability to pass a nasogastric tube
    d. abdominal discomfort

14. Each of the following conditions predisposes to the development of gastric volvulus except:

    a. large hiatal hernia
    b. lax suspensory ligaments of the stomach
    c. eventration of the diaphragm
    d. history of trauma
    e. hepatomegaly

15. Gastric sympathetic efferent nerves emerge from spinal cord segments:

    a. T3 through T5
    b. T2 through T4
    c. T5 through T9
    d. T7 through T12

16. All of the following studies for the diagnosis of retained antrum syndrome are useful except:

    a. basal serum gastrin level
    b. technetium pertechnetate radioisotope scan
    c. secretin stimulation testing
    d. modified sham feeding

17. All of the following are potent acid secretagogues except:

    a. coffee
    b. decaffeinated coffee
    c. milk
    d. alcohol

18. Pepsinogen secretion is increased by each of the following except:

    a. somatostatin
    b. gastrin
    c. histamine
    d. vagal stimulation

19. Which of the following statements regarding serum pepsinogen (PG) levels is not correct?

    a. PG I is derived from chief and mucous cells.
    b. Patients with atrophic gastritis have a decreased PG I:PG II ratio.
    c. PG II is produced only by pyloric, Brunner, and metaplastic glands.
    d. Infection with *Helicobacter pylori* increases serum PG levels.
    e. The ratio of PG I:PG II can predict the presence of atrophic gastritis with 70% accuracy.

20. The gastric acid secretory pump located on the apical surface of the parietal cell uses:

    a. Na^+,K^+-ATPase
    b. H^+,K^+-ATPase
    c. tyrosine kinase
    d. carbonic anhydrase

21. Which of the following statements regarding the regulation of gastric acid secretion is the most accurate?

    a. Basal gastric acid secretion exhibits a circadian variation; the highest secretion occurs in the early morning and the lowest secretion occurs at night.
    b. The cephalic phase of acid secretion is mediated primarily by vasoactive intestinal polypeptide–containing vagal fibers.
    c. The gastric phase of acid secretion consists of two components: a physical component (i.e., distention of the stomach) and a chemical component.
    d. The primary stimulatory factors involved in the intestinal phase of acid secretion include distention and fat.

22. All of the following statements regarding the cellular basis for the regulation of gastric acid secretion are true except:

    a. Parietal cells express cell surface receptors for gastrin, acetylcholine, histamine, and somatostatin.
    b. Transforming growth factor directly inhibits parietal cell activity by epidermal growth factor receptor occupancy.
    c. Occupancy of the muscarinic receptor on parietal cells leads to stimulation of acid secretion by activation of the adenylate cyclase signaling pathway.

    d. Stimulation of parietal cells leads to morphologic transformation, rapid changes in H^+,K^+-ATPase location, and opening of ion channels.

23. All of the following statements about intrinsic factor (IF) are true except:

    a. Pentagastrin stimulates IF release.
    b. Histamine does not stimulate IF release.
    c. Cholinergic agonists stimulate IF release.
    d. Proton pump inhibitors do not stimulate IF release.

24. Which is not a member of the epidermal growth factor family of growth factors?

    a. betacellulin
    b. TGF-α
    c. TGF-β
    d. amphiregulin

25. The gastric source of histamine is:

    a. parietal cells
    b. G cells
    c. ECL cells
    d. D cells

26. The arterial blood supply to the stomach is derived from all of the following except:

    a. right hepatic artery
    b. common hepatic artery
    c. superior mesenteric artery
    d. left gastric artery

27. Which of the following statements regarding gastric cancer is not true?

    a. It is the second most common cancer in the world.
    b. Infection with *Helicobacter pylori* is associated with an increased risk for the development of gastric cancer.
    c. It has been associated with an increase in the consumption of charcoal-grilled meats.
    d. It is associated with elevated levels of *N*-nitroso compounds in the stomach.
    e. The incidence of adenocarcinoma of the gastroesophageal junction is increasing.

28. Which of the following statements regarding gastric malignancies is not true?

    a. Cancers involving the proximal one-third of the stomach have a worse prognosis than more distal tumors.
    b. Chronic atrophic gastritis is associated with both the well-differentiated intestinal type and the diffuse variant of gastric carcinoma.

c. The most common tumors that give rise to gastric metastases are lung carcinoma, breast carcinoma, and melanoma.

d. Hypertrophic gastropathy is a risk factor for gastric carcinoma.

29. Which of the following is not associated with an increased risk of the development of gastric adenocarcinoma?

a. common variable immunodeficiency
b. Billroth II gastrectomy and gastrojejunostomy
c. chronic atrophic gastritis
d. long-term proton pump inhibitor therapy
e. Lynch syndrome II

30. Which statement regarding the epidemiology of gastric cancer is not true?

a. Gastric cancer is directly correlated with the sero-prevalence of *Helicobacter pylori*.
b. It is equally common in men and women.
c. Incidence and mortality rates are higher in groups with lower socioeconomic status.
d. First-generation emigrants have incidence rates similar to those in their country of origin.
e. High-risk areas frequently have high nitrate levels in the water.

31. The prognosis of gastric cancer is worsened by each of the following except:

a. diffuse-type histology
b. penetration beyond the muscularis propria
c. lymph node metastases
d. location in the proximal stomach
e. elevation of the carcinoembryonic antigen level

32. Which of the following statements regarding the pre-operative staging of gastric cancer is not true?

a. Endoscopic ultrasonography is most accurate for T- and N-stage cancers.
b. Computed tomography is best to rule out distant metastases.
c. Laparoscopy can be of value to exclude occult peritoneal involvement.
d. Enlarged celiac nodes render the lesion incurable.
e. Endoscopic ultrasonography can be used to evaluate the extent of both proximal and distal tumors.

33. Which of the following statements regarding surgery for gastric cancer is incorrect?

a. Surgical resection should provide 5-cm tumor-free margins.
b. Perigastric and regional nodes should be removed.
c. Most patients with metastatic disease should have a palliative resection.

d. Routine splenectomy is unnecessary.
e. Adjuvant chemotherapy is of unproved benefit and potential harm.

34. Which of the following statements regarding gastric lymphoma is not true?

a. It can be cured with radiotherapy alone.
b. Most gastric lymphomas are T-cell in origin.
c. Endoscopic ultrasonography is highly accurate in staging.
d. Patients with stages II, III, and IV disease should receive chemotherapy.
e. Subtotal gastrectomy may be adequate treatment and avoids the morbidity of esophagojejunostomy.

35. Which of the following statements regarding gastric lymphoma is not true?

a. It is often associated with *Helicobacter pylori* infection.
b. It is associated with a relatively favorable prognosis if the lymphoma is derived from mucosa-associated lymphoid tissue (MALT).
c. It is not a tumor for which surgical resection is recommended.
d. It may regress after treatment with antibiotics.
e. Diffuse histiocytic lymphoma makes up the largest subgroup.

36. Each of the following statements regarding carcinoid tumors of the stomach is true except:

a. The stomach is the most common site for the development of carcinoid tumors.
b. Gastric carcinoid tumors are usually discovered incidentally.
c. Gastric carcinoid tumors typically synthesize serotonin.
d. Gastric carcinoid tumors occur more frequently in patients with atrophic gastritis and pernicious anemia.

37. The most common type of gastric polyp is:

a. hyperplastic
b. adenomatous
c. fundic gland
d. juvenile
e. carcinoid

38. A 65-year-old man underwent subtotal gastrectomy for advanced gastric adenocarcinoma. A Borrmann type III lesion was resected from the proximal third of his stomach. He was noted to have 15 of 17 positive paraaortic lymph nodes. The depth of invasion was to the muscularis propria. Which of the following statements regarding his prognosis is not correct?

a. The most important predictors of prognosis include the depth of tumor invasion and the extent of lymph node metastasis.

b. The histologic degree of tumor differentiation is independently predictive of prognosis.

c. Increased p53 expression in cancers is associated with a reduced 5-year survival rate.

d. Cancers involving the proximal stomach tend to have a worse prognosis than distal lesions.

39. Which statement regarding the association between *Helicobacter pylori* infection and gastric malignancy is false?

a. *H pylori* has been linked to both mucosa-associated lymphoid tissue lymphoma and gastric carcinoma.

b. In patients infected with *H pylori,* epidemiologic studies suggest an inverse association between duodenal ulcer and gastric cancer.

c. *H pylori* has been linked to the intestinal type but not the diffuse type of gastric adenocarcinoma.

d. *H pylori* infection alone is probably not sufficient to cause gastric cancer.

40. A 55-year-old man presents with a new onset of epigastric pain. He reports mild postprandial nausea but denies vomiting, weight loss, gastrointestinal bleeding, and use of nonsteroidal antiinflammatory drugs. What is the most appropriate diagnostic study for this patient?

a. upper gastrointestinal tract radiologic examination

b. upper endoscopy

c. noninvasive test for *Helicobacter pylori*

d. trial with a proton pump inhibitor and follow-up in 4 weeks

41. A 51-year-old woman is referred to you for the evaluation of a recent upper gastrointestinal hemorrhage from peptic ulcer disease. She brings records indicating that a local physician performed endoscopy and gastric biopsies. Review of these studies reveals that a duodenal ulcer was documented and that *Helicobacter pylori* was discovered in the gastric biopsy specimens. Each of the following statements regarding *H pylori* is correct except:

a. *H pylori* is a gram-negative, microaerophilic, flagellated, urease-producing rod, which is found in the gastric antrum in over 50% of patients with peptic ulcer disease.

b. This organism appears to play an important role in the pathogenesis of peptic ulcer disease.

c. Eradication of this organism with the appropriate antibiotic regimen will lead to ulcer healing; however, it will not alter the recurrence rate of duodenal ulcers.

d. Examination at 1 month or more after cessation of therapy is necessary to verify the eradication of *H pylori.*

42. At upper endoscopy, this patient is found to have a round, 1.5-cm ulcer in the gastric body. Which of the following diagnostic procedures would you recommend?

a. Obtain biopsy specimens from the gastric body and antrum and submit them for a rapid urease test only.

b. Obtain biopsy specimens from the base and rim of the ulcer, and from normal tissue, and submit them for histologic examination.

c. Test for serologic evidence of *Helicobacter pylori* and no biopsy.

d. No biopsy; start the patient on a proton pump inhibitor to facilitate ulcer healing.

43. A 42-year-old woman requests a second opinion regarding management of a newly diagnosed duodenal ulcer. Her main concern is related to the dietary and lifestyle recommendations. After reviewing the records, you agree with the diagnosis of a duodenal ulcer secondary to *Helicobacter pylori* infection, and with the eradication treatment recommended. She is presently asymptomatic, tolerating her medications and participating in normal levels of activity. Which course of action would you recommend?

a. Adhere to a diet consisting of bland food (e.g., mashed potatoes, soup, cooked vegetables) and milk for the next 4 weeks in an effort to accelerate ulcer healing.

b. Eliminate all caffeine-containing beverages from the diet for the next 4 weeks, because studies have demonstrated that consumption of these can result in delayed ulcer healing.

c. Eliminate cigarette smoking because studies have suggested that smokers are at an increased risk for delayed ulcer healing and ulcer-related complications.

d. Change her job since emotional stress is an established risk factor for delayed ulcer healing.

44. A 45-year-old woman was evaluated by her primary care physician for intermittent epigastric pain over the course of 1 month. The result of an office-based serology test was positive for *Helicobacter pylori* and the patient was treated with proton pump inhibitor (PPI)–based triple therapy. The patient initially did well; however, 3 months later she returned to the office with epigastric pain. The primary care physician obtained another serology test, which remained positive. The patient is referred to you for further treatment. The best approach to the management of this case is:

a. endoscopy with biopsy-based testing for *H pylori*

b. PPI therapy for presumed reflux disease caused by *H pylori*

c. repeat therapy to eradicate *H pylori* with bismuth-triple therapy

d. abdominal computed tomography

45. Which of the following characteristics describes the lymphoid follicles that accompany infection with *Helicobacter pylori*?

    a. They are common in noninfected individuals.
    b. They may precede the development of mucosa-associated lymphoid tissue (MALT) lymphoma.
    c. They are rare in children.
    d. Their presence does not correlate with *H pylori* antibody titer.

46. Select the best answer regarding gastrin and gastric acid secretion in the pathogenesis of *Helicobacter pylori*–induced duodenal ulcer disease.

    a. Basal and gastrin-releasing peptide (GRP)–stimulated gastric acid secretion is normal in patients with *H pylori*–associated duodenal ulcer disease as compared to asymptomatic, infected controls.
    b. Patients infected with *H pylori* have significantly higher basal, 24-hour, meal-stimulated, and GRP-stimulated gastrin levels than individuals cured of the infection.
    c. It appears that proinflammatory cytokines such as tumor necrosis factor and interleukin-8 do not play a role in the gastric secretory abnormalities seen in patients with *H pylori*–induced duodenal ulcer disease.
    d. Serum gastrin is increased by the oral administration of urea, thus explaining the mechanism for the observed abnormalities in the regulation of this peptide in *H pylori*–infected patients with duodenal ulcer.

47. A 38-year-old man is referred to you for the evaluation of abdominal pain and a duodenal ulcer that has failed to heal after an 8-week regimen of full-dose H_2 blockers. Serology and antral biopsy confirm that his *Helicobacter pylori* status is negative. The patient denies cigarette smoking and the ingestion of non-steroidal antiinflammatory drugs (NSAIDs). Each of the following statements regarding his condition is true except:

    a. The majority of duodenal ulcers that fail to heal after 8 weeks of therapy are associated with Zollinger-Ellison syndrome.
    b. A careful history regarding the patient's compliance with the antiulcer medication must be performed before recommending further diagnostic evaluation or therapy.
    c. The likelihood that NSAID ingestion (inadvertent or surreptitious) is contributing to the persistence

of this patient's ulcer may be as high as 40% or higher.

    d. Gastric acid hypersecretion may be a contributing factor in this clinical picture.

48. After performing a complete evaluation of the patient presented in the previous question, including medication history, esophagogastroduodenoscopy biopsy specimens, salicylate screen, and serum gastrin and gastric acid analyses, you fail to identify or explain the refractory ulcer. Each of the following statements regarding therapy for this patient are true except:

    a. There is a 50% to 60% chance of this ulcer healing with an additional 8 weeks of H_2-receptor antagonists.
    b. Maintenance therapy with full-dose or half-dose H_2 blockers yields a 1-year symptomatic recurrence rate of less than 20%.
    c. Virtually all refractory ulcers can be healed with omeprazole (40 mg/day) or its equivalent.
    d. Omeprazole at 20 mg/day appears to be less effective in maintaining ulcer remission than is the dose of 40 mg/day.

49. Which of the following is not an important mechanism in the pathogenesis of both nonsteroidal anti-inflammatory drug– and *Helicobacter pylori*–induced injury of the gastric mucosa?

    a. altered mucus barrier
    b. reduced mucosal hydrophobicity
    c. impaired mucosal regeneration
    d. decreased microvascular blood flow
    e. neutrophilic infiltration

50. All of the following statements regarding cyclooxygenase (COX) isoenzymes are true except:

    a. The expression of COX is the rate-limiting catalytic step in the production of prostaglandins from membrane-esterified arachidonic acid.
    b. COX-1 is expressed in a constitutive manner and plays a housekeeping role in macrophages, leukocytes, fibroblasts, and endothelial cells.
    c. COX-2 is the inducible form of the enzyme, which is up-regulated in areas of inflammation.
    d. The expression of COX-1 is regulated by physiologic stimuli and leads to the synthesis of thromboxane A_2, PG_{I2}, and PGE_2.

51. A 70-year-old woman with osteoarthritis is referred to you for the evaluation of anemia. Colonoscopy reveals no abnormality and upper endoscopy reveals a 1-cm benign-appearing gastric ulcer. Evaluation of the surrounding mucosa confirms *Helicobacter pylori*–induced gastritis. The patient has been taking

ibuprofen to alleviate severe arthritis symptoms unresponsive to acetaminophen. She is unwilling to stop her antiinflammatory therapy. What therapy would you recommend?

a. proton pump inhibitor therapy only
b. *H pylori* eradication therapy only
c. proton pump inhibitor therapy and *H pylori* eradication therapy followed by maintenance H_2 blocker therapy (150 mg twice a day)
d. proton pump inhibitor therapy and *H pylori* eradication therapy followed by continued proton pump inhibitor therapy
e. switch to a cyclooxygenase-2–specific inhibitor

52. Which of the following conditions is not a risk factor for nonsteroidal antiinflammatory drug–associated ulcers and their complications:

a. age older than 60
b. previous ulcer disease
c. concomitant steroid therapy
d. alcohol use
e. cardiovascular disease

53. A 45-year-old woman with osteoarthritis has been taking 2400 mg ibuprofen per day. She began experiencing epigastric pain and consulted her primary care physician who prescribed cimetidine, 400 mg twice a day. The patient had initial resolution of the pain; however, it returned 6 weeks later despite therapy with cimetidine. Her primary care physician obtained a serology test for *Helicobacter pylori* and found the patient to be seropositive. The best management option that the gastroenterologist could suggest is:

a. treatment for *H pylori* infection and reevaluation thereafter
b. endoscopy
c. proton pump inhibitor twice a day
d. switch to cyclooxygenase-2–specific inhibitor
e. switch to Arthrotec

54. The relative incidence of gastric ulcers resulting from the use of nonsteroidal antiinflammatory drugs can be significantly reduced by all of the following except:

a. standard-dose H_2-receptor antagonists
b. nonacetylated salicylates
c. misoprostol
d. cotherapy with a proton pump inhibitor

55. Select the best answer regarding nonsteroidal antiinflammatory drug (NSAID)–related gastroduodenal mucosal injury.

a. There is no difference among NSAIDs in their likelihood to cause mucosal injury.

b. The potency and duration of cyclooxygenase-2 inhibition by an NSAID correlates with the risk of the development of ulcers and the risk of ensuing complications.
c. Nonacetylated NSAIDs may be associated with a decreased incidence of mucosal injury compared to acetylated compounds.
d. Nonacetylated NSAIDs are associated with less gastrointestinal toxicity because of the relative selectivity of these agents for the different cyclooxygenase isoenzymes.

56. All of the following statements regarding nonsteroidal antiinflammatory drugs (NSAIDs) and acid peptic disease are true except:

a. Short-term use of aspirin leads to acute mucosal lesions in 100% of patients.
b. Chronic NSAID users show a 2- to 3-fold increase in mortality due to gastrointestinal complications.
c. NSAIDs are a strong risk factor for the development of peptic ulcer disease.
d. NSAID-related complications are usually antedated by warning symptoms.

57. A 42-year-old man seeks a second opinion regarding medication-induced peptic ulcer disease. He has a history of steroid-dependent asthma. He is presently taking prednisone (30 mg/day), and is concerned about developing an "ulcer." He is otherwise healthy. Which of the following courses of action would you recommend?

a. Initiate therapy with a proton pump inhibitor to prevent ulcers from developing.
b. Recommend high-dose H_2-receptor antagonists as prophylaxis against ulcer development.
c. Prescribe the coadministration of misoprostol with the prednisone to prevent ulcer development.
d. Reassure the patient that there is no indication for the routine use of prophylactic antiulcer medications in his clinical situation.

The following case pertains to questions 58 through 60.

A 67-year-old woman is admitted as an inpatient after receiving emergency care for melena. Endoscopy reveals antral gastritis and a 1.5-cm duodenal ulcer without evidence of active bleeding. Her history is significant for rheumatoid arthritis, for which she was taking prednisone (10 mg/day) and ibuprofen (800 mg twice per day).

58. Which of the following regimens would you recommend for this patient?

a. Initiate therapy with sucralfate, 1 g 4 times a day, and allow continuation of ibuprofen.
b. Initiate an H_2-receptor antagonist at a standard dose and allow continuation of ibuprofen.

c. Begin treatment with omeprazole at a standard dose and allow continuation of the nonsteroidal antiinflammatory drug (NSAID).

d. Discontinue the NSAID and begin therapy with omeprazole, 20 mg per day.

59. The primary care team looking after the above patient informs you 24 hours later that the result of the patient's serology test for *Helicobacter pylori* was positive. They now seek your recommendations for further therapy. Select the best answer.

a. No further treatment recommended because the ulcer was probably caused by nonsteroidal antiinflammatory drugs, not *H pylori* infection.

b. Treat the *H pylori* infection and document its eradication with a urea breath test or a stool antigen test.

c. Initiate therapy for the *H pylori* infection and document eradication by serology 4 weeks after the patient completes an antibiotic regimen.

d. Initiate treatment for the *H pylori* infection; no need to document eradication.

60. All of the following statements regarding complications of peptic ulcer disease are true except:

a. Hemorrhage is the most common complication of peptic ulcer disease.

b. Ulcer hemorrhage is more common in the elderly.

c. The specificity and the sensitivity of pain as markers of peptic ulcer disease are very high.

d. Penetrating duodenal ulcers involving the pancreas are usually located at the posterior duodenal bulb.

61. Each of the following features represents a component of mucosal defense at the epithelial level except:

a. cell resistance
b. surface active phospholipids
c. growth factors
d. restitution

62. Strong associations have linked gastric or duodenal ulcer disease to each of the following disorders except:

a. chronic pulmonary disease
b. diabetes mellitus
c. α_1-antitrypsin deficiency
d. hepatic cirrhosis
e. chronic renal failure

63. All of the following statements concerning risk factors for the development of peptic ulcer disease are true except:

a. Cigarette smokers are at increased risk of developing ulcer disease.

b. Genetic factors play an important role in ulcer pathogenesis.

c. Alcohol is an important ulcerogenic substance.

d. Diet does not play an important role in the pathogenesis of peptic ulcer disease.

64. All of the following statements regarding proton pump inhibitors are true except:

a. Proton pump inhibitors inhibit the H^+,K^+-ATPase pump.

b. Proton pump inhibitors are activated in an acidic environment.

c. Proton pump inhibitors cause a rise in the serum gastrin level.

d. Use of proton pump inhibitors leads to enterochromaffin-like cell hyperplasia in most patients.

65. All of the following statements regarding the treatment of peptic ulcer disease are true except:

a. All H_2-receptor antagonists are equally effective in healing peptic ulcer disease.

b. Twice daily versus once at bedtime regimens of H_2-receptor antagonists have demonstrated equivalent healing rates.

c. Proton pump inhibitors relieve ulcer pain more rapidly than do H_2-receptor antagonists.

d. Proton pump inhibitors and H_2-receptor antagonist regimens produce identical rates of ulcer healing at 2 and 4 weeks.

66. All of the following statements regarding peptic ulcer disease are true except:

a. H_2-receptor antagonists and proton pump inhibitors are ineffective in treating nonsteroidal antiinflammatory drug (NSAID)–related ulcerations in patients who are maintained on NSAIDs.

b. Misoprostol is an effective agent for the prevention of chronic NSAID–associated gastric ulcerations.

c. Dyspeptic symptoms in patients receiving long-term NSAID therapy are very common and do not usually warrant endoscopic evaluation.

d. Patients with iron-deficiency anemia and/or hemoccult-positive stools should undergo gastrointestinal endoscopic examination.

67. Each of the following medications requires dosage adjustment or is contraindicated in patients with renal failure except:

a. magnesium hydroxide
b. ranitidine
c. omeprazole
d. cimetidine

68. Each of the following statements regarding recurrent peptic ulcer disease is true except:

a. The major predictor of ulcer recurrence is the successful eradication of *Helicobacter pylori*.

b. Annual recurrence rates may reach as high as 30% to 40% in patients in whom *H pylori* is not eradicated.

c. Annual recurrence rates for gastric and duodenal ulcers fall to 10% to 20% when *H pylori* is eradicated.

d. Cigarette smoking appears to contribute to ulcer recurrence.

69. In what region of the stomach is intestinal metaplasia most frequently found in cases of environmental metaplastic atrophic gastritis type B?

   a. body
   b. incisura angularis
   c. antrum
   d. cardia
   e. pylorus

70. Which of the following statements regarding acute hemorrhagic gastritis is true?

   a. Patients with acute hemorrhagic gastritis usually present with abdominal pain.
   b. Acute hemorrhagic gastritis has a characteristic pathology caused by the inciting agent (e.g., non-steroidal antiinflammatory drugs, ethanol).
   c. It is typically associated with significant inflammation.
   d. Regenerative epithelium is often seen.

71. A 53-year-old man is admitted to the hospital complaining of epigastric pain, lower extremity edema, and diarrhea. The laboratory evaluation reveals iron-deficiency anemia. Upper endoscopy reveals giant gastric folds. Acid secretory studies are consistent with diminished secretion of gastric acid. Deep mucosal biopsy specimens show pit hyperplasia without signs of malignancy. Which of the following is the most likely diagnosis?

   a. Ménétrier disease
   b. gastric lymphoma
   c. Zollinger-Ellison syndrome
   d. scleroderma

72. True statements regarding autoimmune atrophic gastritis include all the following except:

   a. It exhibits a male-to-female ratio of approximately 1:3.
   b. It is associated with pernicious anemia by virtue of decreased vitamin B_{12} absorption.
   c. It is associated with markedly diminished or absent gastric acid production.

   d. It is associated with markedly elevated serum gastrin levels.
   e. It is associated with a 200-fold increased risk of gastric cancer, requiring endoscopic surveillance and biopsy every 6 months.

73. Each of the following statements regarding acute erosive gastritis are true except:

   a. Cushing ulcers are associated with central nervous system trauma.
   b. Stress gastritis is uncommon in patients in the intensive care unit who are not dependent on a ventilator.
   c. Sucralfate is an effective agent for the prophylaxis of stress gastritis bleeding.
   d. Mucosal ischemia is thought to be a major factor in the pathogenesis of stress gastritis.

74. Conditions associated with gastroparesis include each of the following except:

   a. multiple sclerosis
   b. diabetes mellitus
   c. hypokalemia
   d. Parkinson disease
   e. rheumatoid arthritis

75. Which statement about erythromycin is most accurate?

   a. The effects of erythromycin on gastric emptying are thought to be secondary to dopamine receptor antagonism.
   b. The effects of erythromycin on gastric emptying are mediated through motilin receptor antagonism.
   c. Gastric sieving of a solid meal is impaired by erythromycin.
   d. Plasma cholecystokinin levels are elevated after the administration of erythromycin.

76. Which statement regarding the role of gastric motor, myoelectric, and sensory dysfunction in functional dyspepsia is not true?

   a. Gastric emptying is delayed in 30% to 82% of patients.
   b. Dynamic antral scintigraphy reveals increased non-propulsive and uncoordinated distal gastric contractions in patients with functional dyspepsia.
   c. Impaired relaxation of the gastric fundus following meal ingestion has been correlated with symptom induction in patients with functional dyspepsia.
   d. Patients with functional dyspepsia often exhibit reduced symptomatic tolerance to balloon distention of the proximal stomach, which is consistently associated with altered fundic wall compliance.

77. Which of the following statements concerning motor activity of the distal stomach is correct?

    a. Specialized conduction bundles transmit electrical slow-wave activity from the gastric pacemaker to the antrum and the pylorus.
    b. Phase III activity of the antral migrating motor complex can persist after bilateral vagotomy.
    c. The fed motor pattern in the antrum is characterized by regular, intense, phasic contractions that occur with every slow-wave cycle.
    d. The fed motor pattern in the antrum persists until all indigestible residue from the previous meal is evacuated from the stomach.
    e. Migrating motor complex activity decreases in regularity and periodicity with advanced age.

78. Characteristics of pyloric motor responses include all of the following except:

    a. During terminal antral contractile activity, the pylorus closes before the antral ring contraction reaches the pylorus.
    b. In contrast to the fed period when the pylorus exhibits prolonged periods of closure, the pylorus is widely patent during phase III of the antral migrating motor complex.
    c. Perfusion of the duodenum with lipid solutions leads to inhibition of both antral and pyloric motor activity resulting in delayed gastric emptying.
    d. Vagal stimulation may produce either pyloric contraction or relaxation depending on the stimulus parameters.
    e. Coordination of antral and duodenal motor activity is facilitated by preservation of electrical conduction across the longitudinal muscle layer of the pylorus.

79. All of the following statements concerning gastric emptying of liquids are true except:

    a. A 500-mL bolus of normal saline will empty from the stomach at the same volume per minute as a 250-mL bolus of normal saline.
    b. Emptying of nutrient liquids across a broad range of concentrations occurs at a rate of approximately 3 kcal per minute, regardless of whether the nutrient is lipid, carbohydrate, or protein.
    c. Of all the amino acids that might be ingested in a liquid meal, L-tryptophan is the most potent inhibitor of gastric emptying, leading investigators to postulate the presence of specific L-tryptophan receptors in the intestine.
    d. A fatty acid of 12 to 14 carbons is optimal to inhibit the gastric emptying of liquids; fatty acids of longer or shorter chain lengths are not as potent.
    e. Increases in duodenal contractile activity correlate with delays in liquid emptying from the stomach.

80. Which of the following statements concerning external control of gastric motor activity is correct?

    a. Intestinal nutrient perfusion delays the gastric emptying of solids by slowing the linear phase of solid emptying.
    b. Ileal perfusion of lipid solutions results in acceleration of liquid- but not solid-phase gastric emptying.
    c. Cholecystokinin (CCK) is an important physiologic modulator of gastric emptying in response to a meal. Exogenous CCK infusion accelerates the emptying of liquids from the stomach by stimulating antral and pyloric motility.
    d. Mechanical stimulation of the colon does not affect the rate of solid-phase gastric emptying.
    e. Animal models suggest that the effects of many forms of stress on gastric emptying are reversed by pretreatment with receptor antagonists for corticotropin-releasing factor.

The following case pertains to questions 81 and 82.
A 25-year-old woman who has had type I diabetes for 12 years has a 2-year history of intermittent nausea and vomiting that has worsened in the past 3 months. A scintigraphic scan to evaluate solid-phase gastric emptying shows 8% emptying at 2 hours (normal, 42% to 80%).

81. All of the following statements are true except:

    a. This condition is usually associated with other peripheral and/or autonomic neuropathies.
    b. Delays in gastric emptying correlate well with symptoms of nausea and vomiting in this condition.
    c. Findings on gastrointestinal manometry may include loss of fed and fasting antral motility and increased phasic and tonic pyloric motility.
    d. A gastric acid analysis may show a reduction in acid production in response to sham feeding.
    e. The delay in gastric emptying may be exacerbated by periods of worsening hyperglycemia.

82. Which of the following statements concerning management of this case is true?

    a. Avoidance of a high-fat diet might reduce symptoms.
    b. Increasing the oral dose of erythromycin might worsen the nausea.
    c. The efficacy of domperidone in reducing nausea may be partially explained by central nervous system effects on dopamine receptors in the brain stem.
    d. Endoscopic destruction of a gastric bezoar may alleviate symptoms temporarily.
    e. All of the above statements are correct.

83. All of the following statements about gastric slow-wave dysrhythmias are true except:

    a. In diabetics with gastroparesis, restoration of slow-wave rhythm is more closely associated with symptom relief than is acceleration of delayed gastric emptying.

b. Tachygastria usually originates in the gastric body and is associated with rapid gastric contractions, which cause nausea.

c. Tachygastria and bradygastria may be caused by neural and/or hormonal factors.

d. Tachygastria and bradygastria may occur with gastroparesis, but they are not prerequisites for inducing delays in gastric emptying.

e. In addition to rhythm disturbances, some patients with gastroparesis exhibit an abnormal blunting of the increase in slow-wave amplitude after a meal.

The following case pertains to questions 84 and 85.

A 53-year-old man develops light-headedness, flushing, abdominal pain, and diarrhea 30 minutes postprandially after Billroth II surgery for peptic ulcer disease.

84. All of the following statements are true except:

a. Clinical evaluation of this patient shows slight increases in hematocrit and plasma osmolarity after ingestion of a liquid glucose meal.

b. The abdominal pain associated with this condition can be reproduced by mechanical distention of the small intestine.

c. These symptoms are probably secondary to a supraphysiologic release of insulin, which causes reactive hypoglycemia 30 to 60 minutes postprandially.

d. Any of the surgical procedures that include vagotomy can lead to this condition.

e. There may be evidence of malabsorption, including mild steatorrhea, in this condition.

85. In treating this patient, which of the following statements is true?

a. Inclusion of pectin in the diet may increase the viscosity of intragastric contents and lead to a reduction in symptoms.

b. A reduction in dietary carbohydrates, particularly liquids, should be beneficial.

c. Octreotide may be effective because it will reduce the postprandial release of vasoactive hormones such as vasoactive intestinal polypeptide, neurotensin, and enteroglucagon.

d. After ingestion of a liquid meal, symptoms may be reduced by assuming the supine position.

e. All of the above statements are correct.

86. All of the following statements regarding the effects of truncal vagotomy on gastric motility are true except:

a. Receptive relaxation of the stomach is enhanced.

b. Gastric accommodation is impaired.

c. Antral contractile force and frequency are reduced.

d. The fed motor pattern is typically of shorter duration compared with that of normal subjects.

87. Truncal vagotomy in the treatment of duodenal ulcer achieves which of the following results?

a. reduces basal acid output by 50% and maximal acid output by 25%

b. reduces acid secretion by decreasing the influence of acetylcholine on G cells

c. reduces the sensitivity of the parietal cell to gastrin and histamine

d. enhances proximal gastric nonphasic motor activity

88. In patients with anorexia nervosa, all of the following statements regarding the gastrointestinal tract are true except:

a. Gastric electrical dysrhythmias often occur.

b. Gastric antral contractions are impaired.

c. Gastric emptying of solid foods is often delayed.

d. Upper gastrointestinal symptoms rarely improve even years after successful refeeding.

e. Gastric electrical and motor abnormalities may be secondary to defects in dopaminergic pathways, either in the central nervous system or in the gastrointestinal tract.

89. Which statement regarding surgery for peptic ulcer disease is true?

a. Patients with a large ulcer and a visible vessel uniformly require surgical intervention.

b. Proximal gastric vagotomy is associated with a lower ulcer recurrence rate compared to truncal vagotomy with antrectomy.

c. Dumping syndrome occurs in 20% of patients after proximal gastric vagotomy.

d. Truncal vagotomy and antrectomy produce a higher mortality rate and an increased incidence of postoperative complications compared to proximal gastric vagotomy.

e. Preoperative gastric acid analysis predicts those patients at highest risk for ulcer recurrence after surgery.

90. What is the best surgical procedure for a perforated anterior ulcer associated with an acutely bleeding "kissing" duodenal ulcer along the posterior wall?

a. closure of perforation

b. closure of perforation, suture ligature of the ulcer bed, and proximal gastric vagotomy

c. total gastrectomy and closure of perforation

d. proximal gastric vagotomy

91. Each of the following conditions is a recognized complication in patients who have had a previous vagotomy and antrectomy except:

a. dumping syndrome

b. diarrhea

c. malabsorption
d. hypocalcemia

92. Which form of anemia most commonly occurs in postgastrectomy patients?

   a. iron deficiency
   b. vitamin B_{12} deficiency
   c. folate deficiency
   d. hemolytic anemia

93. Nonsurgical management of peptic ulcer perforation includes each of the following except:

   a. nasogastric suction
   b. intravenous H_2-receptor antagonists
   c. antibiotics
   d. octreotide

94. Gastrointestinal motor responses associated with the act of vomiting can include each of the following except:

   a. relaxation of the gastric fundus and the lower esophageal sphincter
   b. retrograde contractions beginning in the jejunum
   c. relaxation of the abdominal musculature
   d. arrest of respiratory function just before vomiting
   e. disruption of normal gastric slow-wave activity

95. Each of the following chemotherapeutic agents commonly causes nausea and vomiting except:

   a. cisplatin
   b. 5-fluorouracil
   c. etoposide
   d. dactinomycin
   e. vinblastine

96. True statements regarding nausea and vomiting during pregnancy include all of the following except:

   a. Nausea and vomiting during pregnancy are more common in nonsmokers.
   b. They are more common in primigravidas.
   c. They are more common in those who have taken oral contraceptives.
   d. They are more common in women with less than a tenth-grade education.
   e. They are more common in obese women.

97. Which statement about hyperemesis gravidarum is true?

   a. Hyperemesis gravidarum typically begins in the second trimester.
   b. The incidence is increased with nulliparity and younger age.
   c. Serum human chorionic gonadotropin levels correlate with the degree of symptoms.

d. Nearly one-third of the women with nausea and vomiting during the first trimester of pregnancy will develop hyperemesis gravidarum.

98. The metabolic consequences of severe nausea and vomiting include each of the following except:

   a. hypochloremic metabolic alkalosis
   b. normal anion gap metabolic acidosis
   c. hyponatremia
   d. hypokalemia

The following case pertains to questions 99 through 101.

A 44-year-old man presents to the emergency department after vomiting bright red blood. He denies having prior medical problems, although he has taken calcium carbonate antacids regularly to relieve indigestion for several years. Physical examination reveals a pale, anxious man with a blood pressure of 90/50 mm Hg and a pulse rate of 120 beats per minute. Rectal examination reveals maroon stool on the examining glove.

99. Which of the following statements regarding the passage of a nasogastric tube is the most appropriate?

   a. A nasogastric tube facilitates the assessment of ongoing hemorrhage.
   b. It allows testing for occult blood in the nasogastric aspirate.
   c. It allows treatment of upper gastrointestinal bleeding by ice water lavage.
   d. Passage of a nasogastric tube is contraindicated if the patient has liver disease with possible bleeding varices.

100. The most important step in the resuscitation of this patient is to:

   a. obtain a complete history from the patient's wife
   b. send a blood specimen to the blood bank for typing and crossmatching, so that a transfusion can be performed immediately
   c. replete the intravascular volume with intravenous saline to prevent the consequences of shock
   d. determine the hematocrit to assess the severity of his blood loss and perform urgent endoscopy to determine the etiology of bleeding

101. After this patient has been adequately resuscitated and is hemodynamically stable, upper endoscopy should be performed:

   a. urgently, to allow for possible therapeutic endoscopy
   b. urgently, because findings of diagnostic endoscopy favorably affect the survival of patients with upper gastrointestinal bleeding
   c. only if the bleeding fails to stop spontaneously

d. only if medical therapy (i.e., H$_2$-receptor antagonists) fails to control bleeding

102. Gastric varices:

   a. occur in up to 20% of patients who have portal hypertension.
   b. most commonly are isolated and located in the gastric fundus
   c. do not regress after esophageal variceal obliteration with sclerotherapy, even when they cross the gastroesophageal junction
   d. may be the result of splenic vein thrombosis, which is best treated by surgical portosystemic shunt
   e. are rarely associated with underlying liver disease

103. A 57-year-old man with a long history of alcoholism presents with an upper gastrointestinal hemorrhage from isolated gastric varices in the fundus. No other endoscopic abnormalities are noted. The levels of serum aminotransferases, bilirubin, and albumin are normal, as is the prothrombin time. Treatment of this patient should include:

   a. repeat sclerotherapy until variceal obliteration is achieved
   b. portosystemic shunt surgery
   c. medical therapy with a β-blocker, because sclerotherapy in the gastric mucosa is associated with a high complication rate
   d. angiography to assess splenic vein patency

104. All of the following statements regarding arteriovenous malformations (AVMs) in the upper gastrointestinal tract are true except:

   a. Estrogen-progesterone therapy decreases blood transfusion requirements in some patients.
   b. Rebleeding is rare after endoscopic coagulation therapy in hereditary hemorrhagic telangiectasia.
   c. AVMs have been reported in association with aortic valve disease.
   d. AVMs are a common cause of upper gastrointestinal bleeding in patients with chronic renal failure.

105. Patients presenting with upper gastrointestinal bleeding in whom upper endoscopy reveals a clean ulcer base:

   a. have a 0% to 3% risk of rebleeding.
   b. account for 75% to 80% of patients with significant upper gastrointestinal hemorrhage (i.e., requiring >2 U of red blood cells) when the endoscopy is performed within 24 hours of the initial bleed
   c. have a risk of rebleeding comparable to patients with flat pigmented spots in the ulcer base.
   d. are unlikely to have bled from the ulcer even though the rest of the upper endoscopic evaluation revealed no abnormalities.

106. All of the following statements concerning optimal therapeutic endoscopic technique in the setting of acute upper gastrointestinal hemorrhage are correct except:

   a. Use of a therapeutic endoscope with two suction channels is advantageous.
   b. For electrocoagulation or heater probe treatment, firm tamponade is indicated for artery coaptation in bleeding ulcers.
   c. Follow-up endoscopy is necessary within 24 hours of the initial treatment.
   d. Arterial compression likely contributes to the mechanism of action of epinephrine injection.

107. Although there are some conflicting studies, the thermal techniques of multipolar electrocoagulation and heater probe are generally considered:

   a. superior to injection techniques for obtaining hemostasis in bleeding ulcers
   b. superior to the Nd:YAG laser because they are portable, less expensive, and require less technical support
   c. superior to medical management in the subgroup of ulcer patients with minor stigmata
   d. frequently complicated by perforation when more than 20 seconds of electrocoagulation or more than 90 joules are used per ulcer

108. Lesions other than bleeding ulcers that have been reported to benefit from epinephrine injection or thermal therapy include all of the following except:

   a. gastric varices
   b. Dieulafoy lesion
   c. gastric tumors
   d. Mallory-Weiss tears
   e. upper gastrointestinal angiodysplasia

109. Which of the following statements about the pathogenesis of nonulcer dyspepsia is not true?

   a. Altered vagal function may occur with nonulcer dyspepsia.
   b. Duodenogastric reflux is more common in patients who have nonulcer dyspepsia than in control subjects.
   c. Postprandial antral hypomotility and disorganized patterns of intestinal motility are not specific findings in nonulcer dyspepsia.
   d. *Helicobacter pylori* gastritis occurs in about 30% to 60% of patients with nonulcer dyspepsia.

110. A 4-mm, yellow, submucosal mass with a central umbilication is observed in the antrum along the greater curvature during an endoscopic evaluation of esophageal variceal hemorrhage. Endoscopic biopsy

specimens reveal that the lesion is a pancreatic rest. Correct treatment includes:

a. referral to a surgeon for excision
b. serum measurements of amylase and lipase
c. no treatment
d. endoscopic retrograde cholangiopancreatography to rule out other congenital anomalies of the pancreatic ducts

111. Which statement regarding dyspepsia is incorrect?

a. The most common symptom cluster in patients with dyspepsia is categorized as ulcer-like.
b. Upper endoscopy identifies structural abnormalities in about 75% of patients with dyspeptic symptoms.
c. Of the patients with nonulcer dyspepsia, at least one-third have concurrent symptoms of irritable bowel syndrome.
d. An extended functional workup, including the evaluation of gastric emptying, identifies abnormalities in about 50% of new patients with dyspepsia who have normal findings on upper endoscopy.

112. Which of the following statements regarding percutaneous endoscopic gastrostomy tubes is false?

a. Postprocedural infections are most commonly caused by *Staphylococcus aureus* and β-hemolytic streptococci.
b. Antibiotics must be given for a 48-hour period to reduce the risk of infection.
c. Peritoneal dialysis is an absolute contraindication to percutaneous endoscopic gastrostomy tube placement.
d. Neoplastic seeding to the skin from oropharyngeal and esophageal cancers can occur.

113. Which of the following statements concerning the prevention of recurrent variceal hemorrhage is true?

a. Treatment to prevent rebleeding includes sclerotherapy, rubber band ligation, transjugular intrahepatic portosystemic shunt (TIPS), surgical shunts, and pharmacologic therapy including propranolol and isosorbide mononitrate.
b. Prophylactic portacaval shunt surgery prevents rebleeding and improves survival.
c. β-Adrenergic antagonists are beneficial in treating grade I varices.
d. Mortality is better correlated with variceal size than with a patient's Child-Pugh score.

114. Which of the following statements regarding a Dieulafoy lesion is true:

a. This lesion typically occurs in the proximal stomach, along the lesser curvature.

b. The mean age for presentation of this disorder is the third decade of life.
c. Optimal surgical treatment of this disorder involves oversewing the lesion.
d. Acid reduction therapy (e.g., H$_2$-receptor antagonists) decreases the risk of recurrent hemorrhage.

115. Endoscopic evaluation reveals an anastomotic ulcer in a patient who has undergone antrectomy and gastrojejunostomy in the past. Which of the following test results suggest the presence of retained antral tissue?

a. a positive response on a secretin stimulation test, which is a provocative test for gastrinoma
b. normal acid secretion from the gastric remnant
c. an abnormal increase in the serum gastrin level in response to meal ingestion
d. an increased basal serum gastrin level

116. All of the following statements regarding pernicious anemia are true except:

a. Malabsorption of cobalamin is a characteristic feature of pernicious anemia.
b. Pernicious anemia is caused by an absence of or a reduction in the number of chief cells.
c. Pernicious anemia causes megaloblastic anemia.
d. Absent or dysfunctional terminal ileal absorption leads to pernicious anemia.

TRUE/FALSE

117. _____ Peptic ulcers in patients with Zollinger-Ellison syndrome are most commonly found in the second and third portions of the duodenum.

118. _____ Approximately 5% of gastric ulcers with benign radiographic appearances harbor malignancy.

119. _____ Approximately 20% of H$^+$,K$^+$-ATPase pumps are active during the basal state of gastric secretion.

120. _____ Patients with duodenal ulcer have normal bicarbonate output in the proximal duodenum and decreased bicarbonate output in the distal duodenum.

121. _____ Leukocyte adhesion and extravasation are an important component of the subepithelial level of mucosal defense.

122. _____ Type B gastritis (i.e., chronic gastritis localized to the antrum) is associated with gastric cancer, whereas type A gastritis (i.e., atrophic gastritis that begins in the fundus) is not.

123. _____ The antrum is the best location to obtain gastric biopsy specimens for rapid urease testing if the patient has been taking a proton pump inhibitor or has had recent antibiotic therapy.

124. _____ Proton pump inhibitor therapy should be withheld for 4 weeks before performing a rapid urease test at endoscopy or a urea breath test.

125. _____ Nonendoscopic tests for *Helicobacter pylori*, including the urea breath test, stool antigen test, and serology, can be used to establish a cure 1 month after antibiotic treatment.

126. _____ In developing countries, *Helicobacter pylori* infection is acquired during childhood, whereas in developed countries, acquisition usually occurs in adolescence or adulthood.

127. _____ After successful *Helicobacter pylori* eradication in people living in the United States, the rate of reinfection is about 5% to 10% per year.

128. _____ Forty percent of persons who are infected with *Helicobacter pylori* develop peptic ulcer disease.

129. _____ In the United States, 15% of *Helicobacter pylori* strains are resistant to metronidazole.

130. _____ Absorption of all H_2-receptor antagonists from the small intestine is rapid and not affected by food.

131. _____ The nitrosamide theory provides a potential explanation for why populations in certain geographic regions are at high risk for gastric cancer.

132. _____ Sucralfate 1 g 4 times per day for 8 weeks heals 60% of duodenal ulcers.

133. _____ Long-term use of proton pump inhibitors in humans is associated with an increased incidence of gastric carcinoid tumors.

134. _____ Routine prophylaxis against ulcer disease is recommended for patients who will receive corticosteroids in total daily dosages greater than 1 g for longer than 1 month.

135. _____ Both acidic (pH = 1) and alkaline (pH = 9) solutions cause pain when applied to normal gut mucosa.

136. _____ Trichobezoars typically respond to enzymatic therapy (e.g., papain, cellulase, pancrelipase).

137. _____ If a bezoar is discovered incidentally on radiography or endoscopy in patients without clear-cut symptoms, no therapy (e.g., trial of enzymes or giving a prokinetic agent) may be appropriate.

138. _____ Gastric outlet obstruction is usually not accompanied by significant abdominal pain.

139. _____ The incidence and mortality of gastric adenocarcinoma are increased in lower socioeconomic groups.

140. _____ The Borrmann classification of gastric cancer is useful to predict the clinical outcome of treatment.

141. _____ The risk of gastric carcinoma in patients who have undergone partial gastrectomy for peptic ulcer disease begins to rise 5 years after surgery.

142. _____ Radiographic evidence of the healing of a previously documented gastric ulceration precludes a diagnosis of gastric cancer.

143. _____ Brush cytology, performed before biopsy, increases the diagnostic yield for malignant gastric lesions.

144. _____ Tumor markers such as carcinoembryonic antigen and fetal sulfoglycoprotein are useful in the early diagnosis of gastric cancer.

145. _____ Regional lymph node metastases preclude the resection of gastric carcinoma.

146. _____ Patients with gastric cancer who are younger than 30 have more aggressive disease.

147. _____ Depth of invasion and pattern of lymph node metastasis are the most significant prognostic factors in gastric cancer.

148. _____ Endoscopic ultrasonography provides the best preoperative local staging of gastric cancer.

149. _____ Treatment of *Helicobacter pylori* in patients with mucosa-associated lymphoid tissue (MALT) lymphoma often leads to regression of the lymphoma in patients with low-grade lesions.

150. _____ The generally poor results of surgical treatment for gastric cancer reflect the inability to perform a curative resection at the time the lesion is diagnosed.

151. _____ Following curative resection of gastric cancer, adjuvant chemotherapy with 5-fluorouracil and mitomycin C improves survival.

152. _____ Genetic factors play a more important role in gastric cancer than in colon cancer.

153. _____ About 30% of gastric cancers exhibit microsatellite instability, which is more than in any other type of tumor.

154. _____ Approximately two-thirds of all gastrointestinal stromal tumors occur in the stomach.

155. _____ Endosonography reliably differentiates between benign and malignant stromal tumors.

156. _____ Cholecystokinin release is stimulated by fat, protein, and carbohydrates.

157. _____ Gastric proteolysis is dependent on acid secretion and is proportional to the residence times of ingested proteins in the stomach.

158. _____ In patients with achlorhydria, absorption of aspirin in the stomach is decreased.

159. _____ In healthy subjects, day-to-day variations in gastric emptying of a solid meal at 2 hours after ingestion approaches 30%.

160. _____ Digestible solid material is triturated to a size of 1 mm or smaller prior to delivery into the duodenum.

161. _____ Hyperosmolar solutions in the duodenum enhance gastric emptying.

162. _____ Entry of food into the stomach results in a vagally mediated reduction in fundic tone.

163. _____ Liquid nutrients are emptied into the duodenum primarily by the action of the interdigestive migrating motor complex.

164. _____ All operations for peptic ulcer disease can result in accelerated gastric emptying of liquids.

165. _____ Gastroparesis is typically not present in the setting of chronic idiopathic intestinal pseudoobstruction.

166. _____ Viral gastroenteritis is typically accompanied by altered gastric motility, and this correlates with the severity of nausea and vomiting.

167. _____ In humans, the gastric slow-wave oscillates at 3 cycles per minute, whereas the duodenal slow-wave oscillates at a rate of 11 cycles per minute.

168. _____ In fasting humans, the upper gastrointestinal tract exhibits a cyclical pattern of motor activity that repeats every 45 to 60 minutes.

169. _____ Phase III activity of the interdigestive migrating motor complex corresponds to peaks in plasma motilin levels.

170. _____ Intestinal sensors involved in the feedback regulation of gastric emptying are located almost exclusively in the duodenum.

171. _____ Whereas whole proteins are weak stimulants of gastrin release, peptic digests of proteins, amino acids, and amines are potent gastrin secretagogues.

172. _____ Antral resection with truncal vagotomy or selective vagotomy is associated with the lowest rate of recurrence of duodenal ulcer.

173. _____ The duration and intensity of the fed motor patterns in the stomach and duodenum are dependent on the type, composition, and amount of nutrients consumed.

174. _____ Distal antral receptors respond mainly to gastric contractions.

175. _____ Diagnostic endoscopy with biopsy is usually safe to perform in patients requiring oral anticoagulation therapy.

176. _____ A nasogastric aspirate that is negative for blood rules out an upper gastrointestinal source of hemorrhage.

177. _____ Hematochezia, which is suggestive of bleeding from a lower gastrointestinal source, occurs in 10% to 12% of cases with upper gastrointestinal hemorrhage.

178. _____ For bleeding ulcers, treatment with multipolar electrocoagulation or heater probe should include vessel compression and tamponade by the probe.

179. _____ Duodenal varices, when present, frequently bleed.

180. _____ Diplopia is the most common clinical manifestation of multiple endocrine neoplasia type 1.

181. _____ The most common cause of hypergastrinemia is gastric atrophy.

182. _____ Acid suppression with either continuous intravenous H_2-receptor antagonists or high doses of omeprazole has been shown to improve survival in patients with active upper gastrointestinal hemorrhage.

183. _____ The best predictor of variceal hemorrhage is variceal size.

184. _____ Decreased bleeding from portal gastropathy has been demonstrated during treatments that reduce portal pressure.

185. _____ Mortality in the first week after an index esophageal variceal bleed is 25%.

186. _____ Mortality is more closely associated with the grade of the bleeding esophageal varices than with the underlying Child classification.

187. _____ Endoscopic band ligation has a complication rate equal to that of sclerotherapy.

188. _____ Rebleeding rates are reduced by transjugular portosystemic shunt (TIPS) surgery as compared to sclerotherapy.

189. _____ Bleeding that begins while patients are hospitalized is associated with a lower mortality rate compared to bleeding that started prior to admission.

MATCHING

(each selection may be used once, more than once, or not at all)

Match each medication with one of the following characteristics:

190. _____ scopolamine

191. _____ domperidone

192. _____ cisapride

193. _____ metoclopramide

a. directly stimulates cholinergic neurons

b. dystonia can be a major side effect

c. most effective for motion sickness

d. specific dopamine receptor antagonist that does not cross the blood-brain barrier

Match the following test results with the most likely diagnosis. Secretin stimulation tests of gastrin release were performed with 2 g/kg secretin (Kabi). Maximal acid output (MAO) was determined after pentagastrin stimulation.

	BAO (mmol/h)	MAO (mmol/h)	basal gastrin (pg/mL)	peak gastrin (pg/mL)	
194. _____	12	16	700	580	a. Zollinger-Ellison syndrome
195. _____	0	0	700	800	b. healthy subject
196. _____	18	20	700	1000	c. retained gastric antrum
					d. pernicious anemia

Match the following drugs with the location at which they act to induce nausea and vomiting:

197. _____ benzamides (e.g., metoclopramide)

198. _____ antiparkinsonian drugs (L-dopa, bromocriptine)

a. area postrema

b. vomiting center

199. _____ opiates

200. _____ nonsteroidal antiinflammatory drugs

201. _____ butyrophenones (droperidol)

202. _____ erythromycin

c. peripheral afferents

Match the following physiologic consequences with either early- or late-dumping syndrome:

203. _____ hypoglycemia

204. _____ hyperglycemia

205. _____ release of vasoactive substances such as vasoactive intestinal polypeptide, bradykinin, and serotonin

206. _____ exaggerated insulin release

a. early-dumping syndrome

b. late-dumping syndrome

Match the chemical messengers of parietal cell biology to their second messenger systems:

207. _____ gastrin

208. _____ acetylcholine

209. _____ histamine

210. _____ somatostatin

a. cAMP

b. phosphoinositides

Match the following complications to the surgical procedure with which they most commonly occur:

211. _____ lowest likelihood of ulcer recurrence

212. _____ disorder of calcium absorption, iron deficiency, or B_{12} deficiency

213. _____ lowest likelihood of postoperative gastroparesis

a. subtotal gastrectomy

b. highly selective vagotomy

c. vagotomy and antrectomy

Match the endoscopic findings with the appropriate gastric tumor:

214. _____ observed in gastric body; may be multiple

215. _____ benign, soft, submucosal lesion; usually in the antrum

216. _____ central umbilication or ulceration; dumbell-like shape

217. _____ accounts for 10% to 20% of gastric polyps; harbors malignant potential

a. leiomyoma

b. carcinoid

c. adenoma

d. lipoma

3

Small Intestine

MULTIPLE CHOICE

(one best answer)

1. Which of the following statements regarding tropical sprue is correct?

   a. Involvement of the ileum and deficiency of vitamin B_{12} are rare in tropical sprue.
   b. Tropical sprue is thought to be due to bacterial overgrowth by nontoxigenic anaerobic bacteria.
   c. Essential clinical features of tropical sprue include chronic malabsorptive diarrhea with weight loss.
   d. Tropical sprue is a frequent cause of travelers' diarrhea.

2. The following persons are at increased risk for gastrointestinal tuberculosis except:

   a. persons from endemic areas
   b. persons infected with human immunodeficiency virus
   c. persons with a history of alcohol abuse
   d. persons who have had a splenectomy

3. What is the most frequent site of gastrointestinal tuberculosis infection?

   a. stomach
   b. duodenum
   c. jejunum
   d. terminal ileum and cecum

4. Which of the following mycotic infections of the small intestine affects immunocompetent as well as immunocompromised persons?

   a. histoplasmosis
   b. aspergillosis
   c. candidiasis
   d. mucormycosis

5. All of the following statements concerning gastrointestinal hemorrhage in immunocompromised persons are correct except:

   a. Viral ulcerations represent the most common causes of gastrointestinal hemorrhage in patients following bone marrow transplantation.
   b. Nonhealing peptic-appearing ulcers in the stomach and duodenum may be caused by cytomegalovirus infection.
   c. Herpes simplex virus infection commonly presents endoscopically with large intestinal nodules.
   d. Graft-versus-host disease is a common cause of hemorrhage in bone marrow transplant patients.

6. The most common cause of occult gastrointestinal hemorrhage in the western world is:

   a. acid-peptic disease
   b. colonic neoplasms
   c. vascular malformations
   d. hookworm infection
   e. diverticulosis

7. All of the following statements regarding giardiasis are correct except:

   a. Giardiasis is a major cause of acute diarrhea in patients with acquired immunodeficiency syndrome.
   b. In the United States, *Giardia lamblia* is the leading infectious agent identified in waterborne outbreaks of diarrhea.
   c. Treatment is indicated if cysts or trophozoites are identified in stool specimens from symptomatic patients.
   d. Recommended therapies include quinacrine or metronidazole for 5 to 10 days.

8. All of the following statements regarding diarrhea are true except:

   a. The mean frequency of stools with diarrhea resulting from colonic disease is greater than that resulting from small intestine disease.
   b. Stool volumes are generally smaller with colonic causes of diarrhea compared with small intestine diseases resulting in diarrhea.

c. Stool frequencies are more regular with small intestine diseases that cause diarrhea than with colonic causes of diarrhea.

d. Colonic diseases that cause diarrhea commonly result in positive tests for fecal occult blood.

9. The most prevalent intestinal helminth is:

a. *Ascaris lumbricoides*
b. *Strongyloides stercoralis*
c. *Enterobius vermicularis*
d. *Clonorchis sinensis*

10. The clinical triad associated with visceral larva migrans infection includes each of the following except:

a. eosinophilia
b. hepatomegaly
c. pleuritis
d. hypergammaglobulinemia

11. A 54-year-old man with degenerative joint disease presents with iron deficiency anemia and hemoccult-positive stools. He has been on oral indomethacin 25 mg twice daily for 12 months. Colonoscopy and upper endoscopy have failed to define the cause of his blood loss. Small intestine enteroscopy demonstrates several 0.3- to 0.6-cm shallow ulcers distal to the ligament of Treitz. Which of the following statements regarding this disorder is true?

a. Almost 25% of patients taking nonsteroidal anti-inflammatory drugs (NSAIDs) have evidence of increased intestinal permeability or inflammation.
b. Nonspecific small intestine ulcers are found in 50% of patients who were prescribed NSAIDs during the 6 months prior to death.
c. The presentation of NSAID-induced enteropathy is often similar to that of Crohn's disease, because both disorders are associated with transmural injury that can cause stricture formation.
d. NSAID-associated intestinal injury primarily affects the proximal small intestine.

12. Each of the following medications is associated with intestinal ischemia except:

a. cocaine
b. oral contraceptives
c. angiotensin-converting enzyme (ACE) inhibitors
d. ergotamine
e. dopamine

13. All of the following statements regarding hemorrhage from aortoenteric fistulas are true except:

a. They almost always involve the third portion of duodenum.
b. The classic presentation is a "herald" bleed.

c. Aortography is often helpful in making the correct diagnosis.
d. With a Dacron graft, the fistula usually arises from the proximal part of the graft.

14. A 5-day-old infant presents with increasing abdominal girth, occasional vomiting, and decreased activity. The infant was born 6 weeks prematurely, but had been taking formula until the day prior to presentation. The pediatrician notes blood in the infant's stool. Abdominal radiographs reveal pneumatosis intestinalis. The child is admitted for management of necrotizing enterocolitis (NEC). Which of the following statements is most accurate?

a. Prematurity is a risk factor for the development of NEC.
b. Intestinal pneumatosis is largely caused by aerophagia.
c. Breastfeeding places infants at an increased risk for NEC.
d. The transverse colon is most commonly involved in NEC.

15. All of the following statements regarding radiation enteritis are true except:

a. It is often seen with total radiation doses of 40 Gy.
b. It commonly presents with diarrhea as the only symptom.
c. It may present with nausea and vomiting.
d. Barium radiographic studies are often nondiagnostic.

16. A 21-year-old woman presents to the emergency department with an 8-day history of upper abdominal cramping and vomiting. She has recently returned from New Guinea, where she worked for 2 years in the Peace Corps. On examination, the patient is afebrile but appears dehydrated. Abdominal examination reveals absent bowel sounds, diffuse abdominal tenderness with guarding, and a palpable segment of bowel in the periumbilical region. Rectal examination is negative for masses or tenderness, but reveals maroon-colored stool that is guaiac-positive. A pelvic examination reveals nothing abnormal. Routine laboratory evaluations, including a serum pregnancy test, are negative except for evident leukocytosis (white blood cell count of 17,000 cells/mm³). Abdominal radiographs reveal multiple air-fluid levels with a thickened jejunal wall. The patient undergoes a laparotomy and is found to have patchy, plum-colored jejunal lesions with areas of necrosis. Gram-positive bacilli are observed in the microscopic sections. Which of the following statements is most accurate?

a. *Clostridium perfringens* is the most likely etiologic agent for the jejunal inflammation.
b. Stool cultures are not helpful in the diagnosis of this infection.

c. Infections with this organism rarely respond to antibiotics.

d. Surgical management should include wide resection of any involved segments of intestine.

17. A 26-year-old woman presents to her local physician for an evaluation of peripheral edema. The patient denies having any other symptoms and reportedly has a normal medical history. The laboratory evaluation is remarkable for a serum albumin level of 2.8 g/dL, with normal liver chemistries (aspartate aminotransferase, alanine aminotransferase, alkaline phosphatase, prothrombin time) and normal results from renal function tests and urinalysis. All of the following studies are indicated except:

a. measure the serum angiotensin-converting enzyme level

b. echocardiography

c. small intestine biopsy

d. analyze stool for α_1-antitrypsin concentration

18. A 28-year-old man is referred for the evaluation of recurrent epistaxis and a family history of recurrent gastrointestinal hemorrhage in one sibling. You render a tentative diagnosis after noting abnormal vascular ectasias on his lips. Which of the following statements is most accurate?

a. The most likely diagnosis is Peutz-Jeghers syndrome.

b. The disease is likely to be autosomal recessive.

c. Connective tissue disorders are often associated with this disease.

d. Lower gastrointestinal hemorrhage is more common than upper gastrointestinal bleeding in this disease.

19. A 43-year-old homosexual man with *Pneumocystis carinii* pneumonia is referred for the evaluation of persistent guaiac-positive stools that began with a single episode of melena 10 days ago. Of the following, which disease process is most likely to account for gastrointestinal blood loss?

a. diverticulitis

b. Kaposi sarcoma

c. infection with *Giardia lamblia*

d. infection with *Isospora belli*

20. All of the following statements concerning pneumatosis intestinalis are true except:

a. It is defined as gas-filled cysts in the wall of the small intestine and colon.

b. A linear pattern of gas accumulation may be associated with intestinal ischemia.

c. Cystic-like pneumatosis intestinalis may be seen in scleroderma.

d. Pneumoperitoneum may occur as a result of this disorder.

e. It represents a severe form of enteritis and is usually fatal.

21. Ischemic injury to the gastrointestinal tract is likely to be mediated by all of the following except:

a. free radicals generated by xanthine oxidase

b. superoxide dismutase

c. proteases

d. bacteria and toxins

22. All of the following are thought to modulate gastrointestinal blood flow except:

a. adenosine and oxygen

b. parasympathetic nervous system

c. arteriolar and precapillary sphincters

d. hormones

23. Which of the following statements regarding primary small intestine tumors is most accurate?

a. Most small intestine tumors will eventually become symptomatic.

b. Small intestine tumors account for approximately 10% of all gastrointestinal malignancies.

c. Japanese immigrants to Hawaii acquire the same risk of the development of small intestine tumors as that found in the Hawaiian white population.

d. Small intestine tumors are more common in Asia than in other parts of the world.

24. Each of the following is associated with an increased risk of small intestine adenocarcinoma except:

a. familial adenomatous polyposis coli

b. celiac sprue

c. Crohn's disease

d. acquired immunodeficiency syndrome

e. ileal conduit

25. Which of the following statements regarding the treatment of carcinoid syndrome with octreotide is correct?

a. Octreotide improves symptoms in 90% of patients with carcinoid syndrome.

b. Octreotide reduces plasma serotonin levels in patients with carcinoid syndrome.

c. Octreotide increases the urinary excretion of 5-hydroxyindoleacetic acid (5-HIAA) in patients with carcinoid syndrome.

d. Octreotide decreases tumor bulk but does not affect mortality rates.

26. All of the following statements regarding carcinoid tumors of the small intestine are true except:

    a. They most commonly are found in the appendix.
    b. They may be malignant.
    c. They are often asymptomatic.
    d. They may be associated with desmoplasia.
    e. In the majority of cases, they secrete a variety of peptide and steroid hormones that produce the clinical carcinoid syndrome.

27. Each of the following statements regarding the genetic and environmental etiologies of celiac sprue is true except:

    a. Ten percent to 15% of first-degree relatives of patients with celiac sprue also have the disease.
    b. The prevalence of prior infection with adenovirus serotype 12 is higher in patients with celiac sprue compared with healthy controls.
    c. There is significant amino acid homology between A-gliadin and a cell wall protein of nonpathogenic anaerobes.
    d. Worldwide, HLA-DR and HLA-DQ antigens have the strongest association with celiac sprue.

28. Of the following statements regarding adynamic ileus, which is the most accurate?

    a. Bowel ischemia may result from decreased arterial blood flow secondary to increased intralumenal pressure in adynamic ileus.
    b. The initial presentation of adynamic ileus typically includes focal pain and borborygmi.
    c. The etiology of adynamic ileus often relates to metabolic abnormalities or infection.
    d. The observation of multiple air-fluid levels on upright abdominal radiographs differentiates adynamic ileus from mechanical intestinal obstruction.

29. All of the following are consistent with the diagnosis of chronic intestinal pseudoobstruction except:

    a. abnormal results on esophageal manometry
    b. cachexia
    c. clusters of phasic contractions in the duodenum with preservation of the interdigestive migrating motor complex on small intestine manometry
    d. symptoms of urinary tract disorder and abnormalities observed on intravenous pyelogram
    e. a family history of gastrointestinal symptoms

30. Which one of the following statements regarding chronic intestinal pseudoobstruction is not true?

    a. It can be caused by drugs such as opiates, anticholinergics, and phenothiazines.
    b. If caused by scleroderma or amyloidosis, it can initially be a neuropathic process.
    c. It can affect only the duodenum.
    d. It can be associated with smooth muscle involvement of extraintestinal organs such as the bladder and ureter.
    e. If idiopathic, it is usually a myopathy rather than a neuropathy.

31. Which one of the following studies is most likely to help make the diagnosis of chronic intestinal pseudoobstruction?

    a. small intestine manometry
    b. colonic manometry
    c. pupillary pharmacologic testing
    d. anorectal manometry
    e. endoscopic small intestine biopsy

32. All of the following statements about type I familial visceral myopathy are true except:

    a. It is inherited in an autosomal dominant pattern.
    b. Ten percent of those affected will manifest the full-blown chronic intestinal pseudoobstruction syndrome.
    c. Esophageal manometry is abnormal in 75% of cases.
    d. Gastroparesis occurs in 60% of cases.
    e. Megacystis occurs in approximately 50% of cases.

33. All of the following statements concerning small intestine motor dysfunction in scleroderma are true except:

    a. Small intestine dysmotility results from the replacement of smooth muscle tissue by collagen.
    b. Small intestine involvement is often characterized by lumenal dilation.
    c. The small intestine circular muscle layer is more often involved than the longitudinal muscle layer.
    d. The small intestine is involved less often than the esophagus and stomach.

34. Which one of the following is not a typical complication of small intestine dysmotility?

    a. steatorrhea
    b. malnutrition secondary to poor oral intake
    c. coagulopathy
    d. bacterial overgrowth
    e. ascites

35. A 38-year-old woman with Crohn's disease, obstructive symptoms, and chronic inflammatory changes localized to the terminal ileum underwent a 40-cm resection of her terminal ileum 3 months ago. She presents with nonbloody watery diarrhea, and without systemic symptoms that began soon after her surgery. This patient will most likely respond to a trial of:

a. prednisone 40 mg per day

b. metronidazole 250 mg 4 times per day

c. sulfasalazine 2 g twice per day

d. cholestyramine 4 g once to twice per day

e. a low-fat diet supplemented with medium-chain triglycerides

36. A 23-year-old woman presents complaining of persistent right lower quadrant pain, diarrhea, and a 7-kg weight loss. She appears pale, her temperature is 37.3°C orally, and she has moderate tenderness over the right lower quadrant. The findings of perianal and rectal examinations are normal. Her leukocyte count is 13,000/mm³, her hemoglobin is 10.9 g/dL, and her platelet count is 823,000/mm³. Colonoscopy is normal, but small bowel barium radiography reveals wall thickening and strictures in the terminal ileum consistent with Crohn's disease. All of the following statements are true except:

a. The strictures noted in her ileum may lead to bacterial overgrowth with deconjugation of bile salts and fat malabsorption.

b. Diminished oral intake is the most likely cause of her weight loss.

c. Her elevated leukocyte count is more likely due to active Crohn's disease than to an abscess or other suppurative complication.

d. She is less likely to develop perianal involvement than a similar patient with predominantly colonic disease.

e. She is more likely to develop extraintestinal manifestations of inflammatory bowel disease than a similar patient with predominantly colonic disease.

37. Barium small intestine radiography may display thickening of the valvulae conniventes in each of the following small intestine diseases except:

a. lymphoma

b. amyloidosis

c. Whipple disease

d. celiac sprue

38. Each of the following statements about abetalipoproteinemia is true except:

a. The plasma cholesterol concentration is typically low.

b. There is a positive association with acanthocytosis.

c. Enterocytes appear normal under light microscopy.

d. It exhibits autosomal recessive inheritance.

39. Each of the following statements concerning microfold (M cells) is true except:

a. They are epithelial cells located in the mucosa overlying lymphoid follicles.

b. They selectively "sample" intralumenal antigens.

c. They transport microorganisms and large molecules to the underlying lymphoid tissue.

d. They express class II antigens on their surface.

40. Intraepithelial lymphocytes are predominantly:

a. B lymphoblasts

b. B lymphocytes

c. CD4⁺ T cells

d. CD8⁺ T cells

41. Which of the following statements regarding secretory IgA is true?

a. It facilitates cell-mediated opsonization of infectious organisms.

b. It is protective only when the mucosal barrier is intact.

c. It is protective as a result of its ability to activate complement.

d. It prevents the adherence of bacteria to epithelial cells.

42. The major mucosal defense system against parasitic infection includes each of the following except:

a. eosinophils

b. IgD

c. IgE

d. mast cells

43. Histamine secretion by mast cells can be triggered by each of the following except:

a. gastrin

b. vasoactive intestinal polypeptide

c. substance P

d. somatostatin

44. The following statements regarding selective IgA deficiency are true except:

a. Most patients with selective IgA deficiency are asymptomatic.

b. Selective IgA deficiency is associated with celiac disease and pernicious anemia.

c. IgA deficiency is the most common primary immune deficiency.

d. Jejunal biopsy specimens are usually histologically abnormal.

45. A predisposition to the development of diarrheal illness from *Giardia lamblia* infection exists with each of the following immunodeficiency syndromes except:

a. X-linked or Bruton hypogammaglobulinemia

b. severe combined immunodeficiency syndrome

c. common variable hypogammaglobulinemia

46. Each of the following statements concerning secretory component (SC) is true except:

   a. SC functions as a receptor for J-chain-dimeric IgA complexes on the basal surface of the epithelial cells.
   b. SC serves a protective function for secretory IgA in the intestinal lumen.
   c. SC is not found by itself in mucosal secretions.
   d. SC is transported to the apical surface of the epithelial cells in endoplasmic vesicles.

47. In intestinal epithelia, the rate-limiting barrier restricting the passive movement of hydrophobic solutes through the paracellular space is:

   a. the plasma membrane
   b. the tight junctions
   c. the intestinal mucus
   d. the basement membrane

48. All of the following statements about tight junctions are true except:

   a. The permeability of tight junctions decreases moving distally from the duodenum to the ileum.
   b. Water, small molecules with molecular weights less than 300 d, and electrolytes are unable to pass through the tight junctions.
   c. Tight junctions in the villous regions are less permeable than those in the small intestine crypts.
   d. The intestinal epithelial cell cytoskeleton is connected directly to the tight junctions.

49. Gap junctions:

   a. behave as conduits to allow the direct passage of ions and small molecules between the cytoplasms of adjacent cells
   b. are located on the apical membrane of cells
   c. consist of homologous proteins that are identical in the epithelia of different organs
   d. are also known as desmosomes

50. All of the following statements concerning chloride channels are true except:

   a. There are at least three different chloride channels in intestinal epithelial cells.
   b. The most important channel in the intestine is the calcium-activated chloride channel.
   c. cAMP-activated chloride channels are defective in cystic fibrosis.
   d. Calcium-calmodulin is an important intracellular regulator of one type of chloride channel.

51. Which of the following statements concerning common variable hypogammaglobulinemia is true?

   a. It is the most common primary immunodeficiency in adults.

b. Jejunal biopsy specimens are usually normal.
   c. Nodular lymphoid hyperplasia is a common finding.
   d. Malabsorption is unusual.

52. Each of the following statements about chronic granulomatous disease is true except:

   a. Catalase-negative organisms (e.g., pneumococci and lactobacilli) are not major pathogens.
   b. Staphylococci, *Serratia* species, and *Salmonella* species are common pathogens.
   c. Gastrointestinal symptoms may mimic those of Crohn's disease.
   d. Liver abscess formation is unusual.

53. Hereditary angioedema (C1 esterase inhibitor deficiency):

   a. can be effectively treated with anabolic steroids (e.g., danazol)
   b. is characterized by recurrent, pitting edema of the extremities
   c. commonly presents in association with pruritus
   d. commonly presents with associated leukocytosis

54. Intestinal lymphangiectasia is typically associated with:

   a. a rash resembling dermatitis herpetiformis
   b. skin test anergy
   c. pruritus
   d. decreased α_1-antitrypsin levels in stool

55. A 35-year-old man presents for the evaluation of suspected food allergies. He reports two discrete episodes of periorbital edema and severe wheezing, one of which required management in a local emergency department with bronchodilators. Both episodes occurred shortly after the ingestion of peanuts. His past medical history is remarkable only for eczema. Findings from a review of systems and a physical examination at this time are normal. Which of the following would be the most appropriate method for evaluating this patient for food allergies?

   a. skin tests
   b. radioallergosorbent test (RAST) or enzyme-linked immunosorbent assay (ELISA)
   c. cytotoxicity food allergy test
   d. double-blind, placebo-controlled oral challenge with peanuts

56. Eosinophilic gastroenteritis:

   a. typically is associated with normal or low peripheral eosinophil counts
   b. may be associated with Charcot-Leyden crystals in the stool

c. is characterized by eosinophilic infiltration confined to the mucosa

d. does not affect the colon

57. True statements regarding eosinophilic gastroenteritis include all of the following except:

   a. The differential diagnosis includes amebiasis and giardiasis.
   b. The presentation may be similar to that of Crohn's disease or gastrointestinal lymphoma.
   c. Barium radiographic studies may show cobblestoning of involved mucosa.
   d. The stomach and small intestine are most commonly involved.
   e. Prednisone therapy at 20 to 40 mg per day is effective for most patients.

58. All of the following statements regarding travelers' diarrhea are true except:

   a. Most cases of travelers' diarrhea are caused by enterotoxigenic *Escherichia coli*.
   b. The treatment of choice for adults is trimethoprim-sulfamethoxazole.
   c. Antibiotics decrease the duration of illness as well as the number of stools per day.
   d. Bismuth subsalicylate is an effective prophylaxis for travelers' diarrhea.

59. All of the following statements regarding food-borne illness are true except:

   a. *Shigella* species are the most common causes of food-borne illness in the United States.
   b. The ingestion of fried rice contaminated with *Bacillus cereus* produces an emetic illness.
   c. Botulinum toxin produces an illness characterized by nausea, vomiting, and mild abdominal pain.
   d. Food poisoning caused by a staphylococcal toxin typically occurs 6 to 24 hours after ingestion of the affected food.

60. The Vibrionaceae are a family of bacteria whose members include *Vibrio, Aeromonas,* and *Plesiomonas* species. Members of this family are responsible for a variety of gastrointestinal illnesses. With respect to specific members of this family, all of the following statements are true except:

   a. Decreased gastric acid is associated with an increased risk of acquiring *Vibrio cholerae* infection.
   b. The use of oral rehydration formula in the treatment of *Vibrio cholerae* infection relies on small intestine glucose-sodium cotransport mechanisms to induce sodium and water absorption.

c. *Vibrio parahaemolyticus* is endemic in several North American fresh-water river systems.

d. *Aeromonas* infections are known to cause a chronic diarrheal illness.

61. All of the following are characteristic of *Staphylococcus aureus* food poisoning except:

   a. nausea and vomiting
   b. fever
   c. recovery within 24 to 48 hours after ingestion
   d. abdominal cramping and diarrhea
   e. attack rates after exposure of greater than 80%

62. All of the following statements regarding *Vibrio cholerae* infections are true except:

   a. Patients with blood type O experience more severe clinical symptoms.
   b. Cholera toxin elevates cellular levels of cAMP and alters the net absorptive tendency of the small intestine to one of net secretion.
   c. Person-to-person transmission is thought to play a major role in the propagation of cholera.
   d. A large inoculum is needed to produce disease except in persons who have gastric hypochlorhydria.
   e. Primary infection with the *Vibrio cholerae* subtype O:1 confers long-term immunity to recurrent illness.

63. Each of the following agents has been shown to be an effective prophylaxis for travelers' diarrhea except:

   a. doxycycline
   b. trimethoprim-sulfamethoxazole
   c. metronidazole
   d. norfloxacin
   e. bismuth subsalicylate

64. Neurologic symptoms that can occur in patients with *Clostridium botulinum* food poisoning include each of the following except:

   a. diplopia and ophthalmoplegia
   b. urinary incontinence
   c. postural hypotension
   d. respiratory muscle weakness
   e. dysphagia or dysphonia

65. A 15-year-old, previously healthy girl develops pharyngitis, diarrhea, and abdominal pain localized to the right lower quadrant, which spontaneously resolves after several days. Shortly thereafter, painful red nodular lesions are noted over her lower extremities. The most likely etiology for this patient's illness is:

   a. *Salmonella* species
   b. *Yersinia* species
   c. *Listeria monocytogenes*
   d. *Clostridium perfringens*

The following case pertains to questions 66 through 68.

A 26-year-old man complains of watery diarrhea with weight loss since returning from India 4 months ago. An initial complete blood count reveals a hemoglobin level of 11 g/dL with a mean erythrocyte volume of 106 fl (normal, 80–100 fl). Additional laboratory tests reveal a normal level of vitamin B_{12}, an albumin level of 3.1 g/dL, and a calcium level of 8.2 mg/dL.

66. The most likely diagnosis is:

   a. equally distributed among adults and children
   b. often associated with an underlying defect in the host immune system
   c. postulated to be associated with aerobic and anaerobic bacterial overgrowth in the small intestine
   d. often complicated by malabsorption

67. Which of the following studies would best confirm the diagnosis?

   a. upper gastrointestinal endoscopy with small intestine biopsy
   b. colonoscopy with biopsy of the terminal ileum
   c. a dedicated small intestine barium radiographic series
   d. a 72-hour stool collection for quantitative fecal fat determination
   e. stool cultures

68. Anemia in patients with this disease is secondary to:

   a. pseudosplenectomy
   b. sickling of erythrocytes
   c. malabsorption resulting in vitamin B_{12} and folate deficiencies
   d. chronic disease
   e. loss of appetite

69. Clinical manifestations of *Ascaris lumbricoides* can include all of the following except:

   a. pulmonary hypersensitivity reactions
   b. intestinal obstruction
   c. common bile duct obstruction
   d. granulomatous hepatic inflammation

70. All of the following intestinal nematodes can be associated with pulmonary hypersensitivity reactions except:

   a. *Trichuris trichiura*
   b. *Necator americanus*
   c. *Ascaris lumbricoides*
   d. *Strongyloides stercoralis*

71. All of the following statements regarding hookworm infections are true except:

   a. Iron deficiency is a hallmark of chronic disease.
   b. Abdominal pain is common.

   c. Direct fecal examination for ova is inadequate to detect significant infections.
   d. Eosinophilia is common.

72. The epithelial lining of the intestinal mucosa includes each of the following except:

   a. enterocytes
   b. B lymphocytes
   c. Paneth cells
   d. enteroendocrine cells
   e. goblet cells

73. Congenital atresia of the small intestine:

   a. is associated with an overall mortality of 80%
   b. most often occurs in the distal ileum
   c. is rarely associated with other birth defects
   d. when involving the duodenum, is associated with Down syndrome

74. Malrotation of the midgut is associated with all of the following complications except:

   a. duodenal obstruction
   b. acute intestinal ischemia
   c. Hirschsprung disease
   d. small intestine arteriovenous malformations

75. A 7-month-old boy presents with "currant jelly" stools and a palpable midabdominal mass. His parents report intermittent irritability and crying over the past few days. After the initiation of intravenous hydration and surgical evaluation, the next most useful step would be:

   a. computed tomography of the abdomen
   b. barium enema radiography
   c. scintigraphy, i.e., a Meckel scan
   d. exploratory laparotomy

76. Which of the following statements regarding Meckel diverticula is true?

   a. They result from ectopic evagination of the primitive appendix.
   b. They most commonly present with gastrointestinal obstruction in adults.
   c. They are usually located in the distal jejunum.
   d. They may be falsely diagnosed by a sodium pertechnetate technetium-99m radionuclide scan in patients with Crohn's disease.

77. Congenital lymphangiectasia typically presents with each of the following except:

   a. diarrhea secondary to an opportunistic infection
   b. asymmetric edema of the extremities
   c. steatorrhea
   d. hypoalbuminemia and lymphocytopenia

78. Volvulus of the small intestine is:

    a. most common in adolescents
    b. more common than colonic volvulus
    c. often associated with an underlying anatomic defect
    d. often treated medically with conservative measures

79. Which statement regarding plicae circulares is true?

    a. They are important for generating coordinated peristaltic movement.
    b. They consist of invaginations of the mucosa, submucosa, and muscularis propria.
    c. They enhance the surface area and absorptive function of the small intestine.
    d. They are most prominent in the ileum.

80. Which of the following neurotransmitter candidates is thought to play a role in the descending relaxation component of intestinal peristalsis?

    a. substance P
    b. vasoactive intestinal polypeptide
    c. acetylcholine
    d. somatostatin

81. Which of the following neurotransmitter candidates is thought to play a role in the ascending contraction component of intestinal peristalsis?

    a. vasoactive intestinal polypeptide
    b. substance P
    c. norepinephrine
    d. calcitonin gene–related peptide

82. Which of the following statements regarding the function of autonomic pathways in the gastrointestinal tract is true?

    a. In general, the activation of sympathetic pathways stimulates gastrointestinal motility.
    b. Stimulation of sympathetic pathways relaxes sphincteric regions of the gut.
    c. Sympathetic neurons exert inhibitory control over secretomotor neurons that innervate the gastrointestinal epithelia.
    d. Vagal afferent neurons terminate centrally in the dorsal motor nucleus of the vagus.
    e. Consciously perceived visceral pain is predominantly transmitted through vagal afferent pathways.

83. A 32-year-old, diet-controlled diabetic man presents for a second opinion regarding bloating and increased flatulence for the past 5 years. His symptoms become worse after ingesting pizza and ice cream, but he is able to tolerate milk on his cereal. His primary physi-

cian has done routine blood work, including a complete blood count, electrolytes, and liver chemistries, all of which are normal. He denies having any diarrhea or weight loss. Which of the following statements is correct?

    a. Lactose intolerance is very unlikely in this patient, because he tolerates milk products.
    b. Small intestine biopsy with mucosal lactase determination is the most sensitive and specific method to document disease in this patient.
    c. After the ingestion of 50 g of lactose, a failure of plasma glucose concentration to rise more than 20 mg/dL definitively establishes the presence of lactase deficiency.
    d. A lactose tolerance test involving the measurement of serum glucose 2 hours after an ingestion of oral lactose would be sufficient to exclude or confirm the diagnosis in this patient.
    e. A lactose hydrogen breath test would exhibit abnormally low 20-minute and 2-hour breath hydrogen levels if this patient was lactose intolerant.

84. Which of the following is not associated with an increased incidence of bacterial overgrowth?

    a. Billroth II anastomosis
    b. small cell lung cancer
    c. small intestine diverticuli
    d. advanced age
    e. pancreatic insufficiency

85. A 57-year-old man presents with a 2-week history of diarrhea. He reports passing 4 to 6 loose-to-watery bowel movements per day. He has a long history of insulin-dependent diabetes mellitus complicated by retinopathy and peripheral neuropathy. Although he does report some problems with bloating, he denies having fever, abdominal pain, or bleeding and has not recently used antibiotics or traveled. Which of the following statements is most accurate?

    a. Celiac sprue is the most likely diagnosis.
    b. Small intestine biopsy specimens will probably reveal villous flattening.
    c. A 7- to 10-day course of tetracycline may be curative.
    d. Anal sphincter dysfunction is rarely seen in this setting.

86. All of the following are risk factors for the development of small bowel lymphoma except:

    a. X-linked or Bruton hypogammaglobulinemia
    b. celiac sprue
    c. human immunodeficiency virus
    d. intestinal lymphangiectasia

87. Which of the following statements about *Tropheryma whippelii,* the causative organism of Whipple disease, is true?

    a. The organism is a gram-positive, acid-fast bacillus.
    b. Infection is transmitted by direct person-to-person contact.
    c. Infection is associated with the presence of periodic acid–Schiff (PAS)-positive macrophages on small bowel biopsy specimens.
    d. The organism is commonly acquired by ingestion of contaminated meat products.

88. Patients with extensive ileal resections have an increased incidence of:

    a. cholesterol gallstones
    b. pigment gallstones
    c. both
    d. neither

89. Which of the following patients with Crohn's disease would not be predisposed to the formation of calcium oxalate renal stones?

    a. a patient who has had more than 100 cm of terminal ileum resected
    b. a patient who has had less than 100 cm of terminal ileum resected
    c. a patient with an ileostomy who has had a total colectomy
    d. a patient with extensive terminal ileum disease who has not had any resections

90. Which of the following is not a mechanism by which neutrophils contribute to epithelial destruction in inflammatory bowel disease?

    a. release of granule-bound proteases
    b. increased IgG secretion
    c. production of superoxide and other reactive oxygen species
    d. breakdown of the tight junction during migration of neutrophils across the epithelium into the lumen

91. Crohn's disease involving the terminal ileum and right colon is diagnosed in a 28-year-old woman. Olsalazine is started. Within 1 week, profound watery diarrhea develops without constitutional symptoms. How should this case be managed?

    a. prescribe steroids
    b. measure serum gastrin and vasoactive intestinal polypeptide levels
    c. stop olsalazine and start mesalamine
    d. perform enteroscopy

92. The most common presenting symptoms of Crohn's disease are diarrhea and:

    a. bleeding
    b. abdominal pain
    c. perianal disease
    d. arthritis

The following case pertains to questions 93 and 94.

A 36-year-old Turkish man presents with a 6-week history of oral ulcers, arthralgia, abdominal pain, and diarrhea. He had been healthy until 2 months ago, when he developed arthralgia, involving mainly his knees and ankles. Three weeks later, he experienced painful oral ulcers, right lower quadrant abdominal pain, and diarrhea. He has lost 7 kg in the past 2 months. He consumes ibuprofen intermittently for occasional arthralgia. The physical examination is remarkable for multiple aphthous ulcers involving the oral mucosa and mild tenderness in the right lower quadrant. A stool examination is unrevealing. Colonoscopy reveals scattered deep ulcerations in the terminal ileum.

93. Which of the following conditions is not included in the differential diagnosis of terminal ileal ulcerations?

    a. Crohn's disease
    b. Behçet syndrome
    c. histoplasmosis
    d. Whipple disease
    e. nonsteroidal antiinflammatory drug–induced ulcerations

94. The patient presents 3 weeks later complaining of worsening abdominal pain and a painful "cord" over his right thigh. His vision is blurred. Physical examination reveals hypopyon. Multiple oral ulcers are again noted, along with three shallow ulcers in the scrotal area. A warm, painful cord is palpated on the inner aspect of his right thigh consistent with a superficial thrombophlebitis. Which of the following would be helpful in establishing the diagnosis?

    a. pathergy test
    b. HLA antigen typing
    c. small bowel biopsy
    d. culture for *Histoplasma* species
    e. a + b
    f. c + d

95. All the following statements regarding bacterial overgrowth are true except:

    a. It may be associated with vitamin B_{12} deficiency.
    b. An abnormally low level of breath glucose after oral ingestion of ^{14}C-D-xylose is diagnostic.
    c. Achlorhydria and immunodeficiency may be predisposing factors.
    d. It may be seen in patients with scleroderma.
    e. It may be seen in patients with amyloidosis.

96. All the following conditions can potentially lead to short bowel syndrome except:

a. Crohn's disease
b. celiac sprue
c. mesenteric ischemia
d. radiation enteritis
e. volvulus

The following case pertains to questions 97 and 98.

A 24-year-old attorney is referred for the evaluation of a 1-year history of abdominal pain. Her symptoms began as a crampy lower abdominal pain that is alleviated by defecation. She has associated bloating and altered stool frequency (i.e., three to four bowel movements per day) with occasional loose stools. She denies epigastric pain, nausea, vomiting, poor appetite, and weight loss. She cannot recall ever being awoken by pain. She has been seen frequently by her primary care physician. Results of stool studies have been negative. Her lower abdominal pain has worsened in the last 2 weeks, and is a source of frustration because it has affected her ability to concentrate on a highly publicized case she is preparing to defend. She refuses to discuss a history of physical or sexual abuse. She appears well nourished; the only remarkable finding on physical examination is mild lower abdominal discomfort on deep palpation. The values of a complete blood cell count and liver chemistries are normal.

97. The initial evaluation should include which of the following diagnostic studies?

a. plain abdominal radiography
b. gastroduodenal manometry
c. sigmoidoscopy
d. serology for *Helicobacter pylori*
e. examination of stool for parasites

98. Assuming that the findings of the initial evaluation are normal, all of the following recommendations are appropriate except:

a. high-fiber diet
b. prokinetic agents
c. antispasmodic agents
d. anticholinergic agents
e. tricyclic antidepressant drugs

99. Which of the following statements regarding the outcome of patients with irritable bowel syndrome is true?

a. Most persons with irritable bowel syndrome are free of symptoms after 5 years.
b. Female patients with a long history of diarrhea and a good initial response to treatment are most likely to achieve long-term improvement.
c. Patients who receive education regarding the roles of psychologic stress and precipitating factors require fewer physician visits for management of their disorder.
d. Persons with irritable bowel syndrome have higher mortality rates than do unaffected persons.

100. All of the following are extraabdominal symptoms associated with irritable bowel syndrome, except:

a. chronic pelvic pain
b. peripheral neuropathy
c. genitourinary symptoms
d. impaired sexual function
e. primary fibromyalgia

101. All of the following statements regarding the pathophysiology of irritable bowel syndrome are true, except:

a. Colonic motor activity is abnormal in the postprandial but not the fasted state.
b. Patients with irritable bowel syndrome do not exhibit heightened sensitivity to somatic stimulation.
c. Reductions in the small intestine migrating motor complex (MMC) cycle length are characteristic.
d. Irritable bowel syndrome is associated with motor abnormalities in other smooth muscles including the lower esophageal sphincter, sphincter of Oddi, and detrusor muscles.
e. Persons with irritable bowel syndrome have heightened awareness of physiologic motor events in the gastrointestinal tract.

102. Each of the following statements regarding intestinal carbohydrate transport is true except:

a. The end products of lumenal and membrane digestion of ingested carbohydrates are D-glucose, D-galactose, and D-fructose.
b. Fructose is transported by facilitated diffusion by glucose transporter 5 (GLUT5).
c. Galactose influx occurs through the apical Na^+-coupled glucose cotransporter (SGLT1).
d. Enterocytes express numerous Na^+-coupled glucose transporters, including the SGLT1 transport system.

103. Each of the following statements regarding glucose-galactose malabsorption syndrome is true except:

a. It involves more than one missense mutation in the glucose cotransporter gene.
b. Symptoms manifest during the first week of life and include profuse watery diarrhea and hyperosmolar dehydration.
c. Glycosuria is not detected in patients affected by glucose-galactose malabsorption.
d. Unabsorbed carbohydrates contribute to increased osmotic pressure in the intestinal lumen with secondary fluid secretion.

104. Each of the following statements regarding Menkes syndrome is true except:

a. The product of the gene responsible for Menkes syndrome is a transmembrane P–type adenosine triphosphatase.

b. Cells affected by a mutation in the Menkes gene are unable to export copper into the extracellular space.

c. The long-term prognosis of Menkes syndrome is good.

d. Diarrhea secondary to altered enterocyte function is a common feature of the disease.

105. An infant with congenital chloride diarrhea can benefit from treatment with:

a. NaCl supplementation
b. omeprazole
c. glucose supplementation
d. cimetidine

106. Each of the following statements regarding abetalipoproteinemia is true except:

a. Abetalipoproteinemia is an autosomal recessive disease characterized by the absence of apolipoprotein B (apoB) and apoB-containing lipoproteins in the plasma of affected subjects.

b. Symptoms of malabsorption and failure to thrive are characteristic of this disease.

c. Plasma lipid and lipoprotein profiles of patients with abetalipoproteinemia include hypocholesterolemia, low triglyceride levels, and virtually nondetectable chylomicrons, very-low-density lipoproteins, low-density lipoproteins, and apoB.

d. mRNA for apoB and apoB protein are absent in the intestinal mucosa and liver of affected subjects.

107. A 22-year-old Asian student presents with complaints of intermittent abdominal pain, cramps, nausea, flatulence, and diarrhea. He has had these symptoms for several years. He describes his stools as bulky, frothy, and watery. He denies weight loss, blood in the stools, fever, or chills. He has no significant medical history. He recently spent 2 weeks in India visiting relatives. Findings on physical examination and results of laboratory tests are all normal. The most likely cause of this patient's discomfort is:

a. lactose intolerance
b. inflammatory bowel disease
c. sprue
d. amebiasis

The following case pertains to questions 108 through 111.

A 36-year-old woman consumed banana pudding, goat cheese, tuna casserole, and homemade canned pears during a winter holiday party. Twenty-four hours after ingestion, she developed abdominal pain, nausea, vomiting, diarrhea, and dysphasia. Physical examination reveals dysarthria and ophthalmoplegia.

108. Which food is the most likely cause of this woman's food illness?

a. banana pudding
b. goat cheese
c. canned pears
d. tuna casserole
e. local water supply

109. The cause of her symptoms are most likely:

a. preformed spores
b. preformed toxin
c. antibody-mediated
d. lipopolysaccharide

110. Which test would definitively diagnose this woman's illness?

a. measurement of the serum IgA
b. assay of the contaminated food
c. culture of a stool specimen
d. It is not possible to definitively diagnosis this illness.

111. The treatment of choice is:

a. aggressive hydration
b. ciprofloxacin 500 mg twice a day
c. antitoxin
d. supportive

112. Which of the following groups are at greatest risk for developing travelers' diarrhea?

a. persons who have undergone gastrectomy and vagotomy
b. persons over age 65
c. long-term bismuth subsalicylate users
d. persons with a history of gastroparesis

113. All of the following statements regarding nontyphoid salmonellosis are true except:

a. Infection is associated with four different syndromes: gastritis, enteric fever, bacteremia, and an asymptomatic carrier state.
b. Antibiotic use is not recommended for mild illness.
c. Tetracycline is recommended for treatment of severe cases.
d. Infection causes epithelial damage.

The following case pertains to questions 114 through 117.

A 53-year-old midwestern farmer presents for the evaluation of a 6-month history of diarrhea and a 20-kg weight loss. He has had intermittent low-grade fevers, and migratory arthritis involving his small and large joints for 3 to 5 years.

114. The differential diagnosis includes all the following conditions except:

a. celiac sprue
b. tropical sprue

c. Whipple disease

d. infection with *Mycobacterium avium* complex

115. The diagnostic test of choice would be:

    a. serum analysis for antiendomysial antibody
    b. small bowel biopsy
    c. stool culture
    d. quantitative fecal fat test

116. Small bowel biopsy specimens reveal infiltration of the lamina propria by periodic acid–Schiff (PAS)-positive macrophages containing gram-positive, non–acid-fast bacilli, accompanied by lymphatic dilation. This man's illness is caused by:

    a. *Mycobacterium avium* complex
    b. *Giardia lamblia*
    c. *Troheryma whippelii*
    d. *Mycoplasma* species

117. Which of the following statements about the treatment of this disease is true:

    a. Treatment with antibiotics results in gradual improvement; full clinical recovery can take up to 1 year.
    b. Small bowel biopsy to document the absence of bacilli is recommended prior to discontinuing therapy at 1 year.
    c. Relapse is uncommon.
    d. Yearly surveillance with endoscopy is recommended.

The following case pertains to questions 118 through 120.

A 25-year-old woman of short stature with chronic diarrhea, atopic eczema, and amenorrhea is referred for gastrointestinal evaluation. The physical examination reveals a normal liver span with diffuse, mild abdominal tenderness and blistering skin eruptions involving the knees, elbows, buttocks, and back. Laboratory studies confirm hypochromic, microcytic anemia, hypoalbuminemia, and hypocalcemia.

118. This woman's skin disorder is most likely:

    a. dermatitis herpetiformis
    b. dermatomyositis
    c. polyarteritis nodosa
    d. the result of niacin deficiency

119. All of the following statements regarding this condition are true except:

    a. Atopic eczema may respond to treatment of the underlying disease.
    b. Skin biopsy specimens will reveal IgA at the dermoepidermal junction in areas not affected by blisters.
    c. No specific treatment for the skin disorder is warranted if the underlying problem is treated.

d. This patient has a high likelihood of being HLA-DQ2 positive.

120. This patient is at increased risk for all of the following except:

    a. lactose and sucrose intolerance
    b. small bowel lymphoma
    c. adrenal insufficiency
    d. hyposplenism

121. All of the following statements regarding the histology of the small intestine in celiac sprue are true except:

    a. There is a loss of villous architecture with a reduction in the ratio of villous height to crypt depth.
    b. There is a decrease in the total thickness of the mucosa because of crypt atrophy.
    c. Mitotic activity is no longer confined to the base of the crypt.
    d. The cell migration time from the base of the crypt to the villous tip is shortened.

122. All of the following statements regarding celiac sprue are correct except:

    a. There is a 15% prevalence of celiac sprue among first-degree relatives of persons with celiac sprue.
    b. Ten percent of patients with celiac sprue are IgA-deficient.
    c. The combination of positive results of tests for IgA antigliadin and antiendomysial antibodies has both positive and negative predictive values approaching 99% for the diagnosis of celiac sprue.
    d. Patients with celiac sprue have complement deficiency.

123. A woman with celiac sprue confirmed by biopsy has been compliant with her recommended diet. Her most recent laboratory studies reveal hypoalbuminemia. This observation should raise concern for:

    a. gluten in the diet
    b. small bowel lymphoma
    c. pancreatic insufficiency
    d. achlorhydria

124. Gluten shock is best treated with:

    a. immune globulin
    b. systemic corticosteroids
    c. somatostatin
    d. antibiotics

TRUE/FALSE

Which of the following statements (125–128) regarding immunodeficiency syndromes are true?

125. _____ Recurrent episodes of infectious diarrhea is the most common presenting clinical feature in

patients with common variable hypogamma-globulinemia.

126. _____ Achlorhydria is uncommon in most immuno-deficiency syndromes.

127. _____ Chronic infections with *Campylobacter* species are common in immunodeficiency syndromes.

128. _____ Common variable hypogammaglobulinemia is associated with an increased incidence of gastric adenocarcinoma and lymphoma.

Which of the following statements (129–132) regarding schistosomiasis are true?

129. _____ Adult worms live as pairs within the venules of their human hosts.

130. _____ *Schistosoma mansoni* migrates to the inferior mesenteric veins, whereas *Schistosoma japonicum* migrates to the superior mesenteric veins.

131. _____ Chronic infection causes pipestem portal fibrosis with presinusoidal portal hypertension.

132. _____ Thiabendazole is the drug of choice for treating *Schistosoma* infections.

133. _____ Resection of transmural lymphoma involving the small intestine prior to chemotherapy reduces the risk of bleeding and perforation.

134. _____ A second-look laparotomy is usually indicated for patients who have recently undergone bowel resection for mesenteric ischemia resulting from mesenteric venous thrombosis.

135. _____ Malrotation presents in the newborn as bilious emesis without abdominal distention.

Which of the following statements (136–139) regarding thrombotic and embolic mesenteric ischemia are true?

136. _____ Most emboli that cause mesenteric ischemia originate from atheromatous plaques that are dislodged from the aorta.

137. _____ Thrombotic intestinal ischemia commonly results from obstruction in one of the major mesenteric arteries.

138. _____ The presence of cardiac disease represents a significant risk factor for both forms of mesenteric ischemia.

139. _____ The mortality rate for embolic mesenteric ischemia is greater than 50%.

The following case pertains to questions 140 through 143.

An 82-year-old man with a history of atherosclerotic heart disease, peripheral vascular disease, and diverticulitis presents with a 4-month history of weight loss and intermittent severe abdominal pain that is precipitated by eating. His referring physician ordered a barium upper gastrointestinal radiographic series and abdominal computed tomography, both of which revealed nothing abnormal. Based on the working diagnosis, which of the following statements are true?

140. _____ Auscultation of the abdomen during pain in patients with this condition typically reveals hypoactive or absent bowel sounds.

141. _____ The development of acute small bowel infarction in this patient is unlikely.

142. _____ The patient may benefit from surgical bypass of the superior mesenteric artery.

143. _____ Chronic anticoagulation and surgical bypass are of equal benefit.

144. _____ A 54-year-old woman with a documented 9-kg weight loss over 6 months is evaluated. If no specific etiology is identified after a complete evaluation, the patient's prognosis is poor.

145. _____ In a patient with liver metastases on abdominal computed tomography and elevated urinary 5-HIAA levels, the appendix is the most likely site for the primary tumor.

146. _____ The most common location for small intestine adenomas is in the second portion of the duodenum.

147. _____ Patients with celiac sprue are at increased risk for the development of small intestine lymphoma but are at no increased risk for other malignancies.

148. _____ A 49-year-old man with a history of celiac sprue develops abdominal pain without weight loss or diarrhea. A small intestine barium radiographic series reveals multiple small intestine ulcers and several strictures. This disease process is usually corticosteroid-responsive and has a good prognosis.

149. _____ A 61-year-old woman with a 6-month history of diarrhea and a 7-kg weight loss undergoes a

small intestine barium radiographic series that reveals no abnormalities. A small intestine biopsy is performed and the histology is consistent with celiac sprue with the additional finding of a collagen-like material deposited beneath the intestinal epithelium. In this case, the patient will probably not respond to a gluten-free diet or corticosteroids.

Factors influencing intestinal adaptation after small intestine resection in animal models include (150–152):

150. _____ the presence of dietary nutrients in the bowel lumen

151. _____ growth-associated polyamines

152. _____ stimulation by pancreatic and biliary secretions

153. _____ Ischemic damage to small intestine mucosal epithelial cells occurs within minutes after an interruption of blood flow and can result in the denuding of villi within 1 hour.

154. _____ Anorexia and lethargy in a patient with diarrhea are more likely indicative of intestinal mucosal disease than of pancreatic disease.

155. _____ An important first step in gastrointestinal smooth muscle contraction is phosphorylation of myosin light chain by myosin light chain phosphatase.

156. _____ Contraction of gastrointestinal smooth muscle may be mediated by calcium flux across open calcium channels or by the release of intracellular calcium evoked by inositol trisphosphate.

157. _____ The membrane potential of gastrointestinal smooth muscle is largely determined by the activity of the Na^+,K^+-ATPase.

158. _____ In the human small intestine, there is an increasing gradient in the slow-wave frequency from the duodenum to the ileum.

159. _____ The interstitial cells of Cajal initiate rhythmic electrical activity and may act as the pacemakers in certain regions of the gastrointestinal tract.

160. _____ The gap junction, a structure prevalent in the intestinal longitudinal muscle layer, provides a low-resistance pathway for the electrical coupling of adjacent muscle cells.

161. _____ The peptide hormone motilin is believed to be an important mediator of fasting gastroduodenal motor activity, because endogenous motilin release cycles in phase with the migrating motor complex, and exogenous motilin administration evokes premature gastroduodenal phase III activity.

162. _____ Distention of the ileum causes relaxation of the ileocecal sphincter, and distention of the proximal colon leads to an increase in ileocecal sphincter pressure.

163. _____ The most common malignancy responsible for the development of paraneoplastic visceral neuropathy is oat cell carcinoma of the lung.

164. _____ Diarrhea is the most common symptomatic manifestation of gastrointestinal dysmotility in diabetes mellitus, occurring in 50% of patients.

165. _____ In scleroderma, gastrointestinal symptoms may precede the development of skin changes, arthritis, or the Raynaud phenomenon.

166. _____ Intestinal pseudoobstruction in the setting of hypoparathyroidism is a consequence of hypophosphatemia.

167. _____ B lymphocytes in gastrointestinal mucosa are capable of switching from predominantly IgM production to IgA production.

168. _____ B lymphoblasts mature into IgA-secreting plasma cells after homing to mucosal sites.

169. _____ IgA is not transported into bile from the systemic circulation.

170. _____ Lymphocytes in the lamina propria play an important role in spontaneous cell-mediated cytotoxicity tested in vitro.

171. _____ M cells may serve as a portal of entry for human immunodeficiency virus.

172. _____ Endoscopic pinch biopsy specimens from the small intestine commonly contain tissue from the submucosa as well as the mucosa.

173. _____ Components of the basement membrane influence the differentiation of epithelial cells.

174. _____ In patients with protein-losing enteropathy and hypogammaglobulinemia, serum IgG levels are reduced to a greater extent than are IgA or IgM levels.

175. _____ In the proximal small intestine, *Bacteroides* species and coliforms are the predominant organisms.

176. _____ Normally, fewer than 10^5 colony-forming units per milliliter are present in cultures of the lumenal contents of the proximal jejunum in humans. These organisms are primarily gram-negative rods and anaerobes.

177. _____ The gold standard for the diagnosis of bacterial overgrowth is the demonstration of an increased number of bacteria (10^5 colony-forming units per milliliter) in fluid that is obtained from the small intestine during duodenal intubation.

178. _____ The Meissner plexus is located between the circular and longitudinal layers of the muscularis externa.

179. _____ About 80% of the neurons in the vagus nerve are afferent (sensory) rather then efferent (motor).

180. _____ The pH at the microvillus border of the enterocyte is lower than the pH of the remainder of the lumenal contents of the small intestine.

181. _____ Receptors for endogenous regulatory peptide hormones are predominantly located on the apical surface of gastrointestinal epithelia.

182. _____ During the endoscopic evaluation of celiac sprue, at least 3 biopsy specimens should be taken from the crests of the valvulae conniventes in the second portion of the duodenum.

183. _____ Recovery after *Vibrio cholerae* infection does not confer immunity.

184. _____ *Vibrio parahaemolyticus* infection arises from contaminated saltwater.

MATCHING

(each selection may be used once, more than once, or not at all)

Match the following characteristic with the appropriate clinical condition:

185. _____ colicky pain is the cardinal symptom

186. _____ may be treated nonoperatively

187. _____ may be diagnosed by water-soluble contrast radiographic studies

188. _____ commonly results in pneumoperitoneum

a. small intestine obstruction

b. perforated duodenal ulcer

c. both

d. neither

Match the following acquired immunodeficiency syndrome–related infections with the clinical associations:

189. _____ *Cryptosporidia* infection

190. _____ Microsporida infection

191. _____ *Isospora* infection

192. _____ *Salmonella* infection

a. pyrimethamine- and sulfadiazine-responsive

b. bacteremia is common

c. acalculous cholecystitis

d. histologic examination reveals a "meront inclusion"

Match the following infectious agents with the clinical manifestations:

193. _____ cytomegalovirus

194. _____ herpes simplex virus

a. perineal ulcer

b. lymphoma

195. _____ Epstein-Barr virus

196. _____ *Mycobacterium avium* complex

c. intranuclear inclusions

d. jejunal thickening

Match the following protozoa with their associated features:

197. _____ *Trypanosoma cruzi*

198. _____ *Giardia lamblia*

199. _____ *Isospora belli*

a. demonstrated by using Kinyoun acid-fast stain

b. megacolon

c. not usually invasive

Match the following intestinal infections with the appropriate associations:

200. _____ *Entamoeba histolytica*

201. _____ *Cryptosporidium*

202. _____ *Isospora belli*

203. _____ *Endolimax nana*

204. _____ *Giardia lamblia*

a. nonpathogenic commensal of the large bowel

b. trophozoites demonstrable in lumenal aspirate, on biopsy specimen, or both

c. tender, palpable, right lower quadrant mass; apple-core lesion on barium enema radiography

d. no effective therapy

e. trimethoprim-sulfamethoxazole therapy

Match each of the intestinal helminth infections with the following associations:

205. _____ anisakiasis

206. _____ *Taenia saginata*

207. _____ *Diphyllobothrium latum*

208. _____ echinococcosis

a. cysticercosis

b. macrocytic anemia

c. hydatid cyst

d. squid

Match the agent responsible for food poisoning with the appropriate characteristics:

209. _____ rotavirus

210. _____ *Yersinia enterocolitica*

211. _____ *Vibrio cholerae*

212. _____ paralytogenic shellfish

213. _____ *Campylobacter* species

a. complications include development of pseudo-membranous colitis

b. neurotoxin, "red tide" season

c. most commonly affects children

d. enterotoxin-mediated

e. may mimic appendicitis

Match the stool electrolyte pattern with the most likely diagnosis:

214. _____ stool osmolality 178 mOsm, sodium 20 mEq/L, potassium 25 mEq/L

215. _____ stool osmolality 295 mOsm, sodium 97 mEq/L, potassium 36 mEq/L

a. osmotic diarrhea

b. secretory diarrhea

c. inflammatory diarrhea

216. _____ stool osmolality 308 mOsm, sodium 37 mEq/L, potassium 42 mEq/L

d. contamination of specimen with concentrated urine

e. contamination of specimen with water

Match the best answer for each of the following patients who are undergoing evaluation for diarrhea:

217. _____ a 22-year-old man surreptitiously taking ricinoleic acid

218. _____ a 36-year-old man with significant weight loss recently diagnosed with celiac sprue based on results of small intestine biopsy

219. _____ a 48-year-old woman surreptitiously taking 6 ounces of milk of magnesia per day

220. _____ a 19-year-old Asian man complaining of mild gas, abdominal cramps, and diarrhea for the past 4 years that have worsened since he moved into his college dormitory

a. secretory diarrhea

b. osmotic diarrhea

c. both secretory and osmotic diarrhea

d. neither secretory nor osmotic diarrhea

Match the following substances that stimulate intestinal secretion with the appropriate intracellular second messenger:

221. _____ acetylcholine

222. _____ histamine

223. _____ prostaglandins

224. _____ Escherichia coli heat-stable toxin

225. _____ vasoactive intestinal polypeptide

a. increased intracellular calcium

b. cyclic AMP

c. cyclic GMP

Match the following substances with the predominant effect on intestinal fluid and ion movement:

226. _____ dopamine

227. _____ calcitonin

228. _____ somatostatin

229. _____ substance P

230. _____ glucocorticoids

231. _____ motilin

a. intestinal absorption

b. intestinal secretion

Match the following diseases with their typical abnormalities:

232. _____ scleroderma

233. _____ dermatomyositis

234. _____ systemic lupus erythematosus

235. _____ diabetes mellitus

a. small intestine ischemia

b. low internal anal sphincter tone and incompetent external anal sphincter

c. aperistalsis of the distal esophagus and incompetent lower esophageal sphincter

d. dilation and dysmotility of the proximal esophagus

A 32-year-old woman with chronic intestinal pseudoobstruction presents with recent onset of diarrhea. After a careful evaluation, bacterial overgrowth is diagnosed. Match the following clinical problems encountered in the setting of bacterial overgrowth with their most likely pathophysiologic explanation:

236. _____ fat-soluble vitamin deficiency

237. _____ lactose intolerance

238. _____ vitamin B$_{12}$ deficiency

239. _____ excessive flatus

a. bacterial fermentation of carbohydrates

b. bile-salt deconjugation

c. brush-border enzyme deficiency

d. intestinal bacterial utilization

Match each of the following small intestine tumors with one of the angiographic features:

240. _____ leiomyoma

241. _____ carcinoid

242. _____ adenocarcinoma

a. arterial tortuosity and narrowing with a stellate pattern

b. hypervascular; a dense, well-circumscribed blush

c. hypovascular mass with arteries that are occluded or encased

Match the following causes of infectious diarrhea in AIDS patients with the recommended initial therapy:

243. _____ *Salmonella* species

244. _____ *Clostridium difficile*

245. _____ *Mycobacterium avium* complex

a. clarithromycin, rifabutin, and ethambutol

b. ceftriaxone or ciprofloxacin

c. metronidazole

Match the following presentations with the disorders listed:

246. _____ a 34-year-old Peruvian man with a 1-year history of watery diarrhea and weight loss; diarrhea improves when he takes tetracycline

247. _____ a 59-year-old man with right lower quadrant abdominal pain and diarrhea for 3 months; a mass is palpable on examination; patient has a previous diagnosis of common variable immunodeficiency

248. _____ a 40-year-old man with history of prior colectomy for unclear reasons presents with painless jaundice

a. small bowel carcinoid tumor

b. immunoproliferative small bowel disease

c. familial adenomatous polyposis

d. small bowel lymphoma

e. Crohn's disease

Select the best designation for each of the following characteristics of familial visceral neuropathy:

249. _____ autosomal dominant

250. _____ no effective medical or surgical therapies

251. _____ associated with malformation of the central nervous system and with a patent ductus arteriosus

252. _____ hypertrophy of argyrophilic neurons and increase in number of nerve fibers

253. _____ associated with intestinal pseudoobstruction

a. type I only

b. type II only

c. both type I and II

d. neither

Match the following characteristics to the respective therapy for Crohn's disease:

254. _____ efficacy in Crohn's disease not clearly established

255. _____ can lead to acute pancreatitis

256. _____ most effective agent for healing refractory fistulous disease

257. _____ first-pass metabolism in the liver limits systemic toxicity

a. budesonide

b. 6-mercaptopurine

c. methotrexate

d. infliximab

4

Colon

MULTIPLE CHOICE

(one best answer)

1. Standard colonic transit testing:

    a. is performed using radioactive markers and nuclear scintigraphy
    b. is a useful study for elderly patients with mild to moderate constipation characterized by daily straining at stool
    c. may help to distinguish colonic inertia from a functional outlet obstruction
    d. should be performed when the patient is not taking any laxatives or fiber products
    e. when normal in a patient with complaints of infrequent stools is unlikely to be associated with psychologic dysfunction

2. Which one of the following pairs of diseases or medications is not typically associated with constipation?

    a. rheumatoid arthritis and systemic lupus erythematosus
    b. iron sulfate and calcium supplements
    c. anticholinergics and opiate analgesics
    d. hypothyroidism and diabetes mellitus
    e. Parkinson disease and multiple sclerosis

3. A 42-year-old woman with persistent constipation despite a high-fiber diet is evaluated. Anorectal manometry shows normal sphincter function and modestly decreased rectal sensation. Defecography reveals a large rectocele with poor expulsion of barium paste. Expulsion of the paste is improved when the patient manually pushes on the posterior wall of the vagina during attempted defecation. A colonic transit test is abnormal, primarily because of delayed transit in the rectosigmoid colon. The patient responded poorly to fiber therapy and saline laxatives. Which one of the following treatments is indicated?

    a. surgical repair of the rectocele
    b. segmental resection of the rectosigmoid colon
    c. subtotal colectomy with ileoproctostomy

    d. constipation biofeedback therapy
    e. posterior division of the puborectalis muscle

4. A 63-year-old man presents with a 3-month history of severe constipation. Which one of the following statements is most accurate?

    a. This patient would be best evaluated with a combination of anorectal manometry, defecography, and colonic transit testing.
    b. Barium enema radiography or an endoscopic procedure of the colon should be performed to rule out a structural lesion.
    c. A flexible sigmoidoscopy should be performed, and if no lesions are noted, a rectal biopsy specimen should be taken.
    d. A short trial of stimulant laxatives is indicated. An evaluation can be performed at a later date if there is no significant benefit.

5. Which one of the following contractile patterns is not seen in the human colon?

    a. quiescent periods
    b. individual phasic contractions of short and long duration
    c. organized groups of nonpropagating and propagating contractions
    d. giant migrating contractions preceded by a transient relaxation
    e. propagative patterns of the interdigestive migrating motor complex

6. Which one of the following statements concerning the gastrocolonic response is true?

    a. The response is defined as an increase in motility in the colon induced by gastric pathology.
    b. The response is partially mediated by cholinergic pathways; this is known because the response is blunted by atropine.
    c. The response is mediated by cholecystokinin (CCK) released following a meal; selective CCK receptor antagonists abolish the response.

d. Motor responses to eating are abolished following gastrectomy.

e. The response is defined as an increase in gastric activity induced by distention of the colon.

7. Which one of the following statements regarding colonic motor function is most accurate?

a. The predominant pattern of contraction in the right colon is rhythmic peristalsis.

b. Tonic circular contractions in the colon can be seen radiographically as haustral markings.

c. The predominant contraction pattern in the left colon is antiperistaltic.

d. The internal anal sphincter tonically contracts during defecation.

8. Which one of the following statements concerning the mechanisms of fecal incontinence is most accurate?

a. The external sphincter muscle contributes to the majority of resting anal canal tone.

b. During acute increases in intraabdominal pressure (i.e., coughing), the internal sphincter has the primary responsibility for maintaining continence.

c. Abnormal straightening of the anorectal angle predisposes to fecal incontinence.

d. Chronic constipation can cause fecal incontinence except when fecal impaction occurs.

9. A 28-year-old man reports episodes of rectal pain that are unrelated to defecation. The pain occurs once or twice per month and is described as severe and "stabbing," but it lasts for only several seconds. The patient is otherwise healthy, and a review of systems reveals nothing abnormal. Findings on physical examination, including anorectal examination, are normal. The most likely diagnosis is:

a. proctalgia fugax

b. intermittent coccygodynia

c. anal fissure

d. levator ani syndrome

10. A 78-year-old man complains of incomplete fecal evacuation and tenesmus, and says that "part of my insides push out when I have a bowel movement." Examination reveals a normal perineum with decreased anal sphincter tone. During attempted defecation, 3 cm of mucosa is seen to emerge from the sphincter in concentric folds. Which one of the follow statements is not true?

a. This lesion is more common in women than men.

b. A voiding defecogram will show intussusception of the rectal mucosa in a downward direction.

c. This lesion cannot be distinguished from prolapsing internal hemorrhoids by appearance alone.

d. Flexible sigmoidoscopy may show changes consistent with solitary rectal ulcer syndrome.

e. An appropriate surgical option for treatment of this lesion is proctopexy and sigmoid resection.

11. A healthy 31-year-old man presents to the clinic with a 2-day history of anorectal pain after a recent diarrheal illness. Examination of the perineum reveals a 5-cm area of erythema, tenderness, warmth, and mild swelling posterolateral to the anus. Which one of the following statements is true?

a. This lesion is caused by *Candida albicans* or a dermatophyte infection.

b. This is a suppurative infection (abscess) caused by a gram-positive organism.

c. The patient probably has Crohn's disease with perianal involvement.

d. This anorectal abscess probably began as an infected anal gland.

e. Anal fissure disease is frequently associated with this condition.

12. A 19-year-old woman requires a large episiotomy during the delivery of her first child. Soon thereafter, she develops persistent symptoms of fecal incontinence. Which one of the following statements is most correct?

a. Flexible sigmoidoscopy should be performed to rule out a structural lesion and mucosal inflammation.

b. Anorectal manometry with biofeedback will probably be helpful in evaluating this patient.

c. The patient should be instructed to keep her stool soft and relatively frequent.

d. Anal sensory testing is indicated.

e. Surgical repair will probably be necessary.

13. A 63-year-old woman complains of a dull, aching rectal pain that lasts for minutes to hours and occurs several times per week. She reports that sometimes she feels like she is "sitting on a ball." Findings from anoscopy and sigmoidoscopy are normal. Which one of the following statements is most accurate?

a. The most likely diagnosis is proctalgia fugax.

b. Digital examination will often yield useful findings despite normal findings from anoscopy and sigmoidoscopy.

c. A trial of antiinflammatory therapy is indicated.

d. Surgery is necessary in the minority of cases that do not respond to medical therapy.

14. All of the following statements concerning anal malignancies are true except:

a. Anal malignancies are most commonly of the squamous cell type.

b. Anal malignancies are associated with receptive anal intercourse in men and genital warts in both genders.

c. Recent investigations suggest a possible causal role for human papillomavirus infection in anal malignancy.

d. Adenocarcinomas are rare tumors that can arise from anorectal fistulas.

e. Anal carcinoma is usually discovered early in the course of the disease because of symptoms of outlet obstruction.

15. A 35-year-old man with a 3-year history of intermittent mild diarrhea develops bright red rectal bleeding with pain on defecation. Anoscopy reveals small internal hemorrhoids and an anal fissure located laterally. Which one of the following statements is true?

a. The lateral location of the fissure should prompt a search for underlying Crohn's disease.

b. Anal fissures are associated with a blunting of the relaxation component of the rectoanal inhibitory reflex.

c. In patients who require a sphincterotomy for fissures, a higher rate of postoperative complications is observed with lateral sphincterotomy compared to posterior midline sphincterotomy.

d. For the treatment of anal fissures, manual anal dilation under anesthesia is associated with a negligible incidence of incontinence and is the preferred surgical treatment.

e. More than 90% of primary fissures are located in the anterior midline.

16. All of the following statements about anorectal fistulas and abscesses are true except:

a. There is an increased incidence of abscesses and fistulas in anal carcinoma, leukemia, and lymphoma.

b. Mortality rates from anorectal infection in acute leukemia can exceed 70%.

c. The most common bacterial isolates from anorectal abscesses are *Pseudomonas* species.

d. Because of the risk of extension into adjacent tissues and the development of necrotizing infection, the presence of an anorectal abscess usually requires immediate surgical action.

e. Infection of the anal glands is believed to be the cause of most anorectal fistulas because the internal orifice is often found at the dentate line.

17. Acute appendicitis is best characterized by which of the following statements?

a. Older patients generally have significantly better outcomes than younger patients.

b. To make an accurate diagnosis of acute appendicitis, ultrasonographic examination of the right lower quadrant is required.

c. Acute appendicitis has a high rate of spontaneous perforation within the first 3 hours of the onset of abdominal pain.

d. Acute appendicitis can be treated nonoperatively if complicated by the development of an appendiceal abscess.

18. Which of the following statements concerning endometriosis is true?

a. The most common location of gastrointestinal involvement is the rectosigmoid colon.

b. The most common gastrointestinal symptoms related to endometriosis are diarrhea, bloating, and rectal bleeding.

c. Most lesions involving the gastrointestinal tract are invasive lesions that can be circumferential and mimic carcinoma on barium enema.

d. Gastrointestinal involvement in patients with documented endometriosis is rare, occurring in less than 5% of affected patients.

e. When gastrointestinal symptoms occur in women with endometriosis, colonoscopy is confirmatory in more than 50% of procedures.

19. Acute colonic pseudoobstruction (Ogilvie syndrome):

a. can occasionally be caused by a left-sided colonic obstruction as a result of tumor or stricture

b. is precipitated by metabolic disturbances, medications, or serious concurrent illnesses

c. has a high mortality related to colonic perforation and peritonitis

d. should be treated with segmental or total colectomy if conservative measures fail

e. should be treated by urgent colonoscopy if cecal distention exceeds 5 to 7 cm

20. An 80-year-old man with Parkinson disease presents at the emergency department with a 3-day history of abdominal distention, pain, and obstipation. Examination reveals the patient has a temperature of 38.8°C, and his abdomen is tympanitic with rebound tenderness. Abdominal radiographs reveal an inverted U-shaped loop of dilated colon. Which of the following is the most appropriate next step in this patient's management?

a. emergent sigmoidoscopy with rectal tube placement

b. emergent diagnostic and therapeutic barium enema

c. prolonged nasogastric suction and avoidance of narcotic analgesic medications

d. surgical consultation for emergency laparotomy

21. Each of the following is a risk factor for the development of megacolon in ulcerative colitis except:

    a. colonoscopy
    b. barium enema radiography
    c. opiates
    d. antibiotics
    e. anticholinergics

22. A 47-year-old previously healthy man presents with fever, right upper quadrant abdominal pain, and leukocytosis. You suspect ascending cholangitis and admit the patient to the hospital for antibiotic therapy. Ultrasonography reveals no evidence of gallstones. The patient improves rapidly, but persistently elevated alkaline phosphatase and total bilirubin levels remain. You perform endoscopic retrograde cholangiopancreatography and find intrahepatic stricturing and segmental strictures in his common hepatic duct which you are able to successfully dilate. You should perform which of the following:

    a. begin a liver transplantation evaluation
    b. obtain a small bowel radiograph to rule out segmental intestinal strictures
    c. perform colonoscopy to rule out ulcerative colitis
    d. obtain a surgical consultation for reconstructive biliary tract surgery
    e. begin a program of rotating outpatient antibiotics

23. You have been treating a 24-year-old woman with ulcerative colitis limited to the distal 30 cm of colon for 2 months. Her symptoms were successfully managed with sulfasalazine, but the development of a rash prompted a change to 5-aminosalicylic acid enemas each night at bedtime. After 1 month on this regimen, the symptoms had completely resolved and she discontinued the enemas completely. Two weeks later, she presents with recurrent symptoms of cramping abdominal pain, tenesmus, and increased stool frequency (6 loose stools per day) with occasional bloody stools. She is afebrile and able to eat without nausea. You should perform the following:

    a. perform colonoscopy to document the extent of disease
    b. institute metronidazole or azathioprine because of the progression of her disease and intolerance to sulfasalazine
    c. reinstitute 5-aminosalicylic acid enemas and consider a slow tapering if the patient stabilizes
    d. begin oral prednisone

24. Chronic radiation–induced proctitis is produced by:

    a. superinfection of the rectal mucosa with common bacterial pathogens
    b. tissue ischemia as a result of obliterative endarteritis

    c. radiation-induced vascular hyperproliferation leading to extensive telangiectasia formation
    d. a direct effect of tissue necrosis as a result of cumulative radiation exposure

25. Which one of the following statements regarding pregnancy and inflammatory bowel disease is true?

    a. Women with Crohn's disease have a slightly increased rate of infertility, which may be closely related to disease activity and nutritional status.
    b. Infertility is greater in patients with ulcerative colitis than in the normal population.
    c. Inflammatory bowel disease management using total parenteral nutrition is detrimental to the fetus.
    d. Steroids should be tapered off and discontinued during pregnancy.

26. All of the following associations regarding collagenous colitis are true except:

    a. female predominance, mean age 55 to 65; frequently associated with arthritis, autoimmune disorders, or celiac disease
    b. chronic, nonbloody diarrhea with occasional nocturnal stools and fecal incontinence
    c. fluctuating clinical course with spontaneous relapses and remissions rather than slowly progressive disease
    d. intraepithelial lymphocyte ratio (lymphocytes to epithelial cells) of 1 : 5
    e. increased subepithelial collagen band between 10 and 100 μm most prominent in the rectum

27. Microscopic colitis/collagenous colitis (MC/CC) is distinguished from inflammatory bowel disease (IBD) by each of the following except:

    a. Typically, the colonic mucosa appears endoscopically normal in MC/CC but not in IBD.
    b. Histologic evaluation of biopsy specimens reveals an increased number of intraepithelial lymphocytes in MC/CC relative to IBD.
    c. Crypt distortion is seen in IBD but is rarely seen in MC/CC.
    d. Ulcerative colitis presents with a more abundant inflammatory cell infiltrate of the lamina propria than does MC/CC.

28. A 67-year-old woman presents with a 4-month history of intermittent colicky abdominal pain, a 7-kg weight loss, and severe watery diarrhea. Empiric trials of loperamide (16 mg/day) are unsuccessful. She has had 15 g of fat in a 72-hour fecal fat collection (i.e., 5 g/24 hours), a normal small intestine biopsy specimen, negative stool examinations for ova and parasites, negative stool bacterial cultures, absent fecal leukocytes, a normal hydrogen breath test after lactose

ingestion, and a colonic biopsy specimen showing increased intraepithelial lymphocytes and a 25-mm subepithelial band. Which of the following is the most appropriate therapy for this patient?

a. sulfasalazine or bismuth and, if no response, corticosteroids in modest doses
b. high-dose oral corticosteroids and broad-spectrum antibiotics
c. pancreatic enzymes and, if no response, a trial of a gluten-free diet
d. conservative therapy with nutritional supplementation as necessary
e. colchicine and a trial of methotrexate

29. Which one of the following statements is true?

a. Approximately 50% of patients with inflammatory bowel disease (IBD) have a first-degree relative with IBD.
b. The risk of developing ulcerative colitis (UC) is increased among smokers, and the incidence of smoking in patients with Crohn's disease is lower than in the general population.
c. Seventy percent of patients with UC are anti-neutrophil cytoplasmic antibody–positive.
d. Patients with IBD have a low incidence of antibodies to cow's milk protein.
e. A person with a first-degree relative with Crohn's disease has the same risk as the general population of developing UC.

30. Regarding the natural history of ulcerative colitis, all of the following statements are true except:

a. Younger patients are more likely than older ones to enter sustained periods of remission.
b. Ulcerative colitis most commonly follows a chronic intermittent course, marked by long periods of quiescence interspersed with acute attacks lasting weeks to months.
c. The rate of colectomy at 2 years from diagnosis for those patients who initially present with severe disease is 50%.
d. The rate of colectomy at 5 years from diagnosis for those patients who initially present with pancolitis is 50%.

31. A small intestine barium radiography series performed on a 34-year-old man with a 6-year history of ulcerative pancolitis reveals a deformed, open ileocecal valve and a mildly dilated terminal ileum with irregular mucosa and no ulcerations. In what percent of patients with ulcerative pancolitis does this process occur?

a. 1%
b. 5%
c. 15%
d. 50%
e. 80%

32. Which one of the following statements is true?

a. Ulcerative proctitis is thought to be a separate pathophysiologic entity from ulcerative colitis (UC).
b. In patients with ulcerative proctitis who are followed up for 10 years, approximately 30% of patients have disease extending proximally to the hepatic flexure.
c. Limited colitis is generally the rule in the initial attack of UC, with 75% of patients having no disease proximal to the sigmoid colon.
d. In approximately 50% of patients with UC, the disease will go into remission after the first attack.
e. Periodic colonoscopies after initiating drug therapy are thought to provide useful information about the severity of disease.

33. All of the following statements are true except:

a. Prostaglandin levels are elevated in the mucosa and serum of inflammatory bowel disease (IBD) patients and can correlate with disease activity.
b. Although nonsteroidal antiinflammatory drugs inhibit prostaglandin synthesis, they fail to induce clinical improvement in patients with IBD.
c. Leukotriene B_4 (LTB_4) is a major neutrophil chemotactic agent in IBD.
d. LTB_4 is found in greater quantities in the colonic mucosa of IBD patients than in controls.
e. Dietary supplements with fish oil containing omega-3 fatty acids reduce colonic inflammation by decreasing prostaglandin production from arachidonic acid.

34. A 34-year-old man with a 5-year history of refractory ulcerative colitis requiring high doses of systemic steroid therapy is scheduled for an elective colectomy with a Brooke ileostomy. Of the following extraintestinal manifestations of inflammatory bowel disease, which one is the least likely to improve following colectomy?

a. uveitis
b. pyoderma gangrenosum
c. peripheral arthritis
d. sclerosing cholangitis
e. erythema nodosum

35. Which one of the following statements regarding immunosuppressive therapy for inflammatory bowel disease is not true?

a. Azathioprine use may allow a tapering or gradual withdrawal of corticosteroids.

b. Azathioprine and 6-mercaptopurine will generally not provide clinical benefit until after 2 months of drug administration.

c. Immunosuppressive therapy is never indicated in ulcerative colitis, because colectomy provides a cure.

d. Pancreatitis and leukopenia are major adverse effects.

36. Which one of the following benign extraintestinal manifestations of Gardner syndrome is most likely to result in substantial morbidity and mortality?

a. osteomas
b. desmoid tumors
c. congenital hypertrophy of the retinal pigment epithelium
d. epidermoid cyst
e. odontomas

37. Which one of the following syndromes is associated with hamartomatous gastrointestinal polyposis and hair loss?

a. Gardner syndrome
b. Peutz-Jeghers syndrome
c. Cronkhite-Canada syndrome
d. familial adenomatous polyposis

38. Which one of the following statements concerning Peutz-Jeghers syndrome is true?

a. The most common location of polyps is the small intestine.
b. There is no significant increased risk of the development of gastrointestinal malignancies.
c. Mucocutaneous pigmentation typically occurs in the third decade of life.
d. Glands often show epithelial invasion into the submucosa, indicating malignancy.

39. Each of the following extracolonic malignancies is associated with familial adenomatous polyposis or Gardner syndrome except:

a. papillary carcinoma of the thyroid
b. duodenal carcinoma
c. biliary neoplasia
d. hepatoblastoma
e. renal cell carcinoma

40. Each of the following statements regarding bacterial infections of the colon is true except:

a. Small-volume diarrhea (1 L/day) is typical.
b. The results of a fecal leukocyte test are considered positive if 3 or more leukocytes per high-power microscopic field are present in four or more fields.

c. The presence of fecal leukocytes makes ulcerative colitis an unlikely diagnosis.
d. Presenting symptoms often include fever and crampy abdominal pain.

41. A 68-year-old man is hospitalized after hip surgery. His postoperative course is complicated by a massive cerebral vascular accident and respiratory insufficiency requiring ventilatory support. He later develops massive abdominal distention. A water-soluble contrast enema radiographic examination excludes mechanical obstruction but shows a massively dilated colon. Appropriate management strategies include all of the following except:

a. correction of underlying metabolic abnormalities
b. placement of a nasogastric tube for decompression
c. a therapeutic trial of a prokinetic agent
d. the performance of a partial colectomy if the cecum diameter exceeds 11 cm
e. colonoscopic decompression if peritoneal signs are absent and medical therapy does not solve the problem

42. Which one of the following statements concerning colonic transit is true?

a. In general, markers ingested within a 48-hour period of time leave the colon in the same order in which they entered.
b. The transit of markers through the colon is dependent upon whether or not they are ingested with a meal.
c. Normally, 80% of ingested markers are passed by the fifth day after ingestion.
d. Segmental colonic transit can be measured by counting the number of markers in the stool.

43. Each of the following statements regarding diverticular bleeding is true except:

a. Hemorrhage arises from an arterial source as a result of a defect in the vasa recta.
b. Histologic studies reveal that most cases of bleeding are not associated with inflammation in the bleeding diverticulum.
c. Bleeding occurs in about 5% of all patients with diverticulosis.
d. Recurrence of bleeding occurs in 20% of patients after one episode and in 50% of patients after recurrent bleeding.
e. Diverticular bleeding is occult in 50% of patients.

44. Each of the following statements regarding diverticulitis is true except:

a. Recurrence of diverticulitis occurs in about 5% of patients.

b. Surgical treatment is necessary in 15% to 30% of patients.

c. Peritonitis, abscess, and fistula are indications for surgery.

d. Broad-spectrum antibiotic coverage for both aerobic and anaerobic organisms is necessary.

45. All of the following statements regarding colonic angiodysplasia are true except:

a. Angiodysplasia occurs in 5% of subjects undergoing colonoscopy for unrelated indications.

b. Angiodysplasia is a frequent cause of recurrent lower gastrointestinal bleeding in elderly subjects.

c. Histologic features of gastric angiodysplasia are distinguishable from those of right colon angiodysplasia.

d. Bleeding from angiodysplastic lesions is usually chronic and low-grade.

46. Which one of the following statements about radiation proctitis is true?

a. Symptoms of acute proctitis occur in 10% of patients receiving greater than 40 Gy of external radiotherapy.

b. Acute radiation injury progresses to chronic injury in approximately 50% of patients.

c. Most patients with chronic radiation injury are identified 6 to 18 months after completion of therapy.

d. The chance of developing chronic radiation proctitis is not related to the total effective dose of radiation received.

e. Acute and chronic radiation proctitis are primarily related to vascular changes within the bowel wall.

47. A 26-year-old man presents to the emergency department with acute bloody diarrhea, crampy abdominal pain, and fever. The differential diagnosis includes infection with each of the organisms listed except:

a. *Shigella* species

b. *Campylobacter* species

c. *Giardia lamblia*

d. *Escherichia coli* O157:H7

48. Each of the following statements concerning *Shigella* infections of the colon is true except:

a. They are endemic in nursing homes and day care centers.

b. Most strains are not highly contagious.

c. The bacteria produce enterotoxins.

d. The most severe infections are usually located in the rectosigmoid region, with infections of diminished severity in the proximal colon.

49. *Escherichia coli* infections have been associated with four diarrheal syndromes, the pathogenic properties of which are under plasmid control. The strain of *E coli* that is associated with the development of hemolytic uremic syndrome and thrombotic thrombocytopenic purpura is:

a. enterotoxigenic *E coli*

b. enteropathogenic *E coli*

c. enteroinvasive *E coli*

d. enterohemorrhagic *E coli*

50. Each of the following statements regarding *Campylobacter jejuni* infections of the colon is true except:

a. They are primarily a disease of children and young adults.

b. Fecal leukocytes and erythrocytes are present.

c. Diagnosis is by culture of stool.

d. Oral antibiotics are required for most patients.

51. Which one of the following statements regarding Hirschsprung disease is true?

a. Symptoms usually present during toilet training.

b. It is diagnosed by deep sigmoid biopsy.

c. It can usually be ruled out if the rectoanal inhibitory reflex is present during anorectal manometry.

d. It requires a subtotal colectomy in the majority of cases.

52. Causes of painful anorectal lesions in AIDS patients include each of the following except:

a. tuberculosis

b. Kaposi sarcoma

c. squamous cell carcinoma

d. *Yersinia enterocolitica*

53. Important functions of the gut microflora include all of the following except:

a. drug metabolism

b. vitamin synthesis

c. suppression of pathogens

d. metabolism of dietary triglycerides

54. Statements that are true concerning pathogenic mechanisms for diarrhea in patients treated with broad-spectrum antibiotics include all of the following except:

a. An accumulation of gastrointestinal mucin, normally hydrolyzed by colonic flora, presents an osmotic load to the colon.

b. The antibiotics and antibiotic metabolites present an osmotic load to the colon.

c. The normal balance between anaerobic and aerobic bacteria is disturbed.

d. Infection with *Clostridium difficile* develops.

55. All of the following statements regarding *Shigella* infections of the colon are true except:

    a. The virulence of *Shigella* infection is related to invasiveness, whereas diarrhea is related to toxin production.
    b. The typical clinical course of shigellosis in adults is onset of fever and diarrhea 4 to 6 days after ingestion of the bacterium, followed by a 5- to 7-day illness.
    c. Hemolytic-uremic syndrome is associated with *Shigella* infection.
    d. Most patients with symptomatic *Shigella* infection should be treated with tetracycline or ciprofloxacin for 5 days.

56. Which one of the following statements regarding *Campylobacter* infections of the colon is true?

    a. *Campylobacter* organisms are found in nearly 50% of positive stool cultures from patients with acute bacillary diarrhea.
    b. The major source of human infection is fecal-oral spread.
    c. Fecal leukocytes are usually found in symptomatic *Campylobacter jejuni* infections.
    d. Abdominal tenderness is rare in patients with *C jejuni* infections.
    e. Treatment of the infection with erythromycin 250 mg four times daily for 5 days reduces both the duration of symptoms and the shedding of bacteria.

57. All of the following statements regarding *Clostridium difficile* infection are true except:

    a. *C difficile* produces two toxins. Toxin A is an enterotoxin thought to be responsible for pseudomembranous colitis, whereas toxin B is a potent cytotoxin.
    b. Diarrhea is present in more than 50% of patients with positive *C difficile* stool cultures.
    c. Pseudomembranous colitis may develop during the first week of antibiotic therapy.
    d. The typical sigmoidoscopic appearance of pseudomembranous colitis is of scattered, 2- to 5-mm, raised, yellow-white plaques.
    e. Only about 15% to 25% of patients with antibiotic-associated diarrhea have *C difficile* toxin in their stool.

58. All of the following statements regarding sexually transmitted rectal, anal, and perianal infections are true except:

    a. Rectal *Neisseria gonorrhoeae* infections are usually asymptomatic.
    b. Diarrhea is the most frequent symptom of gonorrheal proctitis.
    c. *Chlamydia trachomatis* proctitis may mimic Crohn's proctitis.
    d. The differential diagnosis of perianal warts includes secondary syphilis.

59. A 30-year-old woman with chronic extremity aches and pains and a history of a "nervous stomach" presents with abdominal pain and distention, fever, leukocytosis, an elevated sedimentation rate, and proctitis on sigmoidoscopy. All of the following are included in the differential diagnosis except:

    a. antidepressant use
    b. nonsteroidal antiinflammatory drug use
    c. isoretinoic acid use
    d. gold therapy for rheumatoid arthritis
    e. marijuana smoking

60. Pneumatosis cystoides intestinalis has all of the following features except:

    a. There is an equal male-female prevalence.
    b. Secondary cases typically involve the small intestine and ascending colon.
    c. The diagnosis is commonly made on plain radiographs with linear, curvilinear, or cystic lucencies seen in the bowel wall.
    d. Multiple, pale blue, rounded, polyploid masses protruding into the lumen during colonoscopy are seen with cysts that contain a high hydrogen content.
    e. The presence of moderate to large volumes of gas within the intestinal wall warrants surgical exploration, even in asymptomatic patients.

61. Human papillomavirus is associated with all of the following except:

    a. condyloma acuminata
    b. condyloma lata
    c. anal cancer
    d. anal strictures
    e. cervical cancer

The following case pertains to questions 62 through 64.

A 28-year-old man presents with a 3-day history of watery diarrhea and fecal urgency. He reports having up to 10 watery bowel movements per day without blood, fevers, or other systemic symptoms. Recent travel, risk factors for human immunodeficiency virus, antibiotic use, and illness in family members are all denied.

62. Which of the following is the best initial management of this case?

    a. Obtain a complete blood count; examine a stool specimen for fecal leukocyte count, ova and parasites, and culture for bacteria; have the patient return in 1 week, or sooner if his symptoms worsen.

b. Counsel the patient about maintaining proper hydration and advise him to return promptly if he develops bloody diarrhea, fevers, or other systemic symptoms, or if he is not able to maintain proper hydration; schedule a return visit in 2 weeks if the diarrhea persists.

c. Obtain a stool specimen for culture and for fecal leukocyte count; start an empiric regimen of doxycycline 100 mg twice daily; schedule a return visit in 1 week.

d. Measure levels of serum electrolytes, blood urea nitrogen, and creatinine; examine stool specimens for sodium, potassium, osmolality, ova, parasites, and fecal leukocytes, and culture for bacteria; have the patient return in 1 week or sooner if his symptoms worsen; base treatment on the test results.

The patient's diarrhea resolves spontaneously in 5 days, but he returns to your office 3 weeks later describing low back, heel, and knee pain. He denies having fever, dysuria, or urethral discharge. On physical examination, his conjunctivae are "injected."

63. The physical examination should focus on evaluating the following:

a. conjunctivitis
b. urethritis and/or balanitis
c. skin lesions on the palms and soles
d. oral ulcers
e. all of the above

64. Enteric infections associated with this syndrome include each of the following except:

a. *Salmonella* species
b. *Shigella* species
c. *Yersinia enterocolitica*
d. enterohemorrhagic *Escherichia coli*
e. *Campylobacter jejuni*

65. A 67-year-old man presents with diarrhea after a 2-week course of antibiotics. A stool examination is negative for fecal leukocytes, and flexible sigmoidoscopy shows no pseudomembranes but does show friability, erythema, and exudate. Which one of the following statements is true?

a. The lack of fecal leukocytes makes the diagnosis of pseudomembranous colitis unlikely.
b. A stool culture positive for *Clostridium difficile* and *C difficile* cytotoxin would confirm the diagnosis of antibiotic-associated colitis.
c. Lack of pseudomembranes on flexible sigmoidoscopy makes the diagnosis of antibiotic-associated colitis unlikely.
d. If *C difficile* colitis is successfully treated, the likelihood of relapse is 15% to 20%.

66. A 4-year-old girl is admitted for bloody diarrhea and dehydration. She recently ate at a fast-food restaurant. On admission, her creatinine level is 2.0 mg/dL, and her leukocyte count is 22,000/mm³. The next day, after hydration, her creatinine level is 3.4 mg/dL, and her leukocyte count is 18,000/mm³. Which one of the following statements is true?

a. If antibiotics have not been started, they should be started now.
b. The mechanism of disease for this organism is invasiveness rather than toxin production.
c. Cattle appear to be a common reservoir for the agent that causes this infection.
d. Renal insufficiency occurs as a complication in 15% to 20% of cases of this infection.

67. Patient subsets that have a high risk for the acquisition of amebiasis in developed countries include each of the following except:

a. immigrants or travelers from South America, Africa, and India
b. homosexual males and AIDS patients with diarrhea
c. institutionalized individuals
d. individuals with selective IgA deficiency

68. Acute amebic proctocolitis is characterized by each of the following except:

a. progressively more severe and frequent diarrhea
b. abdominal pain and tenderness
c. watery diarrhea with little or no blood
d. weight loss

69. Complications of amebic liver abscess include each of the following except:

a. serous pleural effusions
b. peritonitis
c. pulmonary embolism
d. pericarditis

70. On sensory testing, patients with irritable bowel syndrome (IBS):

a. experience pain in a single, predictable location with balloon inflation of the intestine or colon
b. have heightened perception of electrical or thermal stimulation of the skin, suggesting a generalized sensory abnormality
c. usually exhibit heightened sensitivity to balloon distention of the intestine or colon with normal compliance of the gut wall
d. exhibit sensory abnormalities that can be used as a reasonably sensitive and specific test for the diagnosis of IBS
e. none of the above

71. A 29-year-old woman with a 2-year history of intermittent diarrhea with crampy abdominal pain presents for evaluation. Which of the following sets of data would be most consistent with a diagnosis of irritable bowel syndrome?

   a. hematocrit, 33%; albumin level, 4.4 mg/dL; fecal occult blood, positive; stool volume, 500 mL/day; sigmoidoscopy reveals erythema with aphthous ulcerations with significant pain
   b. hematocrit, 42%; albumin level, 1.8 mg/dL; fecal occult blood, negative; stool volume, 500 mL/day; sigmoidoscopy, normal
   c. hematocrit, 42%; albumin level, 4.3 mg/dL; fecal occult blood, negative; stool volume, 1000 mL/day; sigmoidoscopy, normal with significant pain
   d. hematocrit, 42%; albumin, 4.3 mg/dL; fecal occult blood, negative; stool volume, 250 mL/day; sigmoidoscopy, normal with significant pain
   e. hematocrit, 42%; albumin level, 4.3 mg/dL; fecal occult blood, negative; stool volume, 200 mL/day; sigmoidoscopy reveals loss of vascularity and aphthous ulcerations in the rectum and sigmoid colon

72. Fiber preparations are expected to have the best therapeutic results in which subset(s) of patients with irritable bowel syndrome (IBS)?

   a. diarrhea-predominant
   b. pain-predominant
   c. constipation-predominant
   d. all subsets of patients with IBS
   e. no patients with IBS

73. A 36-year-old woman complains of embarrassment from excessive flatulence. Weight loss and recent dietary changes are denied. In discussing this problem with the patient, which of the following statements would be most accurate?

   a. The expelled gas is largely the result of dietary intake and bacterial fermentation.
   b. Passage of flatus more than 15 times per day is abnormal.
   c. The patient should be evaluated for malabsorption.
   d. Oral simethicone will usually reduce the flatulence.

74. Recommended surveillance colonoscopy with random biopsy for adenocarcinoma in patients with ulcerative colitis involving most of the colon should begin after:

   a. 5 to 7 years of disease
   b. 8 to 10 years of disease
   c. 11 to 15 years of disease
   d. more than 15 years of disease

75. The best estimate of normal daily blood loss from the gastrointestinal tract is approximately:

   a. 0.01 mL/day
   b. 0.7 mL/day
   c. 5.5 mL/day
   d. 10.0 mL/day

76. A 62-year-old man with aortic stenosis is admitted to the hospital with a fever of 39.4°C. Physical examination reveals an aortic insufficiency murmur. Echocardiography reveals vegetations on the aortic valve. Blood cultures grow *Streptococcus bovis.* Which one of the following statements is true?

   a. A search for colonic neoplasia should be undertaken.
   b. A search for gastric neoplasia should be undertaken.
   c. Stool should be collected and examined for *Streptococcus* species.
   d. Telangiectasias in the colon are associated with this infection.

77. With respect to the endoscopic treatment of gastrointestinal lesions, all of the following statements are true except:

   a. Endoscopic strip biopsy allows the removal of a large area of mucosa and limits significant associated complications.
   b. Photodynamic therapy uses photosensitizing agents that are activated by the standard visible light source of the endoscope.
   c. Endoscopic ultrasonography has been shown to add useful diagnostic information to that obtained by computed tomography in the assessment of tumor resectability.
   d. Laser therapy can be used to ablate tumors and recanalize obstructing lesions.

78. The lifelong likelihood of an American developing a colon cancer is approximately:

   a. 1%
   b. 5%
   c. 10%
   d. 25%

79. The following symptoms of colorectal cancer usually suggest advanced disease, with the exception of:

   a. large bowel obstruction
   b. perforation
   c. hematochezia
   d. pneumaturia
   e. abdominal or perirectal pain

80. A 24-year-old man with chronic ulcerative colitis is referred for the consideration of surveillance screening for colon cancer. His disease was diagnosed 15 years ago with inflammation to the level of the

midtransverse colon. His symptoms have been mild, and three sigmoidoscopic examinations over the past 5 years have revealed only quiescent colitis. You should advise the patient that:

a. Mild, well-controlled disease that involves less than the entire colon is not associated with a substantially increased incidence of neoplasia.
b. He should undergo a screening barium enema radiographic examination at this time.
c. The fact that his disease has been mild does not reduce his risk of dysplasia and cancer.
d. If low-grade dysplasia is found, a colectomy will be recommended.

81. A patient with a 15-year history of ulcerative colitis has patchy colitis to the level of the cecum, but the rectum is relatively spared. An irregular, somewhat firm mass is found at the hepatic flexure when biopsy is performed. The pathology report describes high-grade dysplasia in three of the biopsy specimens from the irregular mass, and low-grade dysplasia in the ascending colon as well as in the transverse colon. The sigmoid colon and rectum show stable chronic colitis without active inflammation or dysplasia. You should advise the patient that:

a. The mass at the hepatic flexure is potentially malignant, and a total colectomy should be performed as soon as possible.
b. Colonoscopy should be repeated in 3 months, and if high-grade dysplasia still exists, total colectomy will be recommended.
c. The mass at the hepatic flexure is potentially malignant; a right hemicolectomy is advised to avoid the problems associated with total colectomy.
d. The colonoscopic findings suggest a diagnosis of Crohn's disease, which is associated with a lower risk of cancer.
e. Colonoscopy with biopsy should be repeated in 1 year.

82. A 29-year-old man is referred with a history of juvenile polyposis coli. His father also had the disease. The patient has had 10 polyps, ranging in size from 10 to 20 mm, removed over the past 20 years. The pathology report of the patient's colonic polyps describes large islands of adenomatous tissue in the otherwise characteristic juvenile polyps. You should advise the patient that:

a. Juvenile polyposis is not associated with an increased risk of colon cancer.
b. These polyps are not ordinary juvenile polyps. The risk of colon cancer is increased, and a surveillance program is indicated.
c. This is really a form of familial adenomatous polyposis, and a colectomy is advised.

83. A 63-year-old woman has just undergone a low anterior resection for Dukes stage C cancer of the sigmoid colon. Two of 20 regional lymph nodes are cancerous, but no distant metastases are found. You should advise the patient that:

a. Her prognosis is grim, and she has only a 20% likelihood of long-term disease-free survival.
b. Her likelihood of survival will be improved by taking 1 year of adjuvant chemotherapy with 5-fluorouracil and levamisole.
c. Adjuvant therapy reduces cancer recurrences but does not improve survival because of the serious side effects of 5-fluorouracil and levamisole.
d. Adjuvant therapy should consist of radiotherapy of the pelvis.
e. The best adjuvant therapy for her disease is combined radiotherapy and chemotherapy.

84. A 59-year-old college professor presents with painless hematochezia. Colonoscopy is normal except for a 2.5-cm pedunculated polyp in the sigmoid colon that is completely removed with snare polypectomy. The pathologist reports that the head of the polyp is largely replaced by an invasive cancer that penetrates into the stalk. The stalk is 3 cm long and is examined carefully by the pathologist, who notes that the cancer extends only 5 mm into the stalk and that the margin is free of neoplasm. The cancer is well-differentiated, and no vascular invasion is noted. The patient is otherwise in good health and plans to continue teaching for another 5 to 10 years. You should advise this patient that:

a. The colonoscopic resection of the malignant polyp was adequate, and no additional treatment is needed at this time.
b. A low anterior resection is a low-risk procedure in this patient, and to be safe, the operation should be offered.
c. Recurrence is likely at the polypectomy site, and surveillance is indicated every 6 months.
d. Little information is available on the management of these polyps, and a surgical consultation is the best option.

85. A 66-year-old man comes to your office for advice on the management of recurrent colon cancer. He had a 4-cm cecal adenocarcinoma resected 18 months ago. He has right upper quadrant pain, a carcinoembryonic antigen level of 20 ng/mL (normal, 3.0), and a computed tomography (CT) scan showing a 1.5-cm mass on the right anterior surface of the liver that was not present at the time of surgery 18 months ago. A needle biopsy of the liver mass confirms recurrent adenocarcinoma. No other lesions are detected on the CT scan, and a complete blood count and liver chemistries are all normal. A CT scan of the chest is also normal. You

repeat a colonoscopy to the level of the anastomosis and find no lesions. Your advice to the patient should include each of the following except:

a. A surgical resection of the lesion could be curative.
b. Intraarterial chemotherapy may shrink the tumor and relieve symptoms, but its value in prolonging life is unproven.
c. Although he is interested in pursuing an aggressive approach, you inform him that his condition cannot be improved by interventional measures, and you discuss family support and hospice care.

86. An asymptomatic 50-year-old woman in excellent health undergoes screening sigmoidoscopy, at which time a 7–8 mm submucosal mass is found in the rectum. A colonoscopy is performed, and no other lesions are found. You are able to place a snare around the lesion and excise it completely despite its initial appearance. The pathology report indicates that it is a carcinoid tumor and that it has been completely removed. Your approach to the problem at this point should include which of the following?

a. Order special stains to determine whether the lesion is malignant.
b. Obtain computed tomographic scans of the abdomen and chest to look for metastatic disease.
c. Consult with a surgeon and recommend a proctectomy.
d. Reassure the patient that this lesion is probably benign and likely has been adequately treated by your resection.

87. The following groups of bacteria each account for more than 1% of the fecal flora except:

a. facultative gram-negative organisms (e.g., *Escherichia coli*)
b. *Bacteroides* species
c. *Clostridium* species
d. *Peptostreptococcus* species

88. Which of the following is recognized as a cause of colonic ischemia?

a. digoxin
b. danazol
c. doxycycline
d. dehydration
e. diabetes mellitus

89. Which patient is the least likely to present with colonic ischemia?

a. a 75-year-old lawyer who recently underwent aortic bypass surgery and has blood in his stool
b. a 25-year-old medical student who has a history of substance abuse and complains of chest pain and hematochezia

c. a 55-year-old schoolteacher who is undergoing peritoneal dialysis and has had abdominal pain and diarrhea for 6 hours
d. a 35-year-old executive with a twin pregnancy who has loose stools and rectal bleeding

90. Laxatives composed of docusate sodium:

a. have not been proven to be effective
b. should be taken with other laxatives
c. act as hyperosmolar agents
d. may cause malabsorption of vitamins A, D, and K
e. are systemically absorbed

91. Stimulant laxatives include all of the following except:

a. senna
b. magnesium sulfate
c. castor oil
d. bisacodyl
e. cascara

92. A healthy 33-year-old man presents at the emergency department with rectal pain. He finally sheepishly admits to the inability to extricate a lightbulb from his rectum. Which one of the following statements is true?

a. The lightbulb was probably placed in the rectum in a misguided attempt to relieve a particular rectal symptom.
b. If the object is palpable on digital examination, abdominal radiography is probably unnecessary.
c. Because the object is glass, transanal removal is unsafe.
d. Proctosigmoidoscopy should be performed after the object is successfully removed.

93. Risk factors for anal carcinoma include all of the following except:

a. colorectal cancer
b. lower genital tract tumors
c. cigarette smoking
d. receptive anal intercourse
e. genital warts

94. Which one of the following statements regarding anal cancer is true?

a. It is discovered during a routine examination of asymptomatic patients in 75% of cases.
b. Metastasis is present in 80% of patients at the time of presentation.
c. Abdominoperineal resection for radical excision is usually the treatment of choice.
d. Radiotherapy combined with chemotherapy causes complete tumor regression in most cases.
e. Anal cancer is associated with a 5-year survival rate of approximately 20%.

95. A 29-year-old woman with a long history of laxative abuse and chronic diarrhea now complains of narrow stools, straining at defecation, and small amounts of hematochezia. The most likely diagnosis is:

    a. anal stenosis
    b. solitary rectal ulcer
    c. rectal prolapse
    d. anal fissure
    e. rectal cancer
    f. chemical injection

96. Therapy for diminutive colonic polyps:

    a. Cold snaring is acceptable; however, it is associated with a high rate of hemorrhage.
    b. Hot biopsy forceps are more likely to produce a complication in the left as compared to the right colon.
    c. Cold biopsy is a safe, acceptable technique for polyp removal.
    d. Snare cautery should not be used unless the polyp is larger than 5 mm.

97. Therapy for large sessile polyps:

    a. Saline injection has been associated with tumor seeding.
    b. When assisting polypectomy, an injection with saline should be made directly into the mucosa.
    c. Polyps smaller than or equal to 1.5 cm should be removed by a snare in 2 or 3 pieces, if possible.
    d. The risk of metastasis after snare resection of malignant large sessile polyps is greater than that for pedunculated malignant polyps.

98. The best and most practical way to determine passage of the colonoscope to the cecum is by:

    a. the length of endoscope inserted
    b. finger palpation and transillumination in the right lower quadrant
    c. fluoroscopic confirmation
    d. apparent landmarks in the cecal region (i.e., ileocecal valve, appendiceal orifice)

99. Appropriate preparation for colonoscopy includes:

    a. Discontinue iron preparations for several days prior to the procedure.
    b. Administer antibiotics if biopsy or polypectomy is possible.
    c. Discontinue aspirin for 2 weeks prior to the procedure.
    d. Administer a balanced electrolyte solution, such as oral sodium phosphate.

100. Which of the following is considered a low-yield, usually inappropriate, indication for colonoscopy?

    a. chronic abdominal pain

    b. chronic diarrhea
    c. chronic iron deficiency anemia
    d. acute colonic bleeding
    e. occult gastrointestinal bleeding

101. The difference between the entire transmural thickness of the colonic and small intestine wall is that the colonic wall lacks:

    a. villi
    b. submucosa
    c. inner circular muscle
    d. outer longitudinal muscle
    e. serosa

102. Which portion of the colon is not a retroperitoneal structure?

    a. ascending colon
    b. transverse colon
    c. descending colon
    e. rectum

103. All of the following have a positive association with adenomatous colorectal polyps except:

    a. uretosigmoidoscopy
    b. acromegaly
    c. *Streptococcus bovis* infection
    d. cholecystectomy

104. If one were to characterize adenomas based on their predominant histology, the most common would be:

    a. villous
    b. hyperplastic
    c. tubulovillous
    d. tubular

105. On colonoscopy, the most common site of colorectal adenomas is the:

    a. rectum
    b. descending colon
    c. sigmoid colon
    d. transverse colon
    e. ascending colon

106. In the hereditary nonpolyposis colorectal cancer syndrome, the responsible defect lies in the:

    a. APC gene
    b. K-*ras* gene
    c. p53 gene
    d. microsatellite instability due to DNA mismatch repair

107. Colonoscopy is an appropriate screening tool for all of the following groups of patients except:

    a. patients with multiple first-degree relatives with colon cancer

b. patients with a first-degree relative with a tubular adenoma

c. patients with long-standing, left-sided ulcerative colitis

d. a patient with a large (>1 cm) tubular adenoma on prior colonoscopy

108. Poor prognostic features for a malignant polyp include all of the following except:

a. incomplete resection
b. poorly differentiated carcinoma
c. sessile malignant polyps
d. pedunculated malignant polyp

109. To be considered a malignant polyp, penetration must be into the:

a. mucosa
b. muscularis mucosae
c. submucosa
d. muscularis propria

110. The most prevalent mutation in colorectal adenomas is the:

a. p53 gene mutation
b. K-ras mutation
c. APC gene defect
d. DNA mismatch repair defects

111. All of the following are inherited polyposis syndromes except:

a. hyperplastic polyposis
b. familial adenomatosis polyposis
c. Peutz-Jeghers syndrome
d. Turcot syndrome

112. A 25-year-old man is referred to you for evaluation. He is adopted and knows little of his family history, other than a recollection of "multiple polyps" and "early colon cancer." He does not know his biological parents and is concerned he may be at risk for familial adenomatous polyposis and colon cancer. What type of genetic testing would help identify his risk for familial adenomatous polyposis?

a. flow cytometry of colonic epithelium from biopsy specimens
b. linkage testing
c. in vitro protein synthesis (IVPS)
d. mutation identification

113. The colonic polyps in familial adenomatous polyposis are usually:

a. villous adenomas
b. tubulovillous adenomas

c. tubular adenomas
d. hyperplastic polyps

114. In Gardner syndrome, the extracolonic lesions include all of the following except:

a. ovarian carcinoma
b. osteomas
c. desmoid tumors
d. dental abnormalities, such as unerupted and supernumerary teeth

115. The mutation in familial adenomatous polyposis involves a mutation in:

a. DNA repair enzymes
b. APC protein
c. c282y
d. *ATP7B*

116. The polyps in juvenile polyposis are:

a. tubular adenomas
b. hyperplastic polyps
c. desmoid polyps
d. nonneoplastic hamartomatous polyps

117. Finding nodular lymphoid hyperplasia on colonoscopy should ideally prompt the following treatment strategy:

a. colectomy with mucosal proctectomy and ileoanal pouch pull-through
b. subtotal colectomy with ileorectal anastomosis
c. initiation of this chemotherapy regimen: cyclophosphamide, doxorubicin, vincristine, and prednisone (CHOP)
d. surveillance colonoscopy every 3 years for malignant transformation
e. no specific therapy

118. All of the following have been associated with an increased risk for colorectal cancer except:

a. smoking
b. consumption of alcohol, specifically beer
c. high dietary intake of animal fat
d. radiation for gynecologic cancer

119. Which of the following medications has been shown to promote a regression of adenomas in patients with familial adenomatous polyposis?

a. acetaminophen
b. interferon
c. sulindac
d. mesalamine

120. All of the following characterize hereditary non-polyposis colorectal cancer syndrome except:

a. early-onset colon cancer

b. absence of multiple adenomatous polyps

c. X-linked inheritance

d. linked to germline mutations in DNA mismatch repair genes

121. In colorectal cancer, the best predictor of outcome is:

a. size of tumor

b. pathologic stage

c. well-differentiated tumors

d. presence of K-*ras* mutation

122. The therapy shown to improve the recurrence-free interval and survival in Dukes stage C colon cancer is:

a. levamisole

b. levamisole plus 5-fluorouracil

c. preoperative radiation directed at the tumor bed

d. prophylactic hepatic radiation to prevent metastases

123. The Amsterdam criteria for a diagnosis of hereditary nonpolyposis colorectal cancer in a family include all of the following except:

a. three or more relatives with verified colorectal cancer

b. colorectal cancer involving at least two generations

c. one or more cancers diagnosed before age 50

d. presence in one family member of at least one additional type of carcinoma

124. Which of the following increases the risk for colorectal cancer?

a. cholecystectomy

b. high fiber diet

c. acromegaly

d. skin tags

125. All of the following are acceptable conditions for the performance of an ileal pouch–anal canal anastomosis except:

a. chronic ulcerative colitis

b. familial adenomatous polyposis

c. normal anal sphincter function

d. Crohn's disease

e. age younger than 65

126. A 51-year-old woman presents with a 12-month history of intermittent, crampy abdominal pain, and loose stools occurring 3 to 5 times per day. She denies weight loss, relevant travel, antibiotic use, and consumption of well water. Defecation brings relief of the abdominal pain. Findings on physical examination are normal. Of the following tests, which would be most useful?

a. barium enema

b. culture stool for enteric pathogens

c. colonoscopy with biopsy

d. abdominal ultrasonography

e. computed tomography of abdomen and pelvis

127. Which one of the following is not a hepatobiliary complication of inflammatory bowel disease?

a. fatty liver

b. cholesterol gallstones

c. pericholangitis

d. chronic active hepatitis

e. liver hemangiomas

128. All of the following statements regarding arthritis associated with inflammatory bowel disease are true except:

a. It is usually migratory and affects large joints of the body.

b. It generally parallels disease activity.

c. It is associated with haplotype B27.

d. It responds well to corticosteroid treatment.

e. Deformity with radiologic changes occurs in only a minority of cases.

129. All of the following statements regarding patients with Crohn's disease are true except:

a. Increasing the length (margins) of healthy small intestine resected does not reduce the incidence of local recurrence.

b. The recurrence rate after ileal resection for ileitis, or ileocolic resection for ileocolic disease is about 20% after 10 years.

c. Crohn's disease is more common in people who smoke cigarettes.

d. Growth failure is a major presenting characteristic of 30% of children with Crohn's disease.

e. Hypoalbuminemia is a fairly accurate indicator of disease severity.

130. A 67-year-old woman presents with new-onset diarrhea and occasional hematochezia. In addition, she complains of intermittent, vague, right lower quadrant pain and fullness. She was diagnosed and successfully treated for endometrial carcinoma about 10 months ago with surgery, followed by radiotherapy for 6 weeks. She underwent a colonoscopy with terminal ileum biopsy, which revealed obliterated end arteries, scattered telangiectasias in the rectum, and villous atrophy in the terminal ileum. All of the following statements are true except:

a. Bile acid malabsorption may be the cause of the diarrhea.

b. Bacterial overgrowth may be the cause of the diarrhea.

c. Diphenoxylate or loperamide may be given to control the diarrhea.

d. Mesalamine and corticosteroids are the standard agents for managing diarrhea of this nature.

e. The rectal bleeding may respond to electrocoagulation of the telangiectasias.

131. A 28-year-old woman with a history of Crohn's disease is pregnant for the first time and has been referred from the obstetrics service for further management. She complains of right lower quadrant pain, low-grade fever, joint pains, and mild nonbloody diarrhea. She has been taking mesalamine (2.4 g/day) for maintenance and has been stable until now. Her physical examination was significant only for mild tenderness in the right lower abdomen. Appropriate advice for this patient should include:

a. Take metronidazole to prevent fistula formation, which may be caused by pressure from the growing fetus.

b. Consider termination of the pregnancy, because pregnancy is contraindicated in Crohn's disease.

c. It is safe to increase the dose of mesalamine and to use both intravenous and oral steroids to alleviate disease exacerbations.

d. Deliver baby by cesarean section.

132. The general medical service asks for your evaluation of a 22-year-old college sophomore who presents with lower abdominal cramping, bloody diarrhea, joint pains, and malaise for the past 3 weeks. He denies recent antibiotic use, fevers, and night sweats. His history is unremarkable, although he recalls that while participating in a pharmaceutical trial a year ago, he was found to be a "slow metabolizer." A physical examination shows an anxious nonorthostatic student, without rashes or joint swelling. The results of stool studies for culture and for examination for ova and parasites are negative. A colonoscopy reveals diffuse erythema, friable mucosa with granularity, and loss of the normal vascular pattern. The patient is initially treated with intravenous steroids and sulfasalazine 4 g/day, followed by oral prednisone as he begins to improve. He now complains of headache, abdominal discomfort, nausea, and vomiting. Of the following choices, the most appropriate next step would be to:

a. Perform a colonoscopy and, in addition, perform an esophagogastroduodenoscopy.

b. Measure the sulfapyridine level and decrease the dose of sulfasalazine.

c. Decrease the oral prednisone to 80 mg/day.

d. Discuss with the patient the need for a colectomy and request a consultation with a surgeon.

e. Start a proton pump inhibitor.

The following case pertains to questions 133 and 134.

A third-year gastroenterology fellow reports to the emergency department with the sudden onset of vague abdominal discomfort and diarrhea. He denies fever, chills, nausea, and vomiting. A plain radiograph of the abdomen shows cystic lucencies in the bowel wall. A computed tomographic scan of the abdomen reveals intramural gas that parallels the bowel wall.

133. Complications of this condition may include all of the following except:

a. volvulus

b. intestinal intussusception

c. intestinal perforation

d. renal obstruction

e. tension pneumoperitoneum

134. The above condition is associated with all of the following except:

a. chronic obstructive pulmonary disease

b. systemic amyloidosis

c. viral hepatitis

d. following routine colonoscopy

e. patients with a Crohn's disease flare who are taking steroids

135. All of the following statements about diversion colitis are true except:

a. Hydrocortisone enemas are usually efficacious.

b. It may not develop for many months after fecal diversion.

c. Distinguishing between recurrent Crohn's disease and diversion colitis is sometimes difficult. A computed tomographic scan can be helpful.

d. Diffuse follicular lymphoid hyperplasia with frequent germinal centers is a characteristic feature of diversion colitis.

e. Short-chain fatty acid enemas may induce remission in some patients.

136. A 27-year-old man with Crohn's colitis presents with worsening low back pain, morning stiffness, and a slightly stooped posture. In addition, he complains of fatigue, worsening abdominal cramps, and diarrhea. He has lost 4.5 kg in 3 months. His primary care doctor ordered plain radiographs of the spine, which revealed squaring of the vertebrae and straightening of the spine. Which one of the following statements is true?

a. Medical treatment of the Crohn's colitis will likely help the spine disease.

b. Colectomy will not likely help the spine disease.

c. Administration of nonsteroidal antiinflammatory drugs will halt the spine disease progression.

d. The activity of the spine disease follows that of the bowel disease.

137. The upper (slow) limit of normal colonic transit for most adults is approximately:

a. 24 hours

b. 48 hours
c. 72 hours
d. 96 hours

You are asked to evaluate a patient with a history of significant (at least several diverticula of moderate size) diverticulosis (questions 138 and 139).

138. What percentage of patients with a history of colonic diverticulosis will develop acute diverticulitis?

a. less than 5%
b. 10% to 25%
c. 35% to 50%
d. 60% to 80%

139. What percentage of patients with significant diverticulosis will exhibit diverticular bleeding?

a. less than 5%
b. 5% to15%
c. 20% to 35%
d. 50% to 60%

140. What is the risk of developing arthritis, urethritis, and conjunctivitis (Reiter syndrome) after a case of shigellosis?

a. 1% to 2%
b. 5% to 10%
c. 20% to 30%
d. 50%

141. You are asked to evaluate a patient who has had a recent episode of gastrointestinal bleeding. The history indicates problems with swallowing, and physical examination reveals sclerodactyly and calcinosis. This patient is at increased risk for what cause of gastrointestinal bleeding?

a. hemangiomas
b. angiosarcoma
c. Dieulafoy lesion
d. telangiectasias

The following case pertains to questions 142 through 144.
A 29-year-old woman presents with excess flatulence, bloating, and intermittent loose stools over the past 6 months. A careful dietary history is obtained.

142. Which of the following statements concerning this patient's nutritional practices is true?

a. The pasta this patient frequently eats is efficiently digested and is not a source of carbohydrate malabsorption.
b. The patient switched from chewing gum sweetened with sorbitol to gum sweetened with aspartame, but this produced no improvement; thus, the habit

of chewing gum does not contribute to the gaseousness.
c. Although the patient has stopped eating fresh fruit, she still may be getting enough fructose in her soft drinks to produce symptoms.
d. The patient has tried to cut back on drinking milk and has avoided eating cheese and ice cream, without improvement. This rules out lactose intolerance as a source of her symptoms.

143. The clinician begins a diagnostic evaluation of this patient. Which of the following statements about the assessment of the excess gas and bloating is correct?

a. Most patients with excess gas will have increased quantities of gas concentrated in the hepatic and splenic flexures of the colon, visible on plain abdominal radiographs.
b. Hyperthyroidism is a common cause of bloating in association with constipation.
c. A rise in breath hydrogen excretion of more than 20 PPM after ingestion of lactose is 100% specific for intestinal lactase deficiency as a cause of her symptoms.
d. The patient should be instructed to avoid pasta before hydrogen breath testing, as this may falsely suggest the presence of bacterial overgrowth.
e. Because it is excreted in the breath of most healthy people, methane is the best gas to measure with breath tests.

144. Which of the following statements concerning the management of this patient's symptoms is false?

a. The patient's symptoms may be related to irritable bowel syndrome. Dietary restriction may not alleviate her symptoms.
b. Simethicone is postulated to act via the absorption of excess gas in the intestinal lumen.
c. A transient increase in bloating with the initiation of psyllium therapy is not due to increased gas production, because fiber preparations are inefficiently converted to gas.
d. Oligosaccharides such as stachyose and raffinose are abundant in legumes and may be partially digested by the administration of bacterial β-galactosidase.

145. All of the following statements regarding the pathophysiology of irritable bowel syndrome (IBS) are true except:

a. Mental stress can evoke changes in the small intestine and rectal motor function of healthy volunteers that mimic abnormalities reported in patients with IBS.
b. Exaggerated small intestine motor patterns, such as discrete clustered contractions and prolonged

propagated contractions, are present during some episodes of pain in IBS.

c. Discrete clustered contractions and prolonged propagated contractions are common in healthy volunteers; however, they are not perceived as painful.

d. Meal-evoked colonic motor activity is more prominent in diarrhea-prone patients than in constipated patients with IBS.

e. Discrete clustered contractions and prolonged propagated contractions are more common in patients with diarrhea-prone illness than in those with constipation-predominant illness.

146. All of the following statements regarding the pathophysiology of irritable bowel syndrome (IBS) are false except:

a. Repetitive stimulation of the colon can induce hypersensitivity in patients with IBS who have normal visceral perception on initial testing.

b. Patients with IBS have selective hypersensitivity to colonic distention, whereas patients with functional dyspepsia exhibit hypersensitivity only to gastric distention.

c. Argon washout techniques have shown that patients with bloating have increased volumes of gas that reflux in retrograde fashion into the stomach.

d. Patients with constipation-predominant IBS frequently exhibit decreased rectal compliance that may promote fecal retention.

e. Patients with IBS frequently exhibit generalized hypersensitivity to both painful visceral and somatic stimulation, suggesting a defect in central nervous system pain processing pathways.

147. A 32-year-old woman presents with a history of frequent loose stools associated with meals and relieved by defecation. Results of routine stool and blood studies are negative and findings on sigmoidoscopy with biopsy are normal. All of the following statements regarding therapy for this patient are true except:

a. A trial of a lactose-free diet may provide symptom relief.

b. Ingestion of psyllium is likely to improve stool consistency, reduce urgency, and decrease stool frequency.

c. An opiate-derived antidiarrheal such as loperamide has been advocated as the treatment of choice for patients with similar symptoms.

d. Anticholinergic drugs administered before a meal may reduce postprandial colonic contractions and reduce the cramps associated with this patient's diarrhea.

e. Bran supplements should be avoided as they may increase distention and flatulence.

148. A 42-year-old man presents with the insidious onset of constipation. He reports 1 bowel movement every 3 days associated with straining and the passage of desiccated, pellet-like stools. He has severe left lower quadrant pain that is partially relieved by defecation. This pain forces him to leave work on some days. Results of laboratory studies are normal. Sigmoidoscopy shows no distal obstructing lesions. He has tried bran cereal and prune juice without improvement. Which of the following is not a reasonable recommendation?

a. He should contact his primary physician to change his antihypertensive drug from a calcium channel blocker to a beta blocker.

b. He should begin daily senna to achieve a regular bowel pattern.

c. Calcium polycarbophil should be recommended to provide bulk and increase the water content in the stool.

d. A nonabsorbable electrolyte solution containing polyethylene glycol can be taken safely on a daily basis to provide a gentle laxative effect.

149. A 28-year-old woman has been given a diagnosis of irritable bowel syndrome (IBS) after an initial office visit. Which one of her comments suggests that the diagnosis is incorrect?

a. "I can't possibly have IBS because my lower abdomen hurts for an hour after eating."

b. "I can't possibly have IBS because I pass so much mucus. There must be something more serious causing this."

c. "I can't possibly have IBS. After a bowel movement, I feel like I have to go again."

d. "I can't possibly have IBS because I am awakened from a sound sleep by abdominal pain nearly every night."

e. "I can't possibly have IBS. I can't eat a full meal anymore but I've still gained 20 pounds in the past year."

150. You have just told a mother that her 1-month-old son with nausea, vomiting, constipation, and abdominal distention has Hirschsprung disease. Which of the following statements concerning your diagnosis is correct?

a. Demonstration of an absent rectoanal inhibitory reflex on manometry confirmed the diagnosis of Hirschsprung disease.

b. The infant had a normal proctosigmoidoscopy, an unusual finding in Hirschsprung disease.

c. Mucosal biopsies taken 1 cm proximal to the pectinate line showed an absence of ganglion cells in the submucosal plexus, thereby reliably confirming the diagnosis.

d. The infant's recent problems with diarrhea were caused by pseudomembranous enterocolitis.

e. The infant's recent problems with diarrhea were caused by overflow incontinence.

151. All of the following statements about slow transit constipation are correct except:

a. Straining to evacuate stools of normal consistency is more consistent with slow transit constipation than with pelvic floor disorders.
b. Colonic transit testing using radiopaque markers can be used to detect regional delays in transit.
c. Preoperative comprehensive testing of colonic function is indicated to exclude pelvic floor dysfunction, as outlet disorders respond poorly to subtotal colectomy.
d. Pathologic analyses of colons from patients with slow transit constipation reveal absent or abnormal myenteric neurons, suggesting that the condition may be related to chronic intestinal pseudoobstruction.
e. Many patients with pelvic floor dysfunction will respond to therapy with biofeedback.

TRUE/FALSE

The following characteristics pertain to pruritus ani:

152. _____ is commonly caused by a parasitic infection in adults

153. _____ may be a symptom of fistulous disease or anal carcinoma

154. _____ may respond to treatment of underlying conditions such as hemorrhoids, fecal incontinence, and psoriasis

155. _____ often responds to local massage and vigorous mechanical cleansing measures

The following statements (156–161) pertain to hemorrhoidal disease:

156. _____ External skin tags and external hemorrhoids are different names for the same lesion.

157. _____ Large internal hemorrhoids are equivalent to anorectal varices.

158. _____ Thrombosis of an external hemorrhoid is typically painful and can be treated conservatively or surgically.

159. _____ Internal hemorrhoids can be classified according to the degree of prolapse. First-degree hemorrhoids do not prolapse, and fourth-degree hemorrhoids are not reducible.

160. _____ Most symptomatic third- and fourth-degree internal hemorrhoids require surgery.

161. _____ Rubber band ligation and infrared therapy are appropriate treatment modalities for internal but not external hemorrhoids.

162. _____ The internal anal sphincter is a distal continuation of the longitudinal muscle layer of the rectum.

163. _____ The right colon receives its primary blood supply from the superior mesenteric artery and the left colon from the inferior mesenteric artery.

164. _____ *Clostridium septicum* is a common cause of septicemia and typhlitis (neutropenic enterocolitis) in patients with leukemia or lymphoma.

165. _____ Within the colon, antiperistaltic contractile waves are most commonly seen in the proximal colon.

166. _____ Giant migrating contractions of the colon periodically propagate in a peristaltic manner and are thought to be associated with mass movements of stool and the urge to defecate.

167. _____ The presence of skin tags indicates an increased risk for the development of colonic adenomas.

168. _____ The likelihood of finding a colonic adenoma or carcinoma during colonoscopy in an individual with a positive result on a fecal occult blood test is approximately 50%.

169. _____ Routine screening flexible sigmoidoscopy with a 60-cm endoscope will detect 85% of all colonic neoplasms.

170. _____ Carcinoembryonic antigen measurement is not useful for the initial detection of colonic neoplasms.

171. _____ Carcinoma in situ is routinely cured by simple polypectomy. However, malignant polyps with invasion into the muscularis mucosae should be managed with colonic resection.

172. _____ Diverticulitis and diverticular bleeding characteristically occur concomitantly.

Three days after an uneventful aortic aneurysm repair, a 74-year-old man develops crampy left lower quadrant abdominal pain and is noted to have blood on rectal examination. Expected findings and treatment plans (173–175) can include:

173. _____ Abdominal angiography shows the surgical interruption of the superior mesenteric artery.

174. _____ Colonoscopy shows abnormal mucosa beginning in the anal region and extending for 10 cm.

175. _____ Conservative medical management usually results in a favorable outcome.

176. _____ When mechanical obstruction is suspected, colonic obstruction should be excluded prior to the oral administration of barium.

177. _____ Acute colonic obstruction usually presents with severe abdominal distention but relatively mild pain because of the high compliance of the colonic wall.

178. _____ Most patients with irritable bowel syndrome who complain of excess gas actually do produce greater than normal amounts of intestinal gas.

179. _____ Bran has dual effects: it accelerates colonic transit in persons with slow colonic transit and prolongs the colonic transit time in those with rapid colonic transit.

180. _____ The absence of the rectoanal inhibitory reflex is diagnostic of Hirschsprung disease and precludes the need for additional evaluation.

The following statements (181–184) pertain to fecal occult blood tests:

181. _____ Compliance with fecal occult blood testing in population studies is approximately 75%.

182. _____ Controlled trials have shown a mortality benefit to fecal occult blood testing.

183. _____ Even small to moderate amounts of ethanol induce occult bleeding.

184. _____ Cecal cancers bleed more than sigmoid cancers.

185. _____ The sigmoid colon is the narrowest portion of the colon.

186. _____ In the diagnosis of a volvulus, sigmoidoscopy should be used in favor of barium or Gastrografin enemas if peritonitis is suspected.

187. _____ After nonoperative reduction, recurrence of sigmoid volvulus is very uncommon (10%).

188. _____ Noninvasive (intramucosal carcinoma) carcinomatous polyps require no additional therapy after polypectomy.

189. _____ The adenomatous polyposis syndromes including familial adenomatous polyposis, Gardner syndrome, and attenuated adenomatous polyposis coli are inherited in an autosomal recessive pattern.

190. _____ Overall, colorectal cancers in patients with hereditary nonpolyposis colorectal cancer are associated with a poorer survival rate.

191. _____ For patients with hereditary nonpolyposis colorectal cancer, screening every 5 years with flexible sigmoidoscopy starting at age 25 is adequate to detect early tumors and polyps.

192. _____ In the evaluation of a metastasis of unknown origin, colonoscopy or barium enema is a low-yield procedure in the absence of colorectal symptoms.

193. _____ Radiation therapy has proven to be a useful adjunct in treating colon cancer in terms of survival and disease-free survival.

The following statements (194–198) pertain to surgical procedures for ulcerative colitis:

194. _____ With a Brooke ileostomy, fecal continence is preserved.

195. _____ Anorectal intubations are required for ileal pouch–anal canal anastomosis.

196. _____ Pouchitis is a standard complication of continent ileostomy (Kock pouch).

197. _____ Diarrhea, which may occur as a complication in patients with continent ileostomy, is probably caused by bacterial overgrowth in the pouch.

198. _____ Spontaneous vaginal delivery is contraindicated in pregnant patients with ileal pouch–anal canal anastomosis.

The following case pertains to statements 199 and 200.

A 60-year-old man presents with a history of intermittent low-grade fever, fatigue, and diarrhea for a 6-week duration. He reports 5 watery bowel movements per day; he has noticed small amounts of blood in his stool; and he complains of urgency and tenesmus. There is no history of antibiotic use or recent travel. A physical examination reveals mild pallor, but otherwise, findings are normal. Laboratory studies disclose mild anemia, and a stool culture reveals no pathogens. The patient undergoes a colonoscopy with biopsy and the diagnosis of ulcerative colitis is confirmed. He responds well to treatment.

199. _____ Neither the severity of the first attack nor the degree of colonic involvement at diagnosis predicts the likelihood of recurrence.

200. _____ This patient is more likely to experience long periods without relapse than is a similar patient age 20 to 30.

Collagenous and lymphocytic colitis may be associated with which of the following (201–205):

201. _____ celiac disease

202. _____ Crohn's disease and sclerosing cholangitis

203. _____ autoimmune nongastrointestinal diseases such as diabetes, vitiligo, and thyroid disease

204. _____ perinuclear antineutrophil cytoplasmic antibody (p-ANCA) positivity in approximately 70% of cases

205. _____ certain HLA markers

206. _____ Cocaine use and the nonsteroidal antiinflammatory drugs, including diclofenac, rofecoxib, and celecoxib, have all been implicated as causes of colitis.

207. _____ Stercoral ulcers are primarily located in the rectosigmoid colon and are usually associated with fecal impaction.

208. _____ The mucosa of a patient with melanosis coli may appear endoscopically normal.

209. _____ Motor activity in the human colon is significantly greater during sleep, and especially during the interdigestive migratory motor complex.

210. _____ Dynamic scintigraphic studies of colonic emptying during defecation reveal that nearly all of the marker (>90%) originates from the rectum.

211. _____ Antibiotic-associated *Clostridium difficile* colitis without pseudomembranes rarely occurs.

MATCHING

(each selection may be used once, more than once, or not at all)

For each clinical scenario, pick the one best therapeutic alternative from the list below:

212. _____ A 37-year-old woman presents with a history of mild bloody diarrhea for 1 week. Colonoscopy shows inflammation and ulcers to 30 cm, and biopsy specimens confirm a diagnosis of ulcerative colitis. A trial of sulfasalazine 2 g/day is discontinued because it produced a rash and persistent headaches.

213. _____ A 43-year-old man with a 2-year history of colonic and perianal Crohn's disease required hospitalization 3 times for recurrent anal fistula and abscess formation. Anorectal drainage and diarrhea persist despite the administration of steroids.

214. _____ A 25-year-old woman with a history of repeated hospitalizations for extensive small bowel and colonic Crohn's disease presents for evaluation. She responds well to sulfasalazine

a. azathioprine 1.5 to 2.5 mg/kg/day

b. 5-aminosalicylic acid enema every evening

c. oral corticosteroids

d. surgical resection of the colon

e. metronidazole

and high-dose prednisone, but her condition
flares when the prednisone dose is tapered
below 20 mg/day.

Classify the following examples of ulcerative colitis from the list below:

215. _____ a 62-year-old woman with a temperature of
38°C, a pulse rate of 96 beats/minute, a hemoglobin level of 7.5 g/dL (normal, 14 g/dL), and
8 bloody stools per day

a. toxic megacolon

b. severe ulcerative colitis

c. moderate ulcerative colitis

216. _____ a 25-year-old man with a temperature of 37°C,
a pulse rate of 80 beats/minute, a hemoglobin
level of 13 g/dL (normal, 14 g/dL), and 3 nonbloody stools per day

d. mild ulcerative colitis

217. _____ a 38-year-old woman with a temperature of
39°C, a pulse rate of 120 beats/minute, a hemoglobin
level of 7.5 g/dL (normal, 14 g/dL), lethargy,
absent bowel sounds, rebound abdominal
tenderness, and hypokalemia

Match each complication of colonoscopy to the expected time frame:

218. _____ postpolypectomy bleeding

a. immediate complication of colonoscopy

219. _____ transmural burn syndrome

b. delayed complication of colonoscopy

220. _____ oversedation

c. both

221. _____ colonic perforation

d. neither

222. _____ colonic obstruction

Match the site and amount of gastrointestinal blood loss with the appropriate clinical observation:

223. _____ 20 mL lost from the cecum

a. normal-appearing, guaiac-negative stool

224. _____ 5 mL lost from the anorectum

b. brown, guaiac-positive stool

225. _____ 150 mL lost from the cecum

c. melena

226. _____ 4 mL lost from the duodenum

d. hematochezia

e. melena or hematochezia

Choose the best answer for each statement regarding oral iron therapy for iron deficiency anemia:

227. _____ bone marrow iron stores repleted

a. 3 to 6 months

228. _____ peak reticulocyte count after initiating iron therapy

b. 2 months

229. _____ low hemoglobin normalizes with iron treatment

c. 7 to 10 days

Match the feature with the appropriate fecal occult blood tests:

230. _____ uses antihemoglobin antibodies

a. heme (porphyrin quantitative) assay

231. _____ reacts with any peroxidase, not just blood

232. _____ detects heme and heme-derived porphyrins

233. _____ no need for dietary restrictions

234. _____ most sensitive for upper gastrointestinal blood loss

235. _____ diet should exclude cooked vegetables such as turnips, radishes, broccoli for 72 hours prior to testing

236. _____ can detect 3 mL colonic blood loss per day

b. immunochemical test

c. guaiac test

d. none of the above

e. all of the above

Match the following characteristics with the appropriate polyp or tumor:

237. _____ benign submucosal polyp

238. _____ associated with a syndrome of profuse watery diarrhea

239. _____ associated with inflammatory bowel disease, no malignant potential

a. hyperplastic polyp

b. inflammatory pseudopolyp

c. lipoma

d. villous adenoma

Match the following characteristics with the appropriate diagnosis, agent, or test:

240. _____ locally invasive, benign fibrous tissue tumor that arises in musculoaponeurotic structures

241. _____ central nervous system malignancies occurring together with colonic polyposis

242. _____ inherited disorder expressed as hamartomatous polyposis with a characteristic mucocutaneous pigmentation

243. _____ method of determining presence of relevant DNA mutation by detection of protein truncation

244. _____ colonic adenomatous polyps, colon cancer with high occurrence of extracolonic lesions

245. _____ most common extracolonic malignancies associated with familial adenomatous polyposis

246. _____ multiple hamartomatous polyps of skin and mucous membranes

247. _____ noninherited condition characterized by generalized gastrointestinal polyposis, cutaneous hyperpigmentation, hair loss, and nail atrophy

248. _____ defect is on the long arm of chromosome 5, phenotype manifests more than 100 colonic adenomatous polyps

a. desmoid tumor

b. Gardner syndrome

c. familial adenomatous polyposis

d. linkage testing

e. Turcot syndrome

f. Peutz-Jeghers syndrome

g. mutation identification

h. in vitro protein synthesis

i. hepatoblastoma

j. duodenal carcinoma

k. ovarian carcinoma

l. 5-fluorouracil

m. levamisole

n. Cowden's disease

o. Cronkhite-Canada syndrome

249. _____ test for familial adenomatous polyposis that uses DNA markers near or in the gene in question to identify mutant gene carriers

Match the following characteristics pertaining to colon cancer with the appropriate answer:

250. _____ surgical treatment for colon cancer involving sigmoid colon

a. Dukes stage B

b. APC gene

251. _____ penetrates muscularis mucosae, invades submucosa, but no further

c. p53 gene

252. _____ recurrence rate after curative resection for colon cancer

d. Dukes stage C

e. K-*ras* mutation

253. _____ penetrates muscularis propria and may extend through the serosa into pericolic fat

f. low anterior resection with end-to-end primary colonic anastomosis

254. _____ colon cancer with regional lymph node metastases

g. Dukes stage D

h. Dukes stage A

255. _____ serves as a cell-cycle checkpoint regulator and prevents nuclear replication after injuries likely to damage DNA

i. left hemicolectomy

j. one-third

k. three-quarters

l. total colectomy with ileostomy

Match the following antidiarrheal medications with their side effect:

256. _____ bismuth subsalicylate

a. tardive dyskinesia

257. _____ diphenoxylate

b. intestinal obstruction proximal to preexisting strictures

258. _____ psyllium

c. may precipitate toxic megacolon in patients with inflammatory bowel disease

259. _____ methysergide

d. encephalopathy in patients with chronic renal failure

260. _____ clonidine

e. postural hypotension

Match the following medications with the diarrheal disease for which they are most useful:

261. _____ clonidine

a. AIDS enteropathy

262. _____ indomethacin

b. systemic mastocytosis

263. _____ methysergide

c. Zollinger-Ellison syndrome

264. _____ promethazine

d. diarrhea of opiate withdrawal

265. _____ lansoprazole

e. carcinoid syndrome

5

Pancreas

MULTIPLE CHOICE

(one best answer)

1. A 40-year-old woman with a history of cholelithiasis presents to the emergency department complaining of severe abdominal pain. Results of laboratory studies are:

   aspartate aminotransferase: 180 U/L (normal, 35 U/L)
   alanine aminotransferase: 220 U/L (normal, 40 U/L)
   total bilirubin: 0.8 mg/dL (normal, 0.9 mg/dL)
   amylase: 870 U/L (normal, 100 U/L)
   alkaline phosphatase: 162 U/L (normal, 130 U/L)

   Ultrasonography of the abdomen reveals multiple gallstones, no ductal dilation, and a mildly edematous pancreas.

   Each of the following statements is true except:

   a. A gallstone can be recovered from the stool in up to 85% of these patients.
   b. Biliary pancreatitis is more common in patients with multiple small gallstones.
   c. Chronic morphologic and functional abnormalities of the pancreas sometimes occur after an episode of biliary pancreatitis.
   d. Definitive treatment of persistent biliary obstruction should be performed before discharging the patient from the hospital.

2. Alcohol consumption is the most common cause of chronic pancreatitis in the western world. What is the most common form of nonalcoholic chronic pancreatitis?

   a. hereditary
   b. hypertriglyceridemic
   c. autoimmune
   d. traumatic
   e. idiopathic

3. Which of the following statements regarding alcohol consumption and acute pancreatitis is most accurate?

   a. Alcohol does not result in a direct toxic injury to the pancreas.

   b. The risk of developing pancreatitis is dependent on the amount of alcohol consumed but is relatively independent of the duration of alcohol abuse.
   c. In alcoholic pancreatitis, the pancreas is often morphologically and/or functionally abnormal prior to the first episode of clinical acute pancreatitis.
   d. Diets high in carbohydrates increase the risk of alcoholic pancreatitis.

4. Each of the following statements regarding postoperative pancreatitis is true except:

   a. It is associated with episodes of hypotension during the operative procedure.
   b. It may be a complication associated with common bile duct exploration.
   c. It may be a complication associated with manipulation of the periampullary region.
   d. It is associated with the use of halogenated anesthetic agents.

5. Each of the following statements regarding tropical pancreatitis is true except:

   a. Disease onset occurs in childhood with recurrent abdominal pain, malabsorption, and bilateral parotid gland enlargement.
   b. Malnutrition is believed to be an important factor in the pathogenesis of this disease.
   c. Pancreatic calcifications are uncommon.
   d. Diabetes mellitus develops by puberty in tropical pancreatitis.

6. A 34-year-old man with acquired immunodeficiency syndrome develops an episode of acute pancreatitis without obvious etiology. Computed tomography reveals no evidence of intrapancreatic malignancy. Which opportunistic infectious agent is unlikely to have caused pancreatitis in this patient?

   a. cytomegalovirus
   b. *Cryptococcus* species
   c. *Mycobacterium avium*

d. *Pneumocystis carinii*
e. *Candida* species

7. All of the following drugs used in the treatment of disorders associated with the human immunodeficiency virus may induce acute pancreatitis except:

a. trimethoprim-sulfamethoxazole
b. zidovudine
c. intravenous pentamidine
d. didanosine
e. aerosolized pentamidine

8. All of the following statements regarding the pathogenesis of chronic pancreatitis are true except:

a. There is a linear relationship between the risk of developing chronic pancreatitis and mean daily alcohol consumption.
b. Alcohol-induced pancreatitis occurs more commonly in people who consume low-fat, low-protein diets.
c. Acute hypercalcemia is a potent stimulus for human pancreatic enzyme secretion.
d. Nutritional deficiencies in zinc, copper, and selenium appear to be important in the development of tropical (nutritional) pancreatitis.

9. All of the following statements regarding the genesis of pain in chronic pancreatitis are true except:

a. Histologically, pancreatic nerves appear to be larger and more numerous.
b. Noxious, biologically active materials from the surrounding extracellular matrix may penetrate damaged perineurium and cause pain by continual stimulation of sensory nerve fibers.
c. The organization of intraneural organelles (e.g., microtubules) is disrupted.
d. The amount of the neurotransmitter substance P is decreased in afferent pancreatic nerves.

10. Chronic alcohol ingestion produces chronic pancreatitis by unclear cellular mechanisms. However, distinct changes observed in pancreatic secretion may play an important pathophysiologic role in this condition. Which of the following statements regarding alcohol-induced pancreatic injury is false?

a. Chronic alcoholism causes an increase in the basal secretion of proteases, amylase, and lipase.
b. Rats exposed to chronic ethanol demonstrate a decrease in trypsin inhibitor levels.
c. Pancreatic juice contains large amounts of lipase resulting in the production of free fatty acid.
d. Pancreatic secretion is less responsive than normal to cholecystokinin.

11. All of the following statements regarding serum pancreatic enzyme levels in acute pancreatitis are true except:

a. Amylase elevation in acute pancreatitis results from enhanced release into the bloodstream and decreased renal clearance.
b. The serum half-life of amylase is 12 to 14 hours.
c. Amylase elevation tends to be lower in acute alcoholic pancreatitis than in gallstone pancreatitis.
d. Amylase elevation may be underestimated in lactescent sera.
e. Unlike amylase, lipase levels are usually normal in patients with diabetic ketoacidosis and macroamylasemia.

12. Which of the following statements regarding the treatment of patients with acute pancreatitis is true?

a. Although calcium levels lower than 7.5 mg/dL are associated with a poor prognosis, hypocalcemia should not be treated unless it becomes symptomatic.
b. In patients with resolving acute pancreatitis, an oral diet should be started after normalization of the serum amylase.
c. Nasogastric suction is indicated in patients with pancreatitis to decrease gastric acid–dependent pancreatic stimulation.
d. Intravenous antibiotics should be given routinely until infection has been excluded by cultures.
e. Endoscopic retrograde cholangiopancreatography should always be performed preoperatively in patients undergoing cholecystectomy after an episode of biliary pancreatitis.

13. A 32-year-old man presents to the emergency department with a 6-hour history of progressively increasing, diffuse abdominal pain that radiates to his back. Physical examination reveals ecchymosis involving the flanks. Each of the following statements concerning this physical finding is true except:

a. It represents subcutaneous fatty necrosis.
b. It may be associated with a rise in methemalbumin levels.
c. It is associated with hemorrhagic pancreatitis.
d. It may indicate a poor prognosis.

14. A 50-year-old man presents at the hospital with acute pancreatitis. His serum calcium level on the second day of admission is 7.5 mg/dL (normal, 8.6–10.2 mg/dL). Each of the following statements regarding pancreatitis-associated hypocalcemia is true except:

a. It is associated with a poor prognosis.
b. It may reflect albumin loss.
c. It occurs as a result of an increased release of pancreatic glucagon.
d. It reflects a failure of calcium release from bone in response to circulating parathyroid hormone.

15. Each of the following statements concerning pain associated with chronic pancreatitis is true except:

   a. The onset of painful attacks coincides with the development of pancreatic exocrine insufficiency.
   b. A reduction in intraductal pressure by decompressive surgery may relieve pain in selected patients.
   c. Alterations in the histology of peripancreatic nerves have been demonstrated in patients with chronic pancreatitis.
   d. Celiac plexus blockade provides only limited relief of pain in most patients with chronic pancreatitis.

16. A 48-year-old man is admitted to the hospital with acute pancreatitis. His initial course is uncomplicated, but 4 days after admission, he experiences an exacerbation of abdominal pain. An abdominal ultrasonographic examination reveals a pseudocyst involving the head of the pancreas. Each of the following statements regarding pancreatic pseudocysts is true except:

   a. Pseudocysts larger than 5 cm should be surgically repaired immediately because of the increased risk of rupture.
   b. Hemorrhage caused by erosion of a pseudocyst into a vascular structure is the etiology of up to 40% of deaths associated with this complication.
   c. Pseudocysts may be suspected clinically if serum amylase levels remain persistently elevated.
   d. Pseudocysts that fail to resolve after 6 weeks should be evaluated for surgical drainage.

17. Each of the following statements regarding pancreatic abscesses is true except:

   a. Adult respiratory distress syndrome is mainly due to the damaging effect of free fatty acid.
   b. Recent prospective studies demonstrate a decreased incidence of infectious complications and improved survival in patients with extensive necrosis of the pancreas when given prophylactic antibiotics.
   c. Most abscesses are monomicrobial in nature and can be successfully treated with intravenous antibiotics.
   d. They can be diagnosed by percutaneous fine-needle aspiration of peripancreatic fluid.

18. A 35-year-old alcoholic woman presents with a 2-day history of abdominal pain radiating to the back, a temperature of 40°C, a blood pressure of 140/70 mm Hg, a pulse rate of 100 beats/minute, and a respiratory rate of 16 breaths/minute. Computed tomography (CT) reveals an edematous pancreas and a 3-cm area of low attenuation in the pancreatic body with no air. Which of the following is the most appropriate next step in this patient's management?

   a. emergent surgery
   b. continuation of conservative therapy for acute pancreatitis

   c. follow-up CT scan in 4 to 6 weeks
   d. CT-guided needle aspiration of the pancreas
   e. none of the above

19. A 39-year-old woman hospitalized with acute pancreatitis complains of progressive dyspnea. Arterial blood gas analysis demonstrates marked hypoxemia. This patient is at risk for each of the following except:

   a. atelectasis caused by splinting to avoid pain
   b. adult respiratory distress syndrome
   c. development of a large pleural effusion
   d. acute pulmonary hemorrhage

20. All of the following statements regarding pancreatic pseudocysts are true except:

   a. In the absence of complications, drainage of pseudocysts should be restricted to those that are larger than 6 cm in diameter and that have persisted for more than 6 weeks.
   b. Pseudocysts associated with a normal pancreatic duct can be treated by percutaneous drainage.
   c. Pseudocysts that are proximal to a pancreatic ductal stricture should be drained percutaneously.
   d. Pseudocysts located at the head of the pancreas may be amenable to endoscopic drainage through the major or minor papilla.

21. Each of the following statements regarding malabsorption secondary to chronic pancreatitis is true except:

   a. Steatorrhea due to pancreatic insufficiency does not develop until 90% of the pancreatic exocrine function is lost.
   b. Fat, protein, and starch absorption may be impaired in severe pancreatic disease.
   c. There is a greater increase in fecal weight due to pancreatic insufficiency compared with other etiologies of steatorrhea.
   d. Fat-soluble vitamin deficiency states are less common in association with steatorrhea of chronic pancreatitis compared with celiac sprue.

22. A 42-year-old man with chronic pancreatitis complicated by steatorrhea continues to have oily diarrhea despite taking 4 tablets of pancrelipase (4500 IU lipase/tablet) with each meal. Possible reasons for refractory steatorrhea include each of the following except:

   a. insufficient lipase activity with present dosing
   b. inactivation of lipase by acid in the stomach
   c. presence of undiagnosed bacterial overgrowth
   d. concurrent use of cimetidine

23. A 63-year-old man with chronic diarrhea submits a 72-hour fecal collection while consuming a diet of 100 g/day of fat. Analysis reveals 15 g/day of fecal

fat. Which of the following statements is most accurate?

a. This test is specific for the detection of pancreatic insufficiency.
b. A 72-hour fecal collection detects pancreatic exocrine insufficiency when 50% of lipase activity is lost.
c. A two-stage fecal fat collection (with and without exogenous pancreatic enzymes) can be used to assess the adequacy of pancreatic enzyme replacement.
d. Pancreatic disease typically leads to greater levels of steatorrhea than does small bowel disease.

24. Each of the following statements regarding pancreatic enzymes is true except:

a. The four major enzyme types are amylolytic, lipolytic, proteolytic, and nucleolytic.
b. Pancreatic enzymes are synthesized within ductal cells and packaged into zymogen granules.
c. Trypsinogen is converted into the biologically active trypsin by duodenally secreted enterokinase.
d. All proteolytic enzymes are secreted as inactive proenzymes.

25. The ability of a given lipid to stimulate pancreatic enzyme secretion is dependent on each of the following factors except:

a. chain length of fatty acids
b. presence of acid in the stomach
c. saturation of the fatty acids
d. concentration of bile salts

26. Each of the following is a potent stimulus of pancreatic enzyme secretion except:

a. glucose
b. fatty acids
c. essential amino acids
d. distention of the gastric antrum

27. Each of the following statements concerning the hormone secretin is true except:

a. Secretin is the most potent stimulant of pancreatic juice and bicarbonate secretion.
b. The threshold for secretin release is a duodenal pH of less than or equal to 4.5.
c. Dietary carbohydrate concentration within the duodenum is the major stimulant for secretin release.
d. Secretin-containing cells are present in the proximal small intestine.
e. The stimulatory action of secretin on bicarbonate secretion is potentiated by cholecystokinin.

28. Each of the following statements concerning cholecystokinin (CCK) is true except:

a. Under fasting conditions, plasma CCK levels are low and reach peak concentrations within 10 to 30 minutes postprandially.
b. Factors that influence the plasma CCK response to intraduodenal fatty acids include the chain length of the fatty acids, their degree of saturation, and their concentration in the intestine.
c. Vagotomy does not significantly affect the release of CCK in response to nutrient stimulation.
d. Carbohydrates are more potent stimulants for the release of CCK than are amino acids.
e. CCK plays an important role as a mediator of postprandial pancreatic enzyme secretion.

29. All of the following statements about pancreatic anatomy are true except:

a. The pancreas is a retroperitoneal organ that lies in an oblique orientation behind the peritoneum of the posterior abdominal wall.
b. The pancreatic head is covered by the first portion of the duodenum.
c. Disruption of the pancreatic duct as a result of blunt abdominal injury most commonly occurs in the tail.
d. Because the duodenum and the pancreatic head share a blood supply, a 95% pancreatectomy may compromise blood flow to the duodenum.

30. Regarding pain fibers in the pancreas, each of the following statements is true except:

a. Pain fibers from the pancreas travel through the celiac ganglia and into the sympathetic splanchnic nerves.
b. Pain from the head of the pancreas tends to be broadly localized in the midepigastrium.
c. Pain from the body and tail tends to localize to the left upper quadrant.
d. Visceral pain from the pancreas is usually severe and sharp, because the pancreas is in contact with the parietal peritoneum.
e. Radiation of pain to the back in the area of the lower thoracic vertebrae is common.

31. Which of the following statements concerning pancreas divisum is false?

a. The condition results from noncommunication between the main and accessory pancreatic ducts, caused by abnormal fusion of the dorsal and ventral pancreatic buds during fetal development.
b. Autopsy studies report an incidence of about 7% for this condition in the United States.
c. Patients with pain and chronic pancreatitis are most likely to respond to endoscopic therapy.
d. Endoscopic treatment generally includes sphincterotomy of the minor papilla.

e. A temporary stent is commonly left in place after sphincterotomy to prevent edema from obstructing the papillary orifice.

32. When considering endoscopic therapy for a patient with pancreas divisum, all of the following criteria should be satisfied except:

    a. All other causes of pancreatitis should be excluded.
    b. Evidence of chronic pancreatitis (e.g., pancreatic calcifications) should be documented.
    c. Discrete episodes of proven clinical pancreatitis recur with intervening asymptomatic periods.
    d. Evidence of obstruction of the duct of Santorini (i.e., high sphincter pressures or a dilated dorsal duct) should be provided.

33. Each of the following statements regarding annular pancreas is true except:

    a. Males are more commonly affected than females.
    b. It is frequently associated with other congenital defects, such as tracheoesophageal fistulas and Meckel diverticula.
    c. Over half of all cases are diagnosed in the first year of life.
    d. Plain radiographs of the abdomen often show a "double-bubble" sign.
    e. Division of the annulus in symptomatic individuals is the preferred treatment.

34. Abberant localization of pancreatic tissue, also known as pancreatic rests, is most commonly found in:

    a. stomach and proximal small intestine
    b. colon
    c. appendix
    d. lung
    e. liver

35. Regarding hepatobiliary tract abnormalities in patients with cystic fibrosis, each of the following statements is true except:

    a. Disease of the biliary tract occurs in 50% of patients with cystic fibrosis.
    b. Of the 12% of patients who develop gallstones, most become symptomatic.
    c. A minority of patients develop clinically apparent liver disease.
    d. Clinical manifestations of liver involvement include neonatal jaundice, hypersplenism, bleeding from esophageal varices, and hepatocellular failure.

36. A 2-day-old infant presents with abdominal distention, delayed passage of meconium, and bilious vomiting. Possible therapies for presumed meconium ileus include all of the following except:

    a. N-acetylcysteine
    b. Hypaque or Gastrografin enema
    c. abdominal surgery
    d. observation

37. The majority of pancreatic adenocarcinomas arise from:

    a. ductular cells
    b. acinar cells
    c. islet cells
    d. spindle cells
    e. giant cells

38. A 45-year-old woman with a history of tobacco abuse presents with a history of abdominal pain and a 13.5-kg weight loss over the past 6 months. Her previous medical history is significant for a total abdominal hysterectomy, diabetes mellitus, and recurrent urinary tract infections. She drinks wine occasionally with dinner. Physical examination reveals a tender epigastrium. After routine blood tests, an abdominal computed tomographic scan reveals a mass in the head of the pancreas. Endoscopic retrograde cholangiopancreatography is performed, and cytology obtained at the time of this procedure reveals a ductal adenocarcinoma. Which of the following risk factors in this patient is most strongly associated with pancreatic cancer?

    a. age
    b. diabetes mellitus
    c. smoking
    d. alcohol use

39. All of the following statements concerning pancreatic ductal adenocarcinoma are true except:

    a. Pain from tumors in the body and tail are usually caused by malignant infiltration of the retroperitoneal structures.
    b. Two-thirds of tumors occur in the body and tail.
    c. The majority of adenocarcinomas of the pancreatic head have metastasized to regional lymph nodes at the time of diagnosis.
    d. Most resectable tumors of the pancreatic head have a median diameter of 2.5 to 3.5 cm.

40. Mutation of which of the following genes is most commonly associated with pancreatic adenocarcinoma?

    a. *DPC4*
    b. K-*ras*
    c. *DCC*
    d. p53
    e. *BRCA1*

41. All of the following statements regarding the CA 19-9 tumor-associated antigen and pancreatic cancer are true except:

    a. It is the most sensitive and specific marker available.
    b. The sensitivity and specificity of this marker are not affected by tumor size.
    c. Serum levels of CA 19-9 may be elevated with other cancers and conditions.
    d. It may be a useful surveillance tool to assess response to an intervention or therapy.

42. Which statement regarding therapy for pancreatic cancer is correct?

    a. Treatment with 5-fluorouracil and radiotherapy confers no survival benefit compared to radiotherapy alone for unresectable cancers.
    b. 5-Fluorouracil and radiotherapy provide no survival benefit following curative resection.
    c. Gemcitabine may decrease pain, increase weight, and improve quality of life.
    d. Preoperatively, conditions warranting urgent biliary stenting are preferably treated with a wire mesh stent rather than a plastic stent.

The following case pertains to questions 43 and 44.

A 55-year-old woman presents for an evaluation of watery diarrhea of 1-year duration. Initially, she had diarrhea intermittently for several days at a time that would spontaneously resolve. She was evaluated by her internist, who obtained stool cultures for bacteria and performed stool examinations for ova and parasites. Results of both tests were negative. Colonoscopy with random biopsies revealed no histopathologic cause for her diarrhea. Her internist told her that she had irritable bowel syndrome. She complains of persistent, large-volume, watery, nonbloody diarrhea. She notes no relation between these symptoms and meals and reports frequent nocturnal diarrhea. She also complains of profound weakness. Physical examination is unremarkable. Results of the laboratory studies are:

hemoglobin: 12 g/dL
K^+: 2.8 mEq/L
Na^+: 134 mEq/L
blood urea nitrogen: 12 mg/dL
CO_2: 30 mEq/L
leukocyte count: 8600/mm^3
glucose: 115 mg/dL
Cl: 95 mEq/L
hematocrit: 36%
creatinine: 1.0 mg/dL

43. All of the following studies would be appropriate next steps in the diagnostic evaluation except:

    a. quantitative stool output and electrolytes while the patient is fasting
    b. stool and urine phenolphthalein levels
    c. fasting serum hormone levels (e.g., vasoactive intestinal polypeptide, gastrin, calcitonin, 5-HIAA)
    d. abdominal imaging
    e. hydrogen breath test

44. Which of the following would not be characteristic of this patient's condition?

    a. hypercalcemia
    b. flushing
    c. hypochlorhydria
    d. hypoglycemia
    e. stool output more than 3 L/day

45. Multiple endocrine neoplasia syndrome type I is characterized by each of the following except:

    a. multiple pancreatic tumor foci at time of diagnosis
    b. functional islet cell tumors in 80% of cases
    c. insulinomas are the most common type of islet cell tumor in this syndrome
    d. autosomal dominant inheritance
    e. hypercalcemia is common

46. A number of conditions have been associated with an abnormally elevated plasma glucagon concentration of less than 500 pg/mL. Which of the following conditions can cause the plasma glucagon concentration to be greater than 500 pg/mL?

    a. renal insufficiency
    b. cirrhosis
    c. acute pancreatitis
    d. hyperadrenocorticism
    e. pancreatic adenocarcinoma

The following case pertains to questions 47 and 48.

A 48-year-old female nurse with a 2-year history of emotional irritability, headache, and diaphoresis was evaluated by her internist, who attributed her symptoms to the onset of menopause. She is brought to the emergency department by colleagues because of hostility and progressive confusion that developed around noon while she was at work. On examination, she is noted to be combative and disoriented, both of which resolve dramatically after the administration of 50% dextrose and naloxone. She reports not eating breakfast because she was running late. Results of laboratories studies made prior to the administration of glucose and naloxone are:

hemoglobin: 12 g/dL
Na^+: 140 mEq/L
CO_2: 25 mEq/L
glucose: 30 mg/dL
hematocrit: 36%
K^+: 3.6 mEq/L
blood urea nitrogen: 12 mg/dL
leukocyte count: 10,000/mm^3

Cl: 110 mEq/L
creatinine: 1.0 mg/dL

The patient is admitted to the hospital and placed on a fast with the exception of free access to water. Glucose and insulin levels are checked every 1 to 2 hours with the following results:

Time of day	Glucose (mg/dL)	Insulin (U/mL) (normal, 5–20 U/mL)
Noon	60	30
2 pm	62	30
4 pm	54	26
6 pm	46	20
7 pm	38	20
8 pm	38	24
9 pm	35	30

47. Which of the following conditions should not be considered in the differential diagnosis?

    a. adrenal insufficiency
    b. surreptitious administration of insulin
    c. sulfonylurea ingestion
    d. autoantibodies to the insulin receptor
    e. insulinoma

48. Further studies should include all of the following except:

    a. serum proinsulin levels
    b. serum C-peptide levels
    c. assessment for antibodies to insulin
    d. cosyntropin stimulation test

49. With pancreatic endocrine tumors, all of the following statements are correct except:

    a. The size of the tumor correlates with the severity of the hormonally induced symptoms.
    b. The size of the tumor correlates with the likelihood of malignancy.
    c. Pancreatic endocrine tumors frequently express the α-chain of human chorionic gonadotropin, and it has been proposed that α-chain expression correlates with malignancy.
    d. There is no correlation between the histologic pattern and the associated clinical syndrome.
    e. Histologic classification of these tumors has failed to predict tumor growth patterns and malignant potential.

50. All of the following statements regarding endoscopic ultrasonography (EUS) in pancreatic disease are true except:

    a. Focal chronic pancreatitis and pancreatic adenocarcinoma may have identical appearances on EUS.
    b. EUS is more sensitive than ultrasonography or computed tomography for detecting regional lymph node involvement in patients with pancreatic malignancy.
    c. EUS is the most sensitive test for the detection and localization of endocrine tumors of the pancreas.
    d. EUS may be more sensitive than endoscopic retrograde cholangiopancreatography in the diagnosis of chronic pancreatitis.
    e. EUS reliably identifies neoplastic encasement of the major arterial structures, such as the celiac, hepatic, splenic, and superior mesenteric arteries.

51. With regard to octreotide, all of the following statements are true except:

    a. Insulinomas are generally less responsive to octreotide therapy than are glucagonomas, VIPomas, gastrinomas, and GRFomas.
    b. Octreotide improves the diarrhea associated with VIPoma.
    c. In most patients with glucagonoma, octreotide improves the necrolytic migratory erythema skin rash.
    d. In most patients with glucagonoma, octreotide therapy controls the associated diabetes mellitus.
    e. Octreotide reduces plasma concentrations of GRF in patients with GRFomas.

52. Which of the following statements regarding hereditary pancreatitis and its gene mutation is false?

    a. Hereditary pancreatitis involves a mutation in the cationic trypsinogen gene.
    b. Trypsinogen is activated exclusively by enterokinase in the small bowel under normal physiologic conditions.
    c. Autodigestion and acute pancreatitis may occur in hereditary pancreatitis from autoactivation of trypsin and/or failure to inactivate trypsin within the pancreas.
    d. It is not clear whether other forms of inherited pancreatitis share the gene mutation found in hereditary pancreatitis.

53. All of the following statements regarding pancreatic cancer and diabetes are true except:

    a. Similar to type II diabetics, patients with pancreatic cancer commonly develop hyperinsulinemia and marked peripheral insulin resistance.
    b. Pancreatic tumors may release a substance that stimulates the secretion of islet amyloid polypeptide, which causes insulin resistance and decreased glycogen synthesis.
    c. Islet amyloid polypeptide levels in patients with pancreatic cancer and type II diabetes are elevated compared to those with other cancers and insulin-requiring diabetes.

d. Following tumor resection, the diabetes frequently becomes more severe.

54. Which of the following statements regarding less common exocrine pancreatic tumors is false?

a. Mucinous cystadenomas are premalignant and should be resected.
b. Serous cystadenomas, or microcystic adenomas, may undergo malignant transformation and should be removed if it can be done safely.
c. Mucinous ductal ectasia commonly demonstrates papillary malignant changes in 50% of cases, warranting resection.
d. Solid and papillary epithelial neoplasms have a poor prognosis.

55. Vagotomy has all the following effects on pancreatic function except:

a. It reduces the bicarbonate-secretory response to secretin.
b. It reduces the release of cholecystokinin and secretin.
c. It reduces the sensitivity of the pancreas to enzyme release mediated by submaximal doses of cholecystokinin.
d. It reduces pancreatic enzyme responses to intestinal stimulants and food.

56. An adenocarcinoma in the pancreatic body or tail would most likely invade which venous structure?

a. superior mesenteric
b. inferior mesenteric
c. splenic
d. portal
e. inferior vena cava

TRUE/FALSE

57. _____ Senile idiopathic pancreatitis in patients over age 60 is characterized by the onset of recurrent severe abdominal pain.

58. _____ For a given degree of steatorrhea, the absorption of fat-soluble vitamins (A, D, E, K) is much better in pancreatic insufficiency than in celiac sprue.

59. _____ A plain radiograph of the abdomen should be the first diagnostic test performed in attempting to establish a diagnosis of chronic pancreatitis.

Regarding the complications of chronic pancreatitis:

60. _____ Typically, pancreatic ascites occurs in alcoholic patients with cirrhosis and is thought to be caused by decompensated liver disease.

61. _____ The onset of a pure cholestasis in patients with chronic pancreatitis suggests compression of the distal common bile duct as a result of fibrosis in the head of the pancreas.

62. _____ Patients with chronic pancreatitis and variceal hemorrhage from an isolated gastric varix can often be treated with splenectomy alone, rather than with a portosystemic shunt.

63. _____ Plain abdominal radiographs demonstrate diffuse pancreatic calcifications in the majority (i.e., 60%) of patients with chronic pancreatitis.

64. _____ Most pancreatic pseudocysts that complicate chronic pancreatitis resolve spontaneously.

Endoscopic retrograde cholangiopancreatography should be performed for which of the following reasons in patients with chronic pancreatitis?

65. _____ to evaluate dilation of the pancreatic duct observed on ultrasonography

66. _____ to localize an external pancreatic fistula

The following statements (67–70) pertain to the inhibition of pancreatic enzyme secretion:

67. _____ The presence of lipids in the colon inhibits cholecystokinin-stimulated pancreatic enzyme secretion.

68. _____ Activation of volume receptors in the duodenum inhibits pancreatic enzyme secretion.

69. _____ Hyperglycemia and hyperaminoacidemia induced by intravenous nutrient administration inhibit pancreatic enzyme secretion.

70. _____ Acid entering the duodenum inhibits postprandial pancreatic secretion.

71. _____ Studies of patients with pancreatic divisum show that there is no significant increase in the incidence of pancreatitis compared to persons with normal pancreatic ductal anatomy.

72. _____ Patients with cystic fibrosis and pancreatic insufficiency usually require lower doses of pancreatic enzyme supplementation, because decreased gastric acid output results in less enzyme degradation in the stomach.

The following statements pertain to hereditary pancreatitis:

73. _____ Inheritance follows an autosomal dominant pattern.

74. _____ Progression to diabetes and frank steatorrhea occurs in approximately 20% of cases.

75. _____ The initial onset of abdominal pain occurs most commonly in the second decade of life.

Regarding pancreatic adenocarcinoma and glucose intolerance:

76. _____ Abnormal glucose tolerance is a frequent finding in patients with pancreatic adeno-carcinoma.

77. _____ Glucose intolerance in patients with pancreatic adenocarcinoma may result from an increased secretion of islet amyloid polypeptide.

78. _____ Patients with diabetes mellitus are at increased risk for the development of pancreatic cancer.

The following statements (79–81) pertain to pancreatic carcinoma:

79. _____ Approximately 30% of symptomatic patients have resectable tumors

80. _____ For resectable tumors of the head of the pancreas, pancreaticoduodenectomy (i.e., the Whipple procedure) is the surgical treatment of choice.

81. _____ Neurolytic block of the celiac ganglion may afford pain relief.

82. _____ Glucagonomas are usually benign, well-circumscribed tumors at the time of diagnosis.

83. _____ Insulinomas are commonly benign, well-circumscribed, and associated with a good overall prognosis.

84. _____ Mutations of the cystic fibrosis transmembrane conductance regulator (CFTR) gene may contribute to the development of chronic pancreatitis; however, the mutation occurs exclusively in patients with lung disease.

MATCHING

(each selection may be used once, more than once, or not at all)

Match the hereditary pancreatic disease or syndrome in the first column with the characteristic in the second column to which it best relates:

85. _____ commonly develops in early childhood (ages 1–10 years)

86. _____ autosomal dominant inheritance

87. _____ X-linked inheritance pattern

88. _____ can produce liver disease

89. _____ results in uncontrolled activation of trypsin

a. cystic fibrosis

b. hereditary pancreatitis

c. both

d. neither

Match the following pancreatic neuroendocrine tumors with their characteristic sign or symptom:

90. _____ gastrinoma

91. _____ somatostatinoma

92. _____ glucagonoma

93. _____ growth hormone–releasing factor tumor

a. necrolytic migratory erythema

b. acromegaly

c. cholelithiasis

d. recurrent ulcers of the gastrointestinal tract

For each patient, match the test(s) that are most likely to elucidate the underlying cause of acute pancreatitis:

94. _____ A 27-year-old African American man with a 1-year history of progressive dyspnea and dry cough develops an attack of acute pancreatitis. A recent chest radiograph reveals bilateral adenopathy with parenchymal infiltration.

a. serum triglyceride concentration

b. serum calcium concentration

c. examination of bile for crystals

d. serum antibody for double-stranded DNA

95. _____ A 42-year-old obese woman who has been on a weight-reduction diet over the previous 6 months develops acute abdominal pain and has a serum amylase level of 900 U/L. She denies the excessive use of alcohol. No metabolic abnormalities are detected from routine blood testing. Abdominal ultrasonography is unremarkable.

96. _____ A 35-year-old woman with a history of a malar rash, photosensitivity, and arthritis has recurrent bouts of pancreatitis.

97. _____ A 52-year-old man presents with a 4-day history of severe abdominal pain. Abdominal computed tomography reveals phlegmonous pancreatitis, but his serum amylase level at admission is normal.

For each patient, match the procedure most likely to yield crucial clinical information regarding diagnosis or treatment:

98. _____ A 65-year-old man with a history of "asymptomatic" gallstone disease presents with a 6-month history of progressive, severe abdominal pain and a 9-kg weight loss. Computed tomography shows a mass in the head of the pancreas.

a. abdominal ultrasonography

b. endoscopic retrograde cholangiopancreatography

c. pancreatic function testing

d. computed tomography–guided fine-needle aspiration

e. measure serum CA 19-9 level

99. _____ A 46-year-old man with a history of alcohol abuse and chronic pancreatitis presents with a 1-month history of worsening abdominal pain.

100. _____ A 52-year-old woman is hospitalized with severe abdominal pain. Her serum amylase level is 4500 U/L, aspartate aminotransferase is 156 U/L, and alkaline phosphatase is 360 U/L. Abdominal ultrasonography reveals gallstones. Her abdominal pain worsens over 24 hours, and she develops a temperature of 39.4°C.

6

Biliary Tree

MULTIPLE CHOICE

(one best answer)

1. An 85-year-old man presents with a history of three discreet episodes of severe epigastric pain. The pain occurs suddenly, increases gradually to a peak within 15 minutes of onset, and lasts 1 to 2 hours without fluctuation before slowly resolving. Radiation to the upper back is noted; however, no precipitating events can be recalled. Ultrasonography of the right upper quadrant reveals seven small (<1 cm diameter), buoyant, high-amplitude echoes with postacoustic shadowing within the gallbladder, a normal gallbladder wall, and a nondilated biliary tree. The patient requests that all treatment alternatives be discussed. Reasonable options include all of the following except:

   a. ursodeoxycholic acid
   b. extracorporeal shock-wave lithotripsy
   c. laparoscopic cholecystectomy
   d. contact dissolution with methyl-*tert*-butyl ether (MTBE)

2. Gallstones recur in what percentage of patients following oral dissolution therapy with ursodeoxycholic acid?

   a. 10%
   b. 30%
   c. 50%
   d. 80%
   e. 100%

3. Each of the following statements regarding gallstones is true except:

   a. Pure cholesterol stones are common (approximately 85% of gallstones).
   b. Most gallstones are found incidentally and are not associated with symptoms.
   c. Biliary colic develops in gallstone carriers at a rate of 1% to 2% per year.
   d. Complications of gallstone disease (e.g., pancreatitis, cholangitis) are usually preceded by episodic pain.

4. Risk factors associated with the development of cholesterol gallstones include each of the following except:

   a. ileal resection
   b. clofibrate
   c. estrogenic steroids
   d. marked weight reduction
   e. nonsteroidal antiinflammatory drugs

The following case pertains to questions 5 and 6.

A 70-year-old man with diabetes presents with nausea, vomiting, and abdominal pain of 24-hour duration. Abdominal pain in the right upper quadrant 3 days earlier subsided without intervention. Currently, the abdominal pain is confined to the right lower quadrant and occurs in discrete bouts, each lasting 15 to 20 minutes. His last bowel movement was 2 days ago and was described as normal. Physical examination reveals an obese man in acute distress with an upright blood pressure of 160/100 mm Hg and a pulse rate of 98 beats/minute, and a supine blood pressure of 125/80 mm Hg and a pulse rate of 100 beats/minute. His abdomen is distended and diffusely tender; hyperactive bowel sounds are heard on auscultation. The rectal vault is empty. A brief neurologic examination shows decreased sensation to light touch in both feet. Laboratory studies disclose the following values:

Na^+: 134 mEq/L
K^+: 3.2 mEq/L
Cl^-: 98 mEq/L
CO_2: 13 mEq/L
leukocyte count: 10,200/mm^3
hemoglobin: 15.7 g/dL
hematocrit: 46.3%
platelets: 290,000/mm^3
glucose: 378 mg/dL
aspartate aminotransferase: 40 U/L
alanine aminotransferase: 38 U/L
alkaline phosphatase: 144 U/L
total bilirubin: 0.8 mg/dL
total protein: 6.1 g/dL
albumin: 4.0 g/dL
Ca^{2+}: 9.2 mEq/L
amylase: 130 U/L (normal, 100 U/L)

83

urine ketones: positive
abdominal radiograph: multiple air-fluid levels in the
  intestine
chest radiograph: normal

5. What is the most likely diagnosis?

   a. diabetic gastroparesis
   b. Ogilvie syndrome
   c. gallstone ileus
   d. acute pancreatitis

6. In addition to medical management with fluids, antibiotics, and insulin, what treatment would you
   recommend?

   a. surgery after medical stabilization
   b. endoscopic retrograde cholangiopancreatography
      with sphincterotomy
   c. urgent decompressive colonoscopy after medical
      stabilization
   d. medical management alone will suffice

7. Each of the following is a risk factor for the development of common bile duct stones except:

   a. biliary stasis
   b. cholangitis
   c. juxtapapillary duodenal diverticulum
   d. foreign material in the biliary tree
   e. previous endoscopic retrograde cholangio-
      pancreatography

8. Choledochal cysts may be complicated by any of the
   following except:

   a. pancreatitis
   b. biliary cirrhosis
   c. cholecystitis
   d. hepatitis

9. All of the following statements are true except:

   a. Abdominal radiographs are often helpful in identi-
      fying gallstones in patients with abdominal pain,
      because 50% to 60% of gallstones are radiopaque.
   b. Ultrasonography is highly specific and sensitive
      for diagnosing the presence or absence of chole-
      lithiasis.
   c. The absence of dilated extrahepatic bile ducts on
      ultrasonography does not exclude common bile
      duct or common hepatic duct stones.
   d. Results of biliary scintigraphic scans can be false-
      positive in patients who are fasting, in patients who
      have received long-term total parenteral nutrition,
      and in patients who have chronic cholecystitis.

10. Characteristics of black pigment stones, in contrast to
    brown pigment stones, include all of the following
    except:

   a. prevalent in both western and Asian populations
   b. bacterial infection in bile
   c. recurrent stones are uncommon
   d. most stones are radiopaque

11. Concerning the sphincter of Oddi, all of the following
    statements are true except:

   a. The resting pressure of the sphincter is approxi-
      mately 13 mm Hg above duodenal pressure.
   b. The regulation of bile flow is primarily controlled
      by the sphincter.
   c. Parasympathetic stimulation induces increased
      sphincter tone.
   d. Stimulation with cholecystokinin induces sphincter
      relaxation.

12. The typical pattern of strictures, beading, and dilation
    of intrahepatic and extrahepatic portions of the biliary
    tree as seen on cholangiography with sclerosing
    cholangitis can be seen with all of the following except:

   a. cholangiocarcinoma
   b. trauma to the biliary tree
   c. prior irradiation of the liver
   d. cytomegalovirus cholangitis
   e. prior intraarterial chemotherapy directed at the
      liver

13. A 65-year-old man presents with a history of epigastric
    pain and progressive weight loss over the past 4 months.
    The pain is constant and interferes with sleep. He also
    reports the onset of jaundice and clay-colored stools
    about 1 month ago. The physical examination is no-
    table for jaundice and palpable epigastric fullness.
    Laboratory evaluation disclosed the following data: a
    total bilirubin level of 17 mg/dL, an aspartate amino-
    transferase level of 80 U/L, an alanine aminotransferase
    level of 75 U/L, and an alkaline phosphatase level of
    400 U/L. Considering the most likely diagnosis, which
    of the following statements is most accurate?

   a. Stent placement into the common bile duct will
      significantly reduce the risk of ascending cholangi-
      tis and improve survival.
   b. Stent placement into the common bile duct is effi-
      cacious in the management of pruritus and in
      relieving jaundice.
   c. Biliary drainage will improve the associated abnor-
      malities of gastric emptying.
   d. Stent placement into the pancreatic duct will assist
      in pain control.

14. Which feature characterizes the most common type of
    choledochal cyst?

   a. dilation of the common bile duct without hepatic
      duct involvement
   b. true diverticula of the common bile duct

c. dilation of the distal intraduodenal segment of the common bile duct

d. multiple extra- and intrahepatic cysts

e. intrahepatic cysts only

15. All of the following statements regarding choledochal cysts are true except:

a. They increase the risk of adenocarcinoma of the bile duct.

b. The preferred treatment involves surgery.

c. They are more common in women.

d. They result from distal common bile duct obstruction secondary to choledocholithiasis.

e. There is an increased incidence in Asians.

16. A 49-year-old man underwent open cholecystectomy for symptomatic gallstones. An intraoperative cholangiogram suggested two common bile duct (CBD) stones; these were removed after exploration of the CBD. His recovery was uneventful and he returned several weeks later for a T-tube cholangiogram in preparation for removal of the T tube. Although the patient was asymptomatic, an 8-mm stone was identified in the CBD during cholangiography. What would be the best course of action?

a. repeat laparotomy and CBD exploration to remove the stone

b. endoscopic retrograde cholangiopancreatography with sphincterotomy and stone extraction

c. stone extraction through the T tube

d. remove the T tube as planned and because he is asymptomatic, no further intervention is recommended

17. Which of the following statements is false?

a. A moderate rise in serum amylase is rare following diagnostic endoscopic retrograde cholangiopancreatography (ERCP) and indicates the presence of a complication.

b. Acute pancreatitis following ERCP may occur even when the pancreatic duct has not been cannulated.

c. Addition of sphincter of Oddi manometry to diagnostic ERCP increases the incidence of post-ERCP pancreatitis.

d. ERCP in patients with known pancreatic pseudocysts can be dangerous and should be coordinated with either a surgical or endoscopic drainage procedure in the event of complications.

18. True statements regarding primary sclerosing cholangitis (PSC) in patients with ulcerative colitis include all of the following except:

a. Proctocolectomy will not reverse the course of PSC.

b. Proctocolectomy prevents the development of bile duct cancer.

c. Endoscopic retrograde cholangiopancreatography cannot exclude underlying cholangiocarcinoma in this patient.

d. The patient should be referred for consideration of liver transplantation.

19. The most common complication of diagnostic endoscopic retrograde cholangiopancreatography is:

a. cholangitis

b. pancreatitis

c. bleeding

d. perforation

e. none of the above

20. Increased risks for the development of pancreatitis after endoscopic retrograde cholangiopancreatography (ERCP) include all of the following except:

a. overfilling of the pancreatic duct resulting in acinarization

b. repeated attempts at cannulation

c. repeated pancreatic duct injections

d. performing sphincter of Oddi manometry

e. a history of ERCP-induced pancreatitis

21. The most common cause of a benign bile duct stricture is:

a. surgical injury

b. recurrent pancreatitis

c. choledocholithiasis

d. recurrent cholangitis

e. primary sclerosing cholangitis

22. Which of the following findings is the best predictor of pain relief after endoscopic sphincterotomy in patients with suspected sphincter of Oddi dysfunction?

a. a dilated common bile duct on endoscopic retrograde cholangiopancreatography (ERCP)

b. delayed drainage of contrast after filling the biliary system during ERCP

c. an elevated sphincter of Oddi basal pressure during manometry

d. the presence of a juxtapapillary diverticulum

23. In patients with sphincter of Oddi dysfunction, all of the following findings can be observed except:

a. transient elevations in liver chemistries

b. a dilated common bile duct

c. rapid biliary drainage during endoscopic retrograde cholangiopancreatography

d. increased sphincter of Oddi basal pressure during manometry

24. A 50-year-old woman is referred for evaluation of an asymptomatic elevation of her serum alkaline phosphatase level. Additional laboratory data reveal detectable titers of antimitochondrial antibody and an elevated serum IgM level. Other associated medical problems may include each of the following except:

    a. thyroiditis
    b. renal tubular acidosis
    c. Sjögren syndrome
    d. diabetes mellitus

The following case pertains to questions 25 and 26.

A 67-year-old man presents with a 2-month history of progressive weight loss, decreased appetite, jaundice, and a 2-week history of acholic stools. The patient denies having abdominal pain. Physical examination reveals a soft, palpable mass in the right upper quadrant of the abdomen. Laboratory studies disclose the following values:

    total bilirubin: 7.0 mg/dL (normal, 0.0–0.9 mg/dL)
    alkaline phosphatase: 738 U/L
    aspartate aminotransferase: 34 U/L
    alanine aminotransferase: 42 U/L
    total protein: 6.0 g/dL
    albumin: 3.2 g/dL (normal, 3.5–5.0 g/dL)
    hemoglobin: 13.2 g/dL (normal, 14–18 g/dL)
    leukocyte count: 7000/mm³
    platelets: 237,000/mm³
    electrolytes: normal
    creatinine: 1.0 mg/dL (normal, 1.4 mg/dL)
    blood urea nitrogen: 8 mg/dL (normal, 8–20 mg/dL)
    chest and abdominal radiographs: normal

25. What is the most likely diagnosis?

    a. chronic pancreatitis with stricture
    b. enlarged gallbladder as a result of a tumor of the pancreas or bile duct
    c. cholelithiasis
    d. choledocholithiasis

26. What is the best initial diagnostic imaging technique?

    a. endoscopic retrograde cholangiopancreatography
    b. endoscopic ultrasonography
    c. abdominal ultrasonography
    d. abdominal computed tomography scan

27. Each of the following conditions can result in unconjugated hyperbilirubinemia except:

    a. massive hemolysis
    b. Gilbert syndrome
    c. Crigler-Najjar syndrome type I
    d. Rotor syndrome
    e. hereditary spherocytosis

28. All but one of the following characteristics predict successful dissolution of gallstones:

    a. smaller than 1.5-cm diameter
    b. large surface area in relation to mass
    c. pigment stones
    d. mobile and buoyant gallstones

29. All of the following characteristics of oriental cholangiohepatitis are true except:

    a. occurs mainly in persons older than 50 years
    b. equal prevalence in males and females
    c. commonly recurs after therapy
    d. typically not associated with cholelithiasis
    e. higher incidence in malnourished persons

30. All except one of the following conditions may be associated with primary sclerosing cholangitis:

    a. ulcerative colitis
    b. acquired immunodeficiency syndrome
    c. recurrent pancreatitis
    d. hepatitis B

31. A 32-year-old graduate student presents with fever, chills, right upper quadrant abdominal pain, and a 1-day history of jaundice. He is originally from Taiwan, where he experienced similar symptoms 4 years ago and was treated by cholecystectomy. Physical examination reveals a thin man with a temperature of 39.7°C, scleral icterus, and a positive Murphy sign. Laboratory studies disclose the following values:

    total bilirubin: 4.3 mg/dL
    alkaline phosphatase: 270 U/L
    aspartate aminotransferase: 63 U/L
    alanine aminotransferase: 58 U/L
    albumin: 2.6 g/dL
    total protein: 5.2 g/dL
    leukocyte count: 18,000/mm³
    hemoglobin: 12.1 g/dL
    mean erythrocyte volume: 75.0 (normal, 80–100)

Each of the following statements is true except:

a. Initial management includes intravenous fluid and correction of electrolyte abnormalities, administration of broad-spectrum antibiotics, and surgical evaluation.
b. The hypoalbuminemia may be the result of malnutrition; it may also be secondary to cirrhosis.
c. The most likely diagnosis is oriental cholangiohepatitis.
d. A stool examination may reveal *Clonorchis sinensis* and *Ascaris lumbricoides* ova.
e. The prognosis is excellent if the initial management is successful.

32. A 52-year-old immigrant from Thailand presents with abdominal pain, mild hepatomegaly, diarrhea, and icterus. The presence of which one of the following parasites would be most consistent with this presentation?

    a. *Clonorchis sinensis*
    b. *Diphyllobothrium latum*
    c. *Taenia saginata*
    d. *Enterobius vermicularis*

33. Statements pertaining to human infection with liver flukes include each of the following except:

    a. Adult flukes reside in the lumen of the human gastrointestinal tract.
    b. Fluke lifespans of 10 to 30 years are common.
    c. Bile duct strictures and fibrosis frequently occur.
    d. Ingestion of watercress is associated with human infection.

34. What percentage of cases of acute cholecystitis are associated with cholelithiasis?

    a. 10%
    b. 50%
    c. 75%
    d. 90%

35. Hepatobiliary scintigraphy is useful to evaluate which of the following conditions?

    a. infants with suspected biliary atresia
    b. acute cholecystitis
    c. postoperative bile duct injury
    d. gallbladder ejection fraction
    e. all of the above

36. All of the following clinical situations have been associated with gallbladder stasis except:

    a. pregnancy
    b. diabetes
    c. prior vagotomy
    d. prolonged total parenteral nutrition
    e. high-fat diet

37. All but one of the following have been demonstrated as benefits of laparoscopic cholecystectomy compared with open cholecystectomy:

    a. fewer complications
    b. fewer bile duct injuries
    c. shorter hospital stays
    d. more rapid return to normal activities
    e. minimal use of postoperative analgesia

38. Risk factors for the development of gallbladder carcinoma include all of the following except:

    a. porcelain gallbladder
    b. *Salmonella typhi*

c. alcoholism
d. chronic cholelithiasis (i.e., lasting longer than 40 years)

39. The following forms of biliary disease are associated with AIDS except:

    a. intrahepatic biliary cysts
    b. papillary stenosis
    c. sclerosing cholangitis
    d. combined papillary stenosis with sclerosing cholangitis
    e. long extrahepatic biliary strictures

40. The following are typical features of AIDS-associated cholangiopathy except:

    a. abdominal pain
    b. fever
    c. elevations of total bilirubin (>5 mg/dL)
    d. marked elevations of alkaline phosphatase (>500 U/L)

41. Which of the following statements concerning gallbladder cancer is false?

    a. Metastasis occurs early; more than 50% of patients have lymph node involvement at the time of diagnosis.
    b. Less than 10% of patients with liver metastases have cancer confined to the gallbladder wall.
    c. Jaundice develops in 30% to 60% of patients as a result of obstruction of the extrahepatic ducts.
    d. Jaundice is a favorable prognostic sign, because more than 50% of these patients will be diagnosed earlier in the course of the disease, allowing resection of the tumor.

42. Hepatic conditions associated with AIDS include each of the following except:

    a. granulomatous hepatitis
    b. an illness similar to primary biliary cirrhosis
    c. microvesicular or macrovesicular hepatosteatosis
    d. nodular regenerative hyperplasia

43. The pathogenesis of AIDS-associated cholangiopathy may be related to infection with:

    a. cytomegalovirus
    b. *Cryptosporidium* species
    c. *Enterocytozoon bieneusi*
    d. *Septata intestinalis*
    e. all of the above

44. Conditions associated with bile duct cancer include all of the following except:

    a. primary sclerosing cholangitis
    b. Caroli disease

c. infection with a liver fluke

d. cirrhosis

e. choledochal cysts

45. Which of the following statements concerning bile duct cancer is true?

 a. Preoperative biliary drainage decreases infectious complications prior to resection or diversion.

 b. The location of the tumor is the single most important determinant of resectability; 60% to 70% of tumors in the distal two-thirds of the bile duct are resectable for cure.

 c. Chemotherapy is effective in reducing tumor size and jaundice.

 d. Although resection offers symptomatic and biochemical relief in some patients, the overall mortality rate remains unchanged.

46. All of the following organisms are commonly associated with cholangitis except:

 a. *Klebsiella* species

 b. *Pseudomonas* species

 c. *Enterococcus* species

 d. *Streptococcus pneumoniae*

 e. *Escherichia coli*

47. All of the following statements regarding percutaneous transhepatic cholangiography (PTC) are true except:

 a. A known allergy to iodinated contrast agents is a concern because the contrast agent may enter the vascular space during this procedure.

 b. The success rate of PTC is higher if ductal systems are dilated rather than nondilated.

 c. The effectiveness of PTC drainage for obstructive pancreatic adenocarcinoma is equal to surgical drainage.

 d. PTC is a more effective drainage technique than endoscopic retrograde cholangiopancreatography in patients with obstructive jaundice.

48. Laboratory evaluations of persons with primary sclerosing cholangitis disclose all of the following findings except:

 a. antimitochondrial antibody (AMA)

 b. alkaline phosphatase elevation

 c. increased levels of circulating immune complexes

 d. perinuclear antineutrophilic cytoplasmic antibody (pANCA)

49. All of the following statements regarding laparoscopic cholecystectomy complications are true except:

 a. Bile duct injuries are usually recognized within the first week after surgery.

 b. Duct injury requires either endoscopic stenting or urgent exploratory laparotomy and repair.

 c. Nausea on the first postoperative day is an indication for emergent biliary scintigraphic scanning.

 d. Ileus is rarely seen on the second postoperative day unless there is a complication.

The following case pertains to questions 50 and 51.

A previously healthy 9-year-old girl presents with jaundice and abdominal pain. She reports feeling well until 4 weeks earlier when abdominal pain developed in the right upper quadrant. Since that time, the development of jaundice has been progressive, without fever or chills. The girl has had no exposure to other children with similar complaints, and she has taken no medication. Abdominal examination is notable for a firm, nontender mass in the right upper quadrant. Laboratory studies disclose the following values:

total bilirubin: 5.2 mg/dL (normal, 0–0.9 mg/dL)
alkaline phosphatase: 447 U/L
aspartate aminotransferase: 35 U/L
alanine aminotransferase: 47 U/L
complete blood count: normal

50. Appropriate diagnostic tests may include any of the following except:

 a. endoscopic retrograde cholangiopancreatography

 b. abdominal ultrasonography

 c. hepatobiliary scintigraphy

 d. abdominal computed tomography scan

 e. oral cholecystography

51. The treatment of choice for the majority of patients with this disorder is:

 a. endoscopic retrograde cholangiopancreatography

 b. surgery

 c. percutaneous transhepatic drainage

 d. steroids

52. The following statistics reflect the natural history of gallstones except:

 a. The rate of new-onset biliary colic is 15% to 25% after 10 years.

 b. Once biliary symptoms occur, the rate of recurrence is 60% to 70%.

 c. Less than 50% of complications such as cholecystitis, cholangitis, or pancreatitis are preceded by attacks of pain.

 d. Gangrene or perforation of the gallbladder occurs in about 10% of cases of acute cholecystitis.

53. Which therapy for primary sclerosing cholangitis has been proven to improve survival?

 a. oral bile acids

b. proctocolectomy
c. colchicine
d. liver transplantation
e. all of the above

TRUE/FALSE

54. _____ Biliary sludge is a universal finding in patients on chronic (6 weeks) total parenteral nutrition.

55. _____ Elevation of serum bile acids in cirrhosis most likely results from a defect at the level of the sinusoidal bile acid transport protein.

56. _____ The mechanism for impaired gallbladder emptying observed in patients with celiac sprue is a reversible reduction in cholecystokinin release from the involved intestinal mucosa.

57. _____ Low serum alkaline phosphatase levels are associated with the acute hemolytic anemia that complicates Wilson disease.

58. _____ Fatty infiltration is the most common finding on liver biopsy specimens in patients with asymptomatic mild elevations in serum aminotransferase levels.

59. _____ Prolongation of the prothrombin time is a frequently observed liver function abnormality in patients with congestive heart failure.

60. _____ Hepatocellular injury can be differentiated from cholestatic causes of prothrombin time prolongation on the basis of the response to a parenteral administration of vitamin K.

61. _____ Native Americans have a higher risk of developing symptomatic gallstone disease than the rest of the population of the United States.

62. _____ At the time of cholecystectomy, a concomitant common bile duct stone is discovered in approximately 15% of cases.

63. _____ Spontaneous biliary-enteric fistulas are most commonly produced by gallstones.

64. _____ Most primary common bile duct stones in the western hemisphere are cholesterol stones.

65. _____ Most common bile duct stones in the western hemisphere consist mainly of calcium bilirubinate.

66. _____ Gallstone disease is the most common cause of hemobilia in young men.

67. _____ Typical biliary pain localizes to the right upper quadrant with intermittent episodes lasting 15 to 20 minutes.

68. _____ In acute common bile duct obstruction, elevations in alanine aminotransferase and aspartate aminotransferase levels can sometimes approach the levels observed in patients with acute hepatitis, and then rapidly return to normal upon resolution of the obstruction.

69. _____ The complication rate associated with the use of endoscopic retrograde cholangiopancreatography to evaluate sphincter of Oddi function is 20%.

70. _____ The breakdown of hemoglobin accounts for approximately 80% of the bilirubin in humans.

71. _____ Nonionic and lower osmolality contrast media decrease complications associated with endoscopic retrograde cholangiopancreatography.

72. _____ Early endoscopic retrograde cholangiopancreatography clearly provides a survival benefit in patients with gallstone pancreatitis, even in the absence of biliary obstruction.

MATCHING

(each selection may be used once, more than once, or not at all)

Match the following structures to the correct statement regarding endoscopic retrograde cholangiopancreatography:

73. _____ left hepatic ducts

74. _____ right hepatic ducts

a. may require head-down positioning

b. best images obtained in supine position after endoscope removal

75. _____ gallbladder

76. _____ pancreatic ducts

77. _____ biliary tree

c. the prone position is preferred for filling

d. half-strength contrast agent (e.g., meglumine diatriazoate 25% to 30%) recommended

e. full-strength contrast agent (e.g., meglumine diatriazoate 50% to 60%) recommended

Match the following laboratory studies with the correct finding:

78. _____ alkaline phosphatase

79. _____ γ-glutamyl transpeptidase

80. _____ aspartate aminotransferase

81. _____ ceruloplasmin

a. increased by chronic alcohol consumption

b. increased in pregnancy

c. decreased in severe malnutrition

d. falsely low in uremia

Match each of the following characteristics with the correct type of common bile duct stone:

82. _____ frequent bacterial infection in bile

83. _____ stone composition mostly calcium bilirubinate

84. _____ generally discovered within 2 years of cholecystectomy

85. _____ associated with biliary strictures

a. primary duct stone

b. secondary duct stone

Match the following diseases with the correct laboratory values:

86. _____ brucellosis

87. _____ acetaminophen hepatotoxicity

88. _____ Wilson disease

89. _____ hemochromatosis

aspartate aminotransferase (AST; normal, 35 U/L)
alanine aminotransferase (ALT; normal, 45 U/L)
alkaline phosphatase (AP; normal, 130 U/L)
ferritin (normal, 8–200 ng/mL)
ceruloplasmin (normal, 20–40 mg/dL)

	AST	ALT	AP	ferritin	ceruloplasmin
a.	1390	1602	130	450	35
b.	420	513	45	450	12
c.	245	258	130	5400	35
d.	82	46	986	150	35

Match the following biliary disorders with the correct treatment:

90. _____ biliary stricture secondary to chronic pancreatitis

91. _____ symptomatic AIDS-related papillary stenosis

92. _____ biliary fistula secondary to laparoscopic cholecystectomy injury

93. _____ sump syndrome

a. endoscopic sphincterotomy

b. endoscopic stent

c. either (a) or (b)

Match the following descriptors with the appropriate diagnostic criteria:

94. _____ sphincter of Oddi dysfunction

95. _____ sphincter of Oddi dysfunction, intact gallbladder

96. _____ type I (i.e., definite) sphincter of Oddi dysfunction

97. _____ type II (i.e., probable) sphincter of Oddi dysfunction

98. _____ type III (i.e., possible) sphincter of Oddi dysfunction

a. manometry not necessary, but when performed, results are normal in 14% to 35% of patients

b. biliary-type pain with normal results on liver function tests, nondilated common bile duct, and drainage of contrast agent in less than 45 minutes

c. as demonstrated in a prospective controlled study, elevated basal sphincter pressure is predictive of a good outcome to sphincterotomy

d. impeded transsphincteric bile flow as a result of anatomic stenosis or a motility disorder

e. may overlap with gallbladder microlithiasis or dyskinesia

Match the following associations with the appropriate stone types:

99. _____ associated with hemolytic anemias

100. _____ most commonly seen secondary to infection

101. _____ increased incidence in Asia

102. _____ recurrent stones commonly seen

a. black pigment stones

b. brown pigment stones

c. both

d. neither

7

Abdominal Cavity/Miscellaneous

MULTIPLE CHOICE

(one best answer)

1. Diarrhea is a common complaint in patients with AIDS. Which of the following statements about diarrhea associated with AIDS is not true?

   a. A potential pathogen is more likely to be identified in a patient with weight loss and a CD4 count of fewer than 100 cells/mm, than in a patient with no weight loss and a CD4 count of 500 cells/mm.
   b. A specific pathogen is identified in 50% to 85% of AIDS patients with diarrhea.
   c. *Cryptosporidium parvum* and *Isospora belli* are more common in AIDS patients living in developed countries than in AIDS patients living in developing countries.
   d. Diagnostic evaluation of diarrhea in AIDS patients should begin with a stool culture for *Salmonella, Shigella*, and *Campylobacter* species. If microscopy does not reveal a potential pathogen, an endoscopic examination with biopsy should be performed.

2. A 45-year-old man is referred for an opinion regarding the following liver chemistries:

   aspartate aminotransferase: 265 U/L (normal, 35 U/L)
   alanine aminotransferase: 62 U/L (normal, 45 U/L)
   alkaline phosphatase: 130 U/L (normal, 130 U/L)
   total bilirubin: 5.5 mg/dL (normal, 0.9 mg/dL)

   This pattern of values is most compatible with which of the following hepatitic illnesses?

   a. acute viral hepatitis
   b. alcoholic hepatitis
   c. drug-induced hepatitis
   d. ischemic hepatitis

3. A 28-year-old man undergoes bone marrow transplantation for acute leukemia. He presents 1 year later with odynophagia. The most likely manifestations of chronic graft-versus-host disease in the esophagus include:

   a. desquamation and inflammation of the distal esophagus
   b. biopsy specimens showing an inflammatory infiltrate with no apoptotic figures
   c. observations made on the biopsy specimens are similar to those seen with scleroderma; there is no submucosal fibrosis
   d. endoscopy shows generalized desquamation of the upper and mid esophagus with weblike fibrous bands
   e. all of the above

4. Which of the following statements regarding high-output gastrointestinal fistulas is most accurate?

   a. They are defined by fluid losses greater than 500 mL/day.
   b. They are associated with metabolic alkalosis when they involve the duodenum.
   c. They are associated with a high incidence of spontaneous closure.
   d. They never result in clinically significant dehydration.

5. In cases of peritonitis complicating peritoneal dialysis, each of the following statements is true except:

   a. Gram-positive organisms are the most common causes.
   b. Most patients have abdominal pain or tenderness.
   c. Dialysis catheters must be removed in most cases.
   d. Vancomycin is a reasonable choice for empiric therapy while awaiting results of cultures and sensitivity tests.

6. A 52-year-old man is referred because of abdominal swelling. He has a tattoo, and gives a history of drinking six cans of beer per night—more on the weekends—for the past 25 years. He works in an office and his hobby is bowling. His physical examination is remarkable for moderate ascites and two small spider angiomas on the face. Laboratory stud-

ies disclose the following values: serum bilirubin, 1.0 mg/dL; aspartate aminotransferase, alanine aminotransferase, and alkaline phosphatase levels between 1 and 2 times the upper limit of normal; serum albumin, 3.3 g/dL; and total protein, 6.8 g/dL. To deal with his ascites, which of the following options would you not select?

a. diagnostic paracentesis
b. ascitic fluid white blood cell count and differential
c. ascitic fluid albumin level
d. ascitic fluid lactate dehydrogenase and bilirubin levels

7. Each of the following autoimmune diseases exhibits associated gastrointestinal manifestations except:

a. systemic lupus erythematosus
b. Graves disease
c. psoriasis
d. rheumatoid arthritis
e. Addison disease (i.e., hypoadrenalism)

8. Down syndrome is associated with each of the following conditions except:

a. gastroesophageal reflux
b. duodenal stenosis
c. Crohn's disease
d. Hirschsprung disease

9. Each of the following statements regarding porphyria is true except:

a. The acute porphyrias share an autosomal dominant inheritance pattern.
b. Abdominal pain is a prominent complaint of patients with acute intermittent porphyria, variegate porphyria, and hereditary coproporphyria.
c. Acute intermittent porphyria is associated with skin lesions.
d. Increased coproporphyrin levels in the urine and feces are detected in hereditary coproporphyria.
e. Abnormalities are often seen on liver biopsy specimens from patients with porphyria cutanea tarda and protoporphyria.

10. Each of the following diseases may be associated with the observation of granulomas on liver biopsy specimens except:

a. sarcoidosis
b. polyarteritis nodosa
c. arsenic poisoning
d. Crohn's disease
e. cytomegalovirus

11. A 24-year-old woman in her third trimester of pregnancy presents with thrombocytopenia, hemolysis, an aspartate aminotransferase level of 120 U/L, and an alkaline phosphatase level of 135 U/L. What diagnosis do these features suggest?

a. fulminant liver failure
b. acute fatty liver of pregnancy
c. hemolytic uremic syndrome
d. thrombotic thrombocytopenic purpura
e. HELLP syndrome

12. True statements about systemic amyloidosis include each of the following except:

a. Amyloidosis is a common complication of multiple myeloma.
b. The diagnosis can be established by deep rectal biopsy in 80% of cases.
c. Esophageal involvement occurs in two-thirds of patients.
d. Hepatic infiltration can result in fulminant liver failure.
e. Ascites can result from hypoproteinemia induced by the nephrotic syndrome.

13. Which of the following statements about drug metabolism in the intestine is most accurate?

a. Metabolites generated within enterocytes and excreted into the intestinal lumen may not be subsequently absorbed.
b. The extent of drug metabolism occurring at the level of the intestine has probably been overestimated.
c. Only phase I enzymes are involved in drug metabolism by intestinal enterocytes.
d. Most drug metabolism appears to occur in the intestinal crypt cells rather than in cells at the villus tip.

14. Each of the following statements regarding the etiology of nonmalignant ascites is true except:

a. In most cases, the ascites largely results from fluid weeping from the liver, not from the portal venous bed.
b. Portal vein thrombosis alone usually does not result in the development of clinically significant ascites.
c. Urinary secretion of sodium over a 24-hour period is typically less than 10 mEq.
d. Chylous ascites often develops with fulminant hepatic failure.

15. Each of the following statements concerning malignant ascites is true except:

a. Peritoneal carcinomatosis is a relatively infrequent cause of malignant ascites.

b. In patients with intraabdominal lymphoma or ovarian cancer, malignant ascites may respond to surgical or medical treatment of the primary tumors.

c. In peritoneal carcinomatosis, ascites appears to result from the secretion of fluid and protein by malignant cells.

d. The formation of ascites in patients with advanced liver metastases may be the result of portal hypertension.

16. The serum-ascites albumin concentration gradient:

a. is calculated by dividing the difference between the serum albumin and the ascitic albumin by the volume of fluid removed

b. is calculated by dividing the difference between the serum albumin and the ascitic albumin by the total blood volume

c. will generally discriminate between alcoholic and nonalcoholic chronic liver disease

d. will generally discriminate between ascites due to liver disease and ascites from other causes

17. Each of the following statements regarding spontaneous bacterial peritonitis (SBP) is correct except:

a. Patients with ascites as a result of heart failure rarely develop SBP.

b. SBP most likely results from microperforation of the colon with direct contamination of the ascitic fluid.

c. Patients with malignant ascites resulting from peritoneal carcinomatosis rarely develop SBP.

d. SBP usually results from infection with a single organism.

The following case pertains to questions 18 through 21.

A 50-year-old man presents with complaints of weight gain and abdominal swelling. He has been drinking twelve cans of beer per day for many years, but denies having any other risk factors for liver disease. His physical examination is normal with the exception of shifting dullness. Except for mildly elevated aminotransferase levels, the results of his laboratory studies are normal, including a serum albumin level of 3.6 g/dL. Analysis of ascitic fluid from a diagnostic paracentesis reveals a neutrophil count of 50/mm^3 and an albumin level of 1.8 g/dL.

18. The least likely diagnosis is:

a. cirrhosis of the liver
b. peritoneal carcinomatosis
c. constrictive pericarditis
d. portal vein thrombosis

19. After an appropriate clinical evaluation, a diagnosis is made. Which of the following treatment programs would you institute as a first approach?

a. salt and fluid restriction
b. salt restriction plus oral spironolactone administration
c. salt restriction plus oral furosemide administration
d. salt restriction plus intravenous furosemide followed by oral bumetanide administration
e. salt restriction plus repeated paracentesis

The patient is sent home and does well on the recommended therapy. Six months later, he presents at the emergency department complaining of a distended abdomen, jaundice, and malaise. The emergency department physician reports that the patient appears clinically well, with the exception of moderate ascites, and is afebrile with normal vital signs. Laboratory studies disclose a normal complete blood count, normal electrolyte levels, and a serum ethanol level of 0. His aminotransferase levels are mildly elevated but are essentially unchanged from those recorded at his initial visit to the clinic 6 months earlier. His bilirubin is elevated, measuring 3.2 mg/dL.

20. Which of the following steps is most appropriate?

a. Send the patient home with a program of salt restriction and more diuretics.

b. Perform a diagnostic paracentesis to measure the ascitic fluid albumin level.

c. Perform a diagnostic paracentesis to measure the total leukocyte count and differential, and send the ascitic fluid for culture and sensitivity tests.

d. Perform a diagnostic paracentesis for the measurement of pH, lactate, and glucose levels.

e. Perform a therapeutic paracentesis.

21. The patient is examined and treated appropriately. He returns to the emergency department 6 months later with tense ascites, loss of muscle mass, hyponatremia, mild leukocytosis, and mild abdominal tenderness. His peritoneal neutrophil count is 1000/mm^3. Which of the following statements is most correct?

a. He should receive treatment with ampicillin and gentamicin.

b. He should receive treatment with a third-generation cephalosporin.

c. He should receive treatment with oral norfloxacin.

d. He is good candidate for a Denver shunt.

e. He may require repeated paracentesis as an outpatient.

22. A 65-year-old man comes into your clinic complaining of dysphagia to both liquid and solid food. He reports a high incidence of esophageal cancer in his family. Physical examination reveals thickening of

the skin on the palms and soles of the hands and feet. The presentation suggests:

a. Sweet syndrome
b. psoriasis
c. neurofibromatosis
d. tylosis
e. acromegaly

23. All of the following statements regarding peritonitis are true except:

a. Secondary peritonitis is more common than primary peritonitis.
b. Spontaneous bacterial peritonitis is more common in men than in women.
c. Gram-negative enteric bacteria account for the majority of organisms in ascitic fluid cultures from patients with spontaneous bacterial peritonitis.
d. The mortality from peritonitis has been greatly reduced as the result of medical advances.
e. Gram-negative enteric bacteria account for approximately 25% of all cases of peritonitis associated with chronic ambulatory peritoneal dialysis.

24. Each of the following statements regarding the ascitic fluid leukocyte count is correct except:

a. As a patient undergoes diuresis, the total leukocyte count in ascitic fluid may rise significantly.
b. As a patient undergoes diuresis, the neutrophil count in ascitic fluid may rise significantly.
c. A neutrophil count greater than 250/mm^3 in ascitic fluid strongly suggests peritonitis.
d. In a traumatic paracentesis, the ratio of neutrophils to red blood cells should not exceed 1:250 in uninfected ascitic fluid.

25. You are asked to examine a 24-year-old white-haired, pale, pink-eyed patient of Puerto Rican descent, who complains of recurrent episodes of gastrointestinal bleeding and shortness of breath. A careful history reveals that the patient has other family members with similar symptoms and appearance. The presentation suggests which familial disease?

a. Hermansky-Pudlak syndrome
b. neurofibromatosis type I
c. Peutz-Jeghers syndrome
d. blue rubber bleb nevus syndrome
e. none of the above

26. True statements regarding retractile mesenteritis include each of the following except:

a. Retractile mesenteritis occurs in late adulthood.
b. It is often associated with malignant infiltration of the mesentery.
c. Abdominal pain occurs in one-half of the patients.

d. Laparotomy with biopsy is required to confirm the diagnosis.
e. It can be associated with episodic fevers.

27. The following statements regarding familial Mediterranean fever are true except:

a. It is an autosomal recessive disorder.
b. It has a geographic distribution, but is not more common in any specific ethnic group.
c. It is characterized by recurrent serositis.
d. It is characterized by recurrent painful febrile episodes.
e. It may result in the development of amyloid nephropathy.

28. An 8-year-old girl who recently immigrated from a developing country is brought to your office by her mother. During defecation, the girl occasionally notes moist tissue protruding from the rectum. She is able to reduce this easily with her hand, but is quite embarrassed by it. Examination of the mucosal surface of the rectum reveals white threads. The physical examination suggests:

a. infection caused by *Trichuris trichiura*
b. ascariasis
c. infection caused by a hookworm
d. infection caused by *Schistosoma mansoni*
e. clonorchiasis

29. Each of the following may be a cause of granulomatous peritonitis except:

a. Crohn's disease
b. tuberculosis
c. parasitic infection
d. cellulose fibers
e. talc

30. True statements regarding retroperitoneal fibrosis include each of the following except:

a. Retroperitoneal fibrosis originates in the area of the renal hilus.
b. It may be secondary to an allergic reaction to insoluble lipids.
c. It may be induced by serotonin production from carcinoid tumors.
d. It typically affects middle-aged men.
e. Abdominal or back pain is the most frequent presenting symptom.

31. You are consulted about a patient with recurrent massive upper gastrointestinal hemorrhage. Upper endoscopy has revealed no ulcers or varices. Which of the following statements is most correct?

a. The patient is more likely to be a man than a woman.

b. In 1% to 2% of patients presenting with massive upper gastrointestinal hemorrhage, a Dieulafoy lesion is identified as the source.

c. Endoscopic therapy is a reasonable initial treatment.

d. The lesion is more common in the proximal third of the stomach, especially around the lesser curvature and near the gastroesophageal junction.

e. Angiography rarely confirms the diagnosis.

f. Repeated endoscopic evaluation can be effective in establishing the diagnosis.

g. all of the above

32. A 39-year-old woman with a long-standing history of alcoholic liver disease and ascites presents with vague abdominal pain, vomiting, and bloody diarrhea. Abdominal radiographs, paracentesis, upper endoscopy, and colonoscopy are unremarkable. The patient subsequently develops a fever of 38.3°C and signs of frank peritonitis with a rising hematocrit and leukocyte count. Abdominal radiographs reveal a dilated, edematous intestine. Repeat paracentesis reveals foul-smelling fluid with gram-positive and gram-negative organisms. The most likely diagnosis is:

a. mesenteric arterial thrombosis

b. strangulation

c. mesenteric venous thrombosis

d. nonocclusive mesenteric ischemia

33. Which statement about intestinal ischemia is incorrect?

a. The majority of patients with intestinal ischemia are elderly and they have associated cardiovascular disease such as congestive heart failure or atrial fibrillation.

b. When mesenteric venous thrombosis is diagnosed in a young person, evaluation for an underlying hypercoagulable state should be initiated.

c. If there is strong evidence for small bowel ischemia, abdominal computed tomography and Doppler ultrasonography should be performed immediately. If these procedures do not reveal an occlusion, mesenteric arteriography should be performed.

d. In patients with severe vascular disease and no occlusive lesion, intraarterial vasodilators may be successful and may prevent surgical intervention.

34. Typical angiographic findings in patients with non-occlusive mesenteric ischemia include all of the following except:

a. slowing of the mesenteric arterial blood flow

b. narrowing at the origin of the superior mesenteric artery

c. decreased parenchymal staining with contrast agent

d. diffuse mesenteric arterial constriction

35. All of the following statements regarding splenic artery aneurysms are true except:

a. Splenic artery aneurysms account for 60% of visceral artery aneurysms.

b. They occur more commonly in women than in men.

c. They are often asymptomatic.

d. Pancreatitis is an etiologic factor.

e. They usually require surgical resection when detected.

36. Correct statements concerning splenic vein occlusion include all of the following except:

a. The incidence of gastric variceal bleeding is 11% to 65%.

b. Esophageal varices are a common finding.

c. Splenectomy is the treatment of choice.

d. Venous collaterals involve the short gastric coronary and the gastroepiploic veins.

37. A 60-year-old man is admitted with a gradual onset of right upper quadrant abdominal pain associated with increased liver enzymes and hepatomegaly, documented by physical examination. A radionuclide scan of the liver reveals inhomogeneous uptake in the liver with enhanced uptake in the caudate lobe. All of the following statements regarding this condition are true except:

a. Computed tomography often reveals diffusely hypodense hepatic parenchyma with preservation of a normal density in the caudate lobe.

b. Ultrasonography with color flow Doppler imaging is the preferred diagnostic study.

c. Portal vein occlusion is found in 10% to 20% of patients.

d. Venography often reveals a "spider-web" pattern.

38. A 32-year-old international health worker presents with a clinical history of upper abdominal discomfort, nervousness, vertigo, nausea, vomiting, diarrhea, and weight loss. As one step in an intensive workup, you order a small bowel follow-through, which reveals a 6-meter-long object in the intestinal lumen. You suspect an infection caused by:

a. *Giardia* species

b. *Taenia saginata*

c. *Echinococcus granulosus*

d. *Ascaris lumbricoides*

e. *Enterobius vermicularis*

39. Laboratory studies following paracentesis in a male patient disclosed a white cell count of 1500/mm³ and

a polymorphonuclear leukocyte count of 650/mm³. The patient has cirrhosis that was confirmed by the results of a biopsy. He is asymptomatic except for increased abdominal girth. When should treatment begin?

a. if the results of an ascitic fluid culture are positive for bacteria
b. if the white cell count in the ascitic fluid increases
c. if he becomes symptomatic
d. if he fails to respond to diuretic treatment
e. none of the above

40. Three months after abdominal aortic aneurysm repair, a 64-year-old man presents with one episode of hematemesis. Upper endoscopy, colonoscopy, and aortography all fail to disclose a source of bleeding. The most likely finding on abdominal computed tomography is:

a. identification of a fistula from the aorta to the third portion of the duodenum
b. a thickened loop of duodenum
c. identification of a fistula from the aorta to the jejunum
d. fluid collection at the site of the aortic graft
e. none of the above

41. A 45-year-old homeless man presents with a 6-month history of fever, anorexia, weakness, malaise, and weight loss, as well as abdominal distention secondary to fluid accumulation. You perform a diagnostic paracentesis. Laboratory studies disclose a high protein content (>3 g/dL) and a low glucose concentration (<30 mg/dL). What is your diagnosis?

a. aseptic peritonitis
b. acute bacterial peritonitis
c. end-stage liver disease
d. tuberculous peritonitis
e. none of the above

42. Computed tomography is the test of choice to confirm all of the following diagnoses except:

a. diverticulitis
b. pancreatic pseudocyst
c. recurrence of rectal cancer after abdominoperineal resection
d. small intestine involvement in Crohn's disease
e. intraabdominal abscess

43. A short, obese, 22-year-old woman with a webbed neck comes into your clinic complaining of recurrent gastrointestinal bleeding. Esophagogastroduodenoscopy and colonoscopy have not revealed the source. One likely lesion associated with this phenotype would be:

a. telangiectasia or vascular ectasia of the small bowel
b. chronic ischemia
c. Crohn's disease of the small bowel
d. peptic ulcer disease
e. opportunistic infection of the gastrointestinal tract

44. Which of the following statements about endoscopic ultrasonography imaging is most accurate?

a. Leiomyomas can be reliably distinguished from leiomyosarcomas.
b. Malignant lymph nodes usually have poorly defined margins.
c. Benign lymph nodes are usually hyperechoic.
d. The normal wall thickness of the gastrointestinal tract is 5 to 7 mm.

45. Indications for endoscopic ultrasonography include all of the following except:

a. a submucosal mass in the gastric antrum
b. hypoglycemic symptoms with an insulin-glucose ratio greater than 0.3
c. documented esophageal carcinoma with a normal thoracic computed tomographic scan
d. to differentiate Crohn's disease from ulcerative colitis

46. At the end of a 3-week course of radiation therapy directed at the chest wall, a patient presents with dysphagia and odynophagia. You suggest the most likely diagnosis is:

a. radiation-induced esophagitis
b. radiation-induced motility disorder
c. radiation-induced stricture
d. none of the above

47. Isolated splenic vein thrombosis is most commonly associated with:

a. portal hypertension
b. adenocarcinoma of the stomach
c. hemoglobinopathies
d. acute cholecystitis
e. adenocarcinoma of the pancreas

48. A child walks into your office, complaining of a skin rash, abdominal cramping, vomiting, diarrhea, and bloody urine. On physical examination, the rash is palpable and purpuric. The clinical presentation suggests:

a. giant cell arteritis
b. cryoglobulinemia
c. Wegener granulomatosis
d. polyarteritis nodosa
e. Henoch-Schönlein purpura

49. The following statements regarding common variable hypogammaglobulinemia are true except:

    a. Most patients have a defect in B lymphocyte differentiation.
    b. Patients generally present in the second or third decade of life with recurrent respiratory tract infections or diarrhea.
    c. Nodular lymphoid hyperplasia affects the small intestine in many cases.
    d. The condition is associated with multiple enteric pathogens, particularly *Entamoeba histolytica*.

50. A woman of eastern Mediterranean origin comes into your clinic with volumes of medical records. She states that since childhood she has suffered attacks of fevers, joint aches, abdominal pain, and pain with breathing. She reports that extensive and repeated diagnostic workups in the past, including a laparotomy, have not led to a diagnosis. She is seeking a prescription for Tylox. She is unable to convey a clear family history, as she is adopted. What action do you take?

    a. You diagnose familial Mediterranean fever and prescribe colchicine.
    b. You send her to the pain clinic because she has drug-seeking behavior without obvious organic pathology.
    c. You diagnose Anderson-Fabry syndrome because she has episodes of recurrent abdominal pain.
    d. You diagnose acute intermittent porphyria.
    e. none of the above

51. All of the following statements regarding mesenteric desmoid tumors are true except:

    a. Mesenteric desmoid tumors occur in association with Gardner syndrome.
    b. Desmoid tumors are locally invasive, nonmetastasizing, fibrous tissue masses.
    c. Desmoid tumors have been associated with estrogen therapy.
    d. Desmoid tumors appear as a contrast-enhancing mass on computed tomography.
    e. Mesenteric desmoid tumors can become infiltrative and lead to intestinal perforation.

52. True statements regarding umbilical hernias in infants include all of the following except:

    a. They are more common in African American infants.
    b. They should be surgically corrected before the age of 2 years.
    c. They are more common in male infants.
    d. Adhesive strapping is of no benefit.
    e. They are more common in premature infants.

53. In confirming a diagnosis of spontaneous bacterial peritonitis, the laboratory study of greatest value is:

    a. the total cell count
    b. the polymorphonuclear leukocyte count
    c. the total protein concentration
    d. the concentration of albumin
    e. conventional culture of ascitic fluid
    f. a gram stain of the fluid

54. A 30-year-old woman presents with complaints of recurrent, severe abdominal pain and a history of severe, frequent skin rashes that are often exacerbated by sun exposure. Physical examination reveals no focal abdominal tenderness but shows skin blistering on the extensor surfaces of both hands. Examination of her face and back shows hyperpigmentation and prominent facial hair. An appropriate initial evaluation includes:

    a. colonoscopy
    b. a 24-hour urine sample
    c. HLA typing, antinuclear antibody testing, and rheumatoid factor testing
    d. culture of stool samples for *Yersinia* species
    e. referral to the neurology department for nerve conduction studies

55. All of the following are common symptoms of acute graft-versus-host disease except:

    a. watery diarrhea
    b. skin rash
    c. jaundice
    d. arthritis

56. Each of the following is a common manifestation of acute graft-versus-host disease except:

    a. pancreatitis
    b. cholestasis
    c. diarrhea
    d. gastrointestinal bleeding

57. Each of the following is a common manifestation of chronic graft-versus-host disease except:

    a. cholestasis
    b. small bowel bacterial overgrowth
    c. typhlitis
    d. esophageal stricture

58. Which of the following statements about spontaneous bacterial peritonitis is correct?

    a. More than 10% of patients with spontaneous bacterial peritonitis have no clinical evidence of infection.
    b. The complication rate of abdominal paracentesis is about 5%.

c. Anaerobes rarely cause spontaneous bacterial peritonitis.
d. Patients with ascites due to causes other than cirrhosis may have an elevated polymorphonuclear leukocyte count.
e. All of the above statements are correct.

59. Which of the following antibiotic regimens is the most appropriate for spontaneous bacterial peritonitis when the offending organism has not been identified?

a. aminoglycosides
b. cefotaxime or another third-generation cephalosporin
c. penicillin
d. ampicillin
e. trimethoprim/sulfamethoxazole

60. Chronic graft-versus-host disease is best described by which of the following statements?

a. It most commonly affects persons who have no prior history of acute graft-versus-host disease.
b. It is not associated with mucositis.
c. It typically occurs within 10 weeks of bone marrow transplantation.
d. It has clinical features that resemble scleroderma (i.e., sicca syndrome).

61. A 45-year-old woman has had an aortic valve replacement that was complicated by significant blood loss requiring transfusion. She presents subsequent to the operation with a hoarse voice, complaining of both diarrhea and difficulty swallowing. Esophageal cineradiography reveals several esophageal webs. The patient is noted to have iron deficiency associated with blood-loss anemia. What is the likely diagnosis?

a. Plummer-Vinson-Kelly syndrome
b. achalasia
c. systemic amyloidosis
d. Schatzki ring
e. none of the above

62. Which one of the following therapies is a thermal contact method of tissue destruction?

a. Nd:YAG laser therapy
b. chemical injection
c. bipolar electrocoagulation
d. argon plasma coagulation

TRUE/FALSE

The following studies and procedures are helpful in the evaluation of ascitic fluid that appears milky or opalescent:

63. _____ triglyceride measurement

64. _____ cholesterol measurement

65. _____ refrigerate ascitic fluid for 48 to 72 hours

66. _____ alkaline phosphatase measurement

67. _____ The majority of patients with tuberculous peritonitis do not have radiographic evidence of pulmonary or gastrointestinal tuberculosis.

Visceral pain from the abdomen is characterized by the following features:

68. _____ The pain lateralizes in the direction of the involved organ.

69. _____ Pain originating from the jejunum or the ileum is perceived in the epigastrium.

70. _____ Perception of pain can be produced by distention or contraction of the visceral organs.

71. _____ Referred pain from the pancreas is most commonly perceived in the area of the right scapula.

72. _____ Rebound tenderness is a clinical manifestation of irritation or inflammation of the visceral peritoneum.

73. _____ The gastrointestinal manifestations of acute graft-versus-host disease usually present within 7 to 10 days following bone marrow transplantation.

Mesenteric ischemia is characterized by the following features:

74. _____ It is associated with pathognomonic laboratory findings.

75. _____ It can present with the sudden onset of symptoms, or symptoms can arise in a more insidious manner.

76. _____ It can occur as a result of an angiographic procedure.

77. _____ It can be effectively treated with intraarterial papaverine.

Endoscopic surveillance is recommended for each of the following clinical conditions:

78. _____ chronic gastritis with severe atrophy

79. _____ Barrett esophagus

80. _____ pernicious anemia

81. _____ adenomatous gastric polyps

The following statements relate to intraabdominal abscesses:

82. _____ Pelvic abscesses may cause tenesmus, diarrhea, or urine retention.

83. _____ Postoperatively, clinical signs of abscess typically manifest within 2 to 3 days.

84. _____ The likelihood of abscess formation increases in the presence of barium, feces, necrotic tissue, or hemoglobin.

85. _____ Most chronic intraabdominal abscesses are polymicrobial; anaerobes are cultured in more than 80% of cases.

MATCHING

(each selection may be used once, more than once, or not at all)

Match the following dermatologic findings with the correct gastrointestinal syndrome:

86. _____ scleroderma

87. _____ Behçet disease

88. _____ pyoderma gangrenosum

89. _____ acanthosis nigricans

90. _____ tylosis

91. _____ pseudoxanthoma elasticum

92. _____ hypertrichosis

93. _____ flushing

94. _____ necrolytic migratory erythema

a. pancreatic or colon cancer

b. glucagonoma

c. aphthous ulcers

d. esophageal squamous cell carcinoma

e. inflammatory bowel disease

f. recurrent abdominal adenocarcinoma

g. carcinoid syndrome

h. esophageal dysmotility

i. recurrent upper gastrointestinal hemorrhage

Match the following complications with the appropriate chemotherapeutic agents:

95. _____ mucosal necrosis, abdominal pain, and diarrhea

96. _____ peliosis hepatis

97. _____ hepatic venoocclusive disease

98. _____ dysphagia and colonic pseudoobstruction

a. androgens

b. high-dose cytarabine

c. *Vinca* alkaloids

d. chemotherapy and radiation prior to bone marrow transplantation

Match the clinical characteristic with the appropriate diagnosis:

99. _____ often associated with back pain

100. _____ requires emergent surgical treatment

101. _____ may be diagnosed using ultrasonography

102. _____ diagnosis may be confirmed by scintigraphy

a. ruptured abdominal aortic aneurysm

b. acute cholecystitis

c. both

d. neither

Match the following chronic pain syndromes with the appropriate gastrointestinal manifestations:

103. _____ familial Mediterranean fever

104. _____ hereditary angioneurotic edema

105. _____ Fabry disease

106. _____ hereditary pancreatitis

a. abdominal pain, marfanoid

b. abdominal pain, splenic vein thrombosis

c. abdominal pain, accumulation of lipoid material in numerous organs

d. abdominal pain, C1-esterase inhibitor deficiency

e. recurrent bouts of abdominal pain, chest pain, serositis

8

Nutrition

MULTIPLE CHOICE

(one best answer)

1. The Na$^+$,K$^+$-ATPase pump:

   a. establishes a high intracellular Na$^+$ concentration to drive transport
   b. is electroneutral
   c. is present in all intestinal epithelial cells
   d. is dependent on calcium

2. In addition to the regulatory mechanisms intrinsic to the epithelium itself, electrolyte transport is regulated by all of the following pathways except:

   a. endocrine and paracrine regulation
   b. ATP
   c. enteric neural regulation
   d. intestinal immune system

3. Secretory mechanisms throughout the gastrointestinal tract largely center on the transcellular secretion of:

   a. sodium
   b. potassium
   c. hydrogen
   d. chloride

4. The absorption of hydrophobic compounds is reduced as a result of ineffective micellar concentrations in all of the following conditions except:

   a. Ménétrier disease
   b. biliary obstruction
   c. bacterial overgrowth
   d. Zollinger-Ellison syndrome

5. Each of the following statements regarding intestinal fatty acid–binding proteins is true except:

   a. They are abundant in enterocytes of the small intestine.
   b. They facilitate the intracellular trafficking of fatty acids from the brush border membrane to the smooth endoplasmic reticulum.

   c. They are exported from the cell into the intestinal lumen.
   d. They have been postulated to assist in the formation of chylomicrons and very-low-density lipoproteins for eventual secretion into the portal circulation.

6. The colon is able to readily absorb each of the following except:

   a. monosaccharides
   b. acetate
   c. propionate
   d. butyrate

7. An 18-year-old college freshman presents with a 3-month history of bloating, abdominal pain, and intermittent loose stools. He denies the occurrence of fevers, weight loss, hematochezia, and recent travel. Symptoms date to the start of football camp, at which time he changed his diet to include 4 to 6 glasses of milk per day. Physical examination reveals a healthy African American man. Findings from abdominal and rectal examinations are normal. A clinical diagnosis of primary lactase deficiency is suspected, and a trial of a lactose-restricted diet is advised. The patient, however, is reluctant to refrain from milk ingestion during the football season. The result of a lactose breath hydrogen test is interpreted as normal (i.e., <5 parts per million with no rise in exhaled hydrogen gas following an oral dose of lactose). What is the most appropriate recommendation at this time?

   a. Follow a lactose-free diet for 2 weeks and schedule a follow-up appointment.
   b. Begin an empiric trial of metronidazole.
   c. Undergo flexible sigmoidoscopy with rectal biopsy.
   d. Culture stool for fecal pathogens.

8. Incomplete absorption of each of the following substances has been documented to cause symptoms of carbohydrate malabsorption except:

   a. sorbitol

b. rice starch
c. fructose
d. corn starch

9. Brush border saccharidase activity is decreased by:

a. a diet rich in sucrose
b. fasting
c. diabetes mellitus
d. pancreatic exocrine insufficiency
e. intestinal bacterial overgrowth

10. Folate supplementation is indicated in all of the following situations except:

a. anticonvulsant therapy with phenytoin or carbamazepine
b. celiac sprue
c. chronic sulfasalazine therapy
d. pancreatic insufficiency
e. methotrexate therapy

11. Cobalamin (vitamin B_{12}) absorption may be impaired in each of the following conditions except:

a. pernicious anemia
b. cholestatic jaundice
c. Crohn's ileitis
d. Zollinger-Ellison syndrome
e. small bowel bacterial overgrowth
f. pancreatic insufficiency

12. True statements regarding the Schilling test include each of the following except:

a. The stage I test result is normal in patients receiving acid suppressive therapy.
b. The Schilling test relies on normal renal function for adequate interpretation.
c. The stage II test result is abnormal in healthy patients who have undergone total gastrectomy.
d. Results may be abnormal in patients with small bowel bacterial overgrowth.

13. True statements regarding iron deficiency anemia include each of the following except:

a. Decreased acid production impairs the absorption of nonheme ferric iron.
b. The first stage of iron deficiency is the depletion of iron stores and is manifest by a low serum ferritin level.
c. The level of transferrin saturation is less because the decrease in serum iron concentration is greater than the decrease in transferrin.
d. Dietary iron, in the form of heme iron, has a low bioavailability due to variable absorption.

14. Each of the following conditions is associated with decreased calcium absorption except:

a. celiac sprue
b. chronic cholestasis
c. hyperthyroidism
d. sarcoidosis

15. Laboratory parameters that correlate with postoperative morbidity and mortality include each of the following except:

a. delayed hypersensitivity to common skin test antigens
b. serum transthyretin level
c. triceps skinfold measurement
d. serum albumin level
e. serum transferrin level

16. Complications of excessive calorie administration in patients requiring nutritional support include each of the following except:

a. increased susceptibility to infection
b. hyperglycemia
c. hepatic steatosis
d. excessive carbon dioxide production

17. The most common cause of death in patients with anorexia nervosa is:

a. malnutrition
b. cardiac arrhythmias
c. suicide
d. infection
e. gastrointestinal complications

18. The following statements regarding enteral nutrition are all true except:

a. Parenteral nutrition provides all of the nutrients available from enteral nutrition.
b. Diarrhea is the most common complication, occurring in 30% to 50% of critically ill patients receiving tube feedings.
c. Protein present in oligomeric formulas may be better absorbed than monomeric and polymeric formulas in patients who have impaired intestinal function.

19. Each of the following conditions may explain the presence of abnormal liver chemistries in patients receiving total parenteral nutrition (TPN) except:

a. hepatic steatosis
b. acalculous cholecystitis
c. calculous cholecystitis
d. TPN-associated hemolysis

20. Metabolic responses to illness and injury include all of the following except:

a. thermoregulatory setpoint of the body temperature increases by 1°C to 2°C
b. lipolysis increases

c. glucose production and insulin sensitivity increase
d. protein synthesis and breakdown increase

21. Which statement about the medical complications of obesity is most accurate?

a. Liver disease in nonalcoholic obese patients is common and can be detected reliably by abnormal liver chemistries.
b. Obesity has greater health hazards for men than for women.
c. Obesity is strongly associated with cancer of the lung, prostate, and stomach.
d. During rapid weight loss, the risk of gallstones is less in persons consuming a low-calorie diet with about 1 g of fat per day compared to those consuming 15 g of fat per day.

22. In patients with anorexia nervosa who present at 65% of their ideal body weight, rapid refeeding can cause all of the following except:

a. pancreatitis
b. diarrhea
c. acute mesenteric ischemia
d. edema
e. acute gastric or duodenal dilation

23. A 22-year-old college student presents for evaluation of recurrent sinus infections and amenorrhea. Physical examination reveals a thin woman weighing 36 kg with a height of 1.65 m and an oral temperature of 35.5°C. She denies having a decrease in her energy level and states that she is a member of the track team. When questioned about her weight, she appears disinterested and unconcerned. She reports symptoms of occasional early satiety and emesis. Which of the following statements is true?

a. The most likely diagnosis is bulimia.
b. The amenorrhea is likely caused by reduced end-organ sensitivity to circulating gonadotropins.
c. This disorder likely developed after she began attending college.
d. She probably has significant insight into her condition.
e. She most likely comes from a lower- or middle-class background.

24. Which statement regarding bulimia nervosa is true?

a. It often presents with a greater than 15% loss of body weight.
b. There is often a childhood history of obesity.
c. Patients frequently report symptoms to their physicians.
d. Bulimic patients, unlike anorectic patients, rarely use laxatives or diuretics.
e. Bulimic patients rarely have electrolyte disorders.

25. Which of the following statements regarding large surveys of patients who present for evaluation of weight loss is true?

a. The initial history and physical examination rarely lead to a likely diagnosis.
b. Increased energy consumption from an underlying inflammatory condition is the most common etiology.
c. Of the approximately 25% of patients in which no diagnosis is made, the majority will die of progressive inanition.
d. Gastrointestinal disorders are an uncommon underlying diagnosis.
e. The evaluation of the patient should take into account medication use and age.

26. True statements regarding factors influencing short bowel syndrome include each of the following except:

a. The ileocecal valve serves as a barrier that prevents the migration of colonic bacteria into the distal small bowel.
b. The colon undergoes adaptive changes of dilation, lengthening, and mucosal proliferation to increase the capacity for absorption of fluid and electrolytes.
c. Resection of the distal 100 cm of ileum leads to spillage of bile acids into the colon, producing pure osmotic diarrhea.
d. Patients with massive small bowel resection and fat malabsorption form calcium oxalate renal stones because the free fatty acids in the colon preferentially bind calcium, leaving oxalate free to be absorbed systemically.

27. True statements regarding vitamins and minerals include all of the following except:

a. Vitamin K is fat-soluble; therefore, there are large total body stores of this vitamin.
b. Iron and zinc inhibit copper absorption.
c. High doses of vitamin C (i.e., 3–4 g per day) can produce diarrhea.
d. Vitamin E acts as an antioxidant and free-radical scavenger.

28. Which of the following statements regarding glutamine metabolism by enterocytes is true?

a. Enterocytes obtain glutamine from the intestinal lumen but not from the intestinal circulation.
b. Enterocytes use glutamine primarily as an energy source, not as a substrate for protein synthesis.
c. Glutamine is a poor source of ammonia for enterocytes.
d. Glutamine enters the enterocyte primarily by passive diffusion.

The following case pertains to questions 29 through 31.

A 42-year-old woman presents with an acute abdomen following a motor vehicle accident. At laparotomy, a tear in the superior mesenteric artery is identified and all but 50 cm of her small intestine is resected. Her colon is left intact. Two weeks later, attempts at oral feeding are abandoned when the patient develops severe diarrhea requiring total parenteral nutrition to maintain hydration, electrolyte balance, and nutrition.

29. Each of the following conditions is a likely explanation for the diarrhea except:

    a. increased osmolarity of lumenal contents
    b. increased secretions into the gut
    c. bacterial overgrowth
    d. steatorrhea

30. In addition to total parenteral nutrition, the initial management of diarrhea in this patient should include each of the following except:

    a. H$_2$-receptor antagonist therapy
    b. pancreatic enzyme replacement
    c. antidiarrheal agents (e.g., loperamide)
    d. oral nutrition

One year later, the woman is brought to the emergency department by her friends. She has a fever and a productive cough. There is no history of recent drug or toxin ingestion. She had been stable since the discontinuation of total parental nutrition. She has noted progressive numbness in her feet and difficulty walking. Physical examination reveals tachycardia, ophthalmoplegia, right lung rhonchi, ataxia and findings suggestive of a peripheral neuropathy. A chest radiograph reveals a right lower lobe infiltrate. Laboratory studies are performed, and intravenous antibiotics and 5% dextrose saline are administered, after which the patient becomes unarousable.

31. This acute change in mental status is most likely the result of a:

    a. zinc deficiency
    b. magnesium deficiency
    c. folate deficiency
    d. vitamin B$_{12}$ deficiency

32. A 53-year-old man with short bowel syndrome presents with severe right flank pain and hematuria. Which of the following is most likely to predispose the patient to these symptoms?

    a. short bowel with an ileostomy
    b. short bowel with a subtotal colectomy
    c. short bowel requiring daily total parenteral nutrition and inability to tolerate oral feeding
    d. short bowel with an intact colon

33. Factors stimulating intestinal adaptation after small intestine resection include each of the following except:

    a. dietary nutrients in the intestinal lumen
    b. biliary and pancreatic secretions
    c. trophic effect of hormones
    d. dietary bulking agents
    e. polyamines

34. Which of the following is an absolute contraindication for placement of a percutaneous endoscopic gastrostomy?

    a. ascites
    b. ventriculoperitoneal shunt
    c. morbid obesity
    d. peritoneal dialysis

35. All of the following are possible mechanisms by which the gastrointestinal immune system generates a tolerance to mucosal antigens except:

    a. IgA may mask antigens from exposure to the immune system in the intestine.
    b. Low doses of antigen induce the development of CD4$^+$ T cells capable of inhibiting antigen-specific effector cells.
    c. High doses of antigen induce clonal anergy or apoptosis of antigen-specific effector cells.

36. All of the following enzymes play an important role in carbohydrate digestion at birth except:

    a. maternal mammary amylase
    b. intestinal glucoamylase
    c. pancreatic amylase
    d. salivary amylase

37. Carbohydrates in the diet:

    a. for the most part, are ingested as simple sugars
    b. are the main energy source for humans
    c. are absorbed in their disaccharide form
    d. are nearly completely absorbed in the small intestine
    e. are all composed of six-carbon monosaccharides

38. All of the following statements regarding dietary fiber are true except:

    a. It is rapidly hydrolyzed by amylase.
    b. It can be converted into short-chain fatty acids by colonic bacteria.
    c. It can result in poor absorption of coadministered drugs.
    d. It will increase stool weight with regular ingestion.
    e. It is composed of plant cell wall components.

39. Which of the following statements regarding sucrase-isomaltase is true?

    a. It is secreted into the intestinal lumen after ingestion of a meal.
    b. It is the only enzyme capable of cleaving sucrose to glucose and fructose.
    c. The enzyme is not detectable at birth.
    d. Levels of this enzyme increase with infection and inflammation.

40. All of the following reduce lactase-phlorizin hydrolase activity in adults except:

    a. starvation
    b. infection with human immunodeficiency virus
    c. inflammatory bowel disease
    d. corticosteroid use

41. All of the following statements regarding bile salts are true except:

    a. They are passively absorbed in the proximal small intestine.
    b. They are absorbed by active transport in the ileum.
    c. They are reabsorbed very efficiently in the small intestine.
    d. They result in the generation of short-chain fatty acids within the colon.

42. The gastric phase of protein digestion:

    a. includes the secretion of pepsinogen by parietal cells
    b. is controlled by factors also involved in regulating acid secretion
    c. is a mandatory phase for intestinal protein assimilation
    d. is independent of the gastric pH

43. All of the following statements regarding small intestine assimilation of protein are true except:

    a. It occurs exclusively by absorption of single amino acids.
    b. It can be used as an energy source by the small bowel epithelium.
    c. It involves a sodium-independent transporter.
    d. It results in the delivery of free amino acids into the portal circulation.

44. All of the following statements regarding pernicious anemia are true except:

    a. It occurs primarily in older people of Anglo-Saxon descent.
    b. It is confirmed by a normal result from a stage II Schilling test.
    c. It is the result of a reduced production of intrinsic factor.

    d. It results in a low serum vitamin B_{12} level prior to the development of anemia, macrocytosis, and neuropsychiatric symptoms.
    e. It is treated by oral vitamin B_{12} supplementation at a dose of 10 µg per day.

45. All of the following statements regarding vitamin K are false except:

    a. It is concentrated in the liver.
    b. Vitamin K deficiency related to antibiotic use is unusual.
    c. Vitamin K deficiency is rare because of the presence of large body stores.
    d. It is safely administered intravenously.

46. Each of the following statements concerning calcium are true except:

    a. Calcium supplements should be given to the following patients: those who have undergone gastric surgery, those who have chronic cholestasis, and those who have been taking steroids long-term.
    b. Calcium absorption is regulated by $1,25(OH)_2$ vitamin D_3 at the level of the small intestine.
    c. Calcium absorption is increased in the presence of hypophosphatemia.
    d. Calcium absorption is frequently enhanced in patients with calcium urinary stones.
    e. Calcium absorption is greater with calcium carbonate than with calcium citrate.

47. True statements regarding folate absorption include all of the following except:

    a. Folate supplementation for patients with inflammatory bowel disease may reduce the risk of colorectal cancer.
    b. Patients with celiac disease may have reduced folate absorption.
    c. Folate deficiency in alcoholics is the result of poor absorption.
    d. Oral contraceptives may inhibit enzymes important in folate homeostasis.

48. All of the following statements regarding iron absorption are true except:

    a. Iron absorption increases in response to iron deficiency.
    b. Unlike ferric iron (Fe^{3+}), ferrous iron (Fe^{2+}) remains soluble across a broad pH range.
    c. Dietary substances such as sugars, amino acids, and ascorbate promote iron absorption.
    d. Iron is absorbed at the brush-border membrane by passive diffusion.

49. All of the following statements are true except:

    a. The recommended daily allowance is the minimum intake required to prevent a negative balance.

b. Vegetable oils are rich sources of essential fatty acids.

c. The intake of polyunsaturated fats should be increased.

d. The average intake of fruits and vegetables on a western diet is less than 1 serving per day.

50. Each of the following statements regarding medium-chain triglycerides is true except:

a. Coconut and palm kernel oil are good sources of medium-chain triglycerides.

b. Medium-chain triglycerides are more efficiently absorbed than long-chain triglycerides in patients with decreased amounts of bile salts or decreased small bowel surface area.

c. Medium-chain triglycerides are a good source of essential fatty acids.

d. Medium-chain triglycerides cause less impairment of the reticuloendothelial system than do long-chain triglycerides.

51. Correct statements concerning the role of the gut in electrolyte homeostasis include all of the following except:

a. Hypokalemia in the vomiting patient may result from renal potassium wasting.

b. Hyponatremia rarely occurs as a result of decreased gut absorption.

c. In healthy individuals, only 30% to 35% of ingested calcium is absorbed.

d. Increased fecal losses of magnesium can occur in alcoholics.

52. A patient presents with bone pain, an elevated alkaline phosphatase level, and a history of severe liver disease with presumed vitamin D deficiency. Which of the following is the appropriate treatment?

a. cholecalciferol (vitamin D_3) 8000 IU orally per day

b. cholecalciferol (vitamin D_3) 50,000 IU orally per day

c. ergocalciferol (vitamin D_2) intravenously

d. 25-hydroxycholecalciferol (calcifediol) orally

53. Total parenteral nutrition is indicated for each of the following clinical situations except:

a. elderly patients with decreased oral intake secondary to dysphagia

b. severely malnourished patients requiring surgery

c. severe, active Crohn's disease with malabsorption

d. during prolonged bowel rest resulting from the inability to tolerate oral feeding

54. Which of the following statements concerning the increased risk of serious medical complications associated with obesity is the most correct?

a. Although obesity is a risk factor for developing cardiovascular disease, the degree of obesity does not correlate with the extent of cardiovascular risk.

b. The body mass index (BMI) can be used to assess the degree of an individual's obesity and is calculated as height divided by body weight.

c. For the same BMI, individuals with primarily upper body obesity are at higher risk for developing diabetes, hypertension, and ischemic heart disease.

d. Upper body obesity is more common in women than in men.

55. Which of the following statements regarding food allergy or food hypersensitivity is true?

a. Most cases of immunologically mediated food allergy are IgE-mediated.

b. The majority of cases presenting with "food allergy" are immune-mediated.

c. Most food allergens are of high molecular weight (greater than 150 kd) and are resistant to proteolysis.

d. Skin tests of specific antigens are available for most common food allergens and are helpful in the diagnosis of food allergy in cases of life-threatening anaphylactic reactions.

TRUE/FALSE

56. _____ Caloric supplementation with intravenous lipid emulsions is particularly beneficial for patients with sepsis.

57. _____ Enterocytes along the outer half of the villus (i.e., enterocytes closer to the villus tip) are responsible for the majority of secretory activity within the small intestine.

58. _____ Triglyceride malabsorption is relatively mild in patients with total biliary obstruction.

59. _____ Dietary cholesterol is absorbed into the enterocyte by an active transport process.

60. _____ Small bowel biopsy specimens from patients with abetalipoproteinemia appear normal.

61. _____ Humans absorb approximately 50% of their dietary cholesterol.

62. _____ Lactase deficiency can be prevented (or reversed) by the continued feeding of lactose.

63. _____ Enterocytes are capable of transporting amino acids as well as dipeptides and tripeptides into the cell.

64. _____ The rate-limiting step in the assimilation of dietary sucrose and glucose is transport across the apical membrane of the enterocyte.

65. _____ Serum concentrations of magnesium and zinc are reliable indicators of total body stores.

66. _____ Pancreatic enzymes are largely responsible for the generation of amino acids, dipeptides, and tripeptides from dietary protein.

67. _____ All dipeptides and tripeptides must be hydrolyzed to free amino acids before they can enter the intestinal enterocytes.

68. _____ Proteins such as gluten or casein are relatively easy to digest because of their high proline content.

69. _____ Pancreatic proteases are synthesized, stored in zymogen granules, and secreted as active enzymes.

70. _____ Exocrine pancreatic insufficiency is the most common cause of defective intralumenal proteolysis.

71. _____ Satiety after a meal is primarily mediated by the vagus nerve.

72. _____ Reduced caloric intake with dieting causes a decrease in the body's resting energy expenditure.

73. _____ Pharmacotherapy can be effective in helping patients achieve clinically important weight loss (10% or more of body weight).

74. _____ Cases of a genetic deficiency of the pancreatic enzyme, trypsinogen, have not been described, probably because a lack of trypsinogen is incompatible with life.

75. _____ Both monosaccharides and disaccharides can be absorbed directly across the intestinal epithelial cells of the small intestine.

76. _____ Digestion of dietary proteins begins with proteolysis by pancreatic peptidases in the small bowel.

77. _____ Perioperative antibiotics have been shown to reduce the infectious complications of percutaneous endoscopic gastrostomy tube placement.

78. _____ Patients with as little as 60 cm of residual small intestine may eventually be weaned off total parenteral nutrition.

79. _____ Medium-chain triglycerides are poorly absorbed by patients with short bowel syndrome; thus, this type of fat should be restricted in their diet.

80. _____ The metabolic bone disease and decreased bone mass that occur in patients on total parenteral nutrition are largely the result of inadequate replacement of calcium in the parenteral formula.

81. _____ Results of Shilling tests are abnormal in about 50% of patients with severe pancreatic insufficiency.

82. _____ Hyposensitization with food extracts is useful in the treatment of patients with food allergy.

83. _____ The primary micronutrient deficiency that occurs in small bowel bacterial overgrowth is cobalamin (vitamin B_{12}).

84. _____ Small intestine protein assimilation is an inefficient process.

85. _____ Plant and animal proteins are equally digestible and equally absorbed.

86. _____ Vegetarians who eat eggs will not develop vitamin B_{12} deficiency.

87. _____ The abnormal liver chemistries that frequently occur in patients with anorexia nervosa are secondary to hepatic steatosis and nonspecific periportal infiltrates.

MATCHING

(each selection may be used once, more than once, or not at all)

Match the condition with the most likely deficiency (*use each answer only once*):

88. _____ ulcerative colitis

89. _____ chronic alcoholism

a. vitamin A deficiency

b. vitamin K deficiency

90. _____ pancreatic insufficiency

91. _____ antibiotic therapy

c. zinc deficiency

d. thiamine deficiency

Match the human plasma lipoprotein subclass with the most accurate description:

92. _____ chylomicrons

93. _____ very-low-density lipoproteins

94. _____ low-density lipoproteins

95. _____ high-density lipoproteins

a. primary lipid is cholesterol esters

b. synthesized by both liver and intestine

c. major vehicle for transport of dietary triglyceride

d. major vehicle for transport of endogenous triglyceride

Match these vitamins and minerals with the primary site of absorption:

96. _____ folate

97. _____ cobalamin

98. _____ dietary vitamin K

99. _____ magnesium

100. _____ zinc

101. _____ calcium

a. proximal small intestine (duodenum and jejunum)

b. distal small intestine (ileum)

Match the following micronutrients with the clinical signs of their deficiency:

102. _____ magnesium

103. _____ zinc

104. _____ ascorbic acid

105. _____ vitamin A

106. _____ folate

107. _____ cobalamin

a. weakness, irritability, arthralgia, myalgia, weight loss, petechiae, and gum bleeding

b. thrombocytopenia, leukopenia, anemia, glossitis, and fatigue

c. tremor, myoclonic jerks, ataxia, tetany, delirium, and psychosis

d. anemia, anorexia, muscle weakness, numbness and tingling in the lower extremities, and memory disturbances

e. growth retardation, alopecia, diarrhea, poor wound healing, and loss of taste

f. night blindness, xerophthalmia, follicular hyperkeratosis, and altered taste and smell

Answers

Chapter and page numbers refer to the Textbook of Gastroenterology, third edition.

CHAPTER 1

Multiple Choice

1. b

   The tongue provides the major propulsive force for the transfer of the bolus into the pharynx. Upper esophageal sphincter (UES) relaxation occurs early and precedes pharyngeal contraction. UES pressure increases over the baseline after passage of the bolus. Liquid boluses pass through the esophagus by gravity, whereas esophageal body peristalsis is more important for the transit of solid boluses. (Ch. 9; pg 163)

2. d

   The entire swallowing cycle takes about 1 second to complete. The nasopharynx closes with tongue loading and pulsion. The tongue is most important in clearance, and the most sensitive reflux trigger is the epiglottis. (Ch. 9; pg 164)

3. c

   Upper esophageal sphincter (UES) pressure increases are greater when the stimulus is closer to the UES. Acid causes the highest increase, which is abolished by bilateral vagosympathetic blockade. In contrast to acid, air inflation causes UES relaxation. (Ch. 9; pg 167)

4. d

   Esophageal peristalsis requires both cholinergic innervation and nitric oxide–induced relaxation. Neural innervation of the brain, spinal cord, and esophageal wall is required for normal motor function. The movement of liquid food is primarily a gravity function, whereas the movement of solid food requires intact peristalsis. (Ch. 9; pg 158)

5. c

   Relaxation of the lower esophageal sphincter (LES) requires no central input since vagotomy does not affect LES relaxation. Both vasoactive intestinal polypeptide and nitric oxide are important in LES relaxation, with nitric oxide working through cGMP as a second messenger. LES relaxation is determined by a balance between cholinergic excitatory input and inhibitory neurotransmission. (Ch. 9; pg 179)

6. c

   Depending on the animal studied, cholecystokinin (CCK) can increase both contraction and relaxation of the lower esophageal sphincter (LES) (in humans, CCK induces relaxation); gastrin increases LES contraction, vasoactive intestinal polypeptide increases LES relaxation, and somatostatin has no effect. (Ch. 9; pg 179, Table 9.1)

7. d

   Transient lower esophageal sphincter relaxations (TLESRs) occur spontaneously; however, they can also be induced by pharyngeal stimulation. TLESRs increase in frequency with distention of the stomach. (Ch. 58; pg 1237)

8. d

   Patients who have suffered a recent cerebrovascular accident may experience dysphagia. Dysphagia in this setting is most often the consequence of tongue and pharyngeal muscular weakness or incoordination. Cricopharyngeal achalasia is rare, and upper esophageal sphincter (UES) relaxation in this disorder is typically normal. Barium radiographic studies are more sensitive than esophageal manometry in detecting UES dysfunction. (Ch. 57; pg 1205)

9. a

   Oropharyngeal dysphagia may occur as a consequence of tumors of the medulla, involvement of the vagus nerve, or involvement of the recurrent laryngeal nerve. Mediastinal tumors frequently involve the recurrent laryngeal nerve, especially on the left side where the nerve has a longer course. Unilateral damage results in vocal cord paralysis and laryngeal impairment, thereby allowing aspiration. Primary pharyngeal dysfunction from recurrent laryngeal nerve damage is rare. Soft palate and pharyngeal constrictor dysfunction reflect high vagus lesions that would not be expected in this clinical setting. (Ch. 57; pg 1207)

10. b

A Zenker diverticulum may result from high pharyngeal pressures caused by reduced upper esophageal sphincter compliance. Patients with a Zenker diverticulum have a 0.4% chance of developing squamous cell carcinoma. Zenker diverticula may be missed on upper endoscopy and are best evaluated by barium radiography. Treatment of a Zenker diverticulum usually involves surgical resection. (Ch. 56; pg 1192)

11. b

A Zenker diverticulum is an outpouching of the esophageal wall above the upper esophageal sphincter (UES). As the sac enlarges, symptoms become more apparent: persistent cough, fullness in the neck, regurgitation, and aspiration. Manometric and videofluoroscopic studies suggest that a loss of UES elasticity results in restricted opening of the sphincteric segment of the esophagus during swallowing. UES relaxation is normal and is coordinated with pharyngeal contraction in patients with a Zenker diverticulum. (Ch. 30; pg 685)

12. b

Good responses to cricopharyngeal myotomy are observed in patients with normal innervation but poor upper esophageal sphincter relaxation or cricopharyngeal achalasia. Treatment of a Zenker diverticulum involves removal of the diverticulum, in addition to myotomy. Globus sensation may be associated with esophageal dysmotility or reflux; it usually does not respond to myotomy. (Ch. 57; pg 1204)

13. a

This symptom complex can be seen in patients with diseases affecting proximal striated muscles, including the oropharyngeal musculature. Diseases such as polymyositis (i.e., skin rash, proximal muscle weakness, heliotropic rash) would produce this picture, whereas smooth muscle diseases (e.g., scleroderma) would not. (Ch. 57; pg 1202)

14. b

The most likely diagnosis is achalasia. Although the results of all the diagnostic tests described can be abnormal in this disease, the diagnosis is most reliably established by esophageal manometry. A strict diagnostic criterion for achalasia is esophageal body aperistalsis. Other findings include incomplete lower esophageal sphincter (LES) relaxation, elevated LES pressure, and increased intraesophageal pressure. (Ch. 57; pg 1214)

15. a

Nitrates and calcium channel blockers treat achalasia by decreasing lower esophageal sphincter pressure and esophageal body contractile amplitude. Oral agents, particularly calcium channel blockers, are more effective than sublingual products, and they are most effective in patients with achalasia who have a nondilated esophagus. Initial pneumatic dilation may be more cost-effective than traditional open surgery because of a low initial cost and a low rate (20% to 30%) of recurrent symptoms. The cost-effectiveness of laparoscopic therapy for achalasia requires evaluation. (Ch. 57; pg 1218)

16. d

Most patients older than 50 with these symptoms have primary achalasia rather than pseudoachalasia. Esophageal manometric findings in achalasia and pseudoachalasia are identical. Adenocarcinoma of the gastric cardia is the most common gastric malignancy resulting in pseudoachalasia. Paraneoplastic achalasia with small cell carcinoma of the lung is believed to result from antibodies directed at enteric neurons in the lower esophageal sphincter. Intestinal pseudoobstruction may also occur with small cell carcinoma of the lung. (Ch. 57; pg 1218)

17. c

Both pneumatic dilation and surgical myotomy give comparable initial responses; more than 80% of patients achieve good to excellent symptomatic relief. Esophageal perforation occurs in 4% to 6% of patients after pneumatic dilation. Gastroesophageal acid reflux occurs in less than 1% of patients after pneumatic dilation and in 5% to 10% of patients after surgical myotomy. Pneumatic dilation may have to be repeated in up to 25% of patients. (Ch. 57; pg 1220)

18. c

Sphincter relaxation and peristaltic function are not significantly changed with pneumatic dilation. A lower esophageal sphincter pressure less than 10 mm Hg is an excellent predictor of prolonged remission, whereas a pressure greater than 20 mm Hg is associated with minimal relief. It is not unusual for patients to require 2 to 3 dilation sessions. (Ch. 57; pg 1220)

19. c

Chagas disease is still endemic in parts of South America. It is caused by *Trypanosoma cruzi*. Autonomic ganglion nerves are destroyed with chronic infection. Cardiomyopathy, megaduodenum, megacolon, and megaureter may also occur. Serologic tests with complement fixation can be diagnostic. Treatment has no proven efficacy in chronic disease or in acute infection. (Ch. 57; pg 1217)

20. d

Diffuse esophageal spasm accounts for less than 10% of esophageal dysmotility syndromes. Nutcracker esophagus most commonly occurs in patients with chest pain, whereas nonspecific esophageal dysmotility syndromes are the most common motor causes of dysphagia after achalasia has been excluded. The response to medical therapy often correlates poorly with improvement in manometric parameters. Gastroesophageal reflux may produce symptoms identical to those produced by primary esophageal dysmotility. Furthermore, acid reflux may induce esophageal dysmotility. (Ch. 57; pg 1221)

21. d

The manometric criteria defined are classic for the diagnosis of diffuse esophageal spasm. However, this diagnosis should be made only if clinical symptoms are evident. Unlike achalasia, symptoms are usually not progressive, and peristalsis is preserved between episodes of spasm. The results of a methacholine challenge may be positive in either condition. (Ch. 30; pg 690)

22. e

The localization of symptoms associated with oropharyngeal dysphagia is reasonably accurate. However, the ability of patients to localize proximal versus distal etiologies for esophageal dysphagia is clearly poor. Mechanical and inflammatory etiologies are much more common causes of dysphagia than are motility disorders; therefore, endoscopic or radiographic procedures should be the initial tests of choice to rule out the common etiologies. Deglutitive inhibition refers to the phenomenon of suppressed striated esophageal contractions during swallows and is intended to promote esophageal transit during sequential swallows. In achalasia, esophageal pH monitoring demonstrates acidic conditions only from fermentation of retained esophageal food, not from acid reflux from the stomach. Solid food dysphagia frequently improves after esophageal dilation, even if the findings of an esophageal evaluation are normal. (Ch. 57; pgs 1210, 1216)

23. b

All of the listed medications will help to control the symptoms of esophageal spasm. However, reflux may induce symptoms of spasm, and in fact, reflux-induced esophageal spasm is a very common disorder. Therefore, reflux therapy may aid many patients, and reflux may actually be worsened when the listed smooth muscle relaxants are used first. (Ch. 57; pg 1226)

24. a

This is a case of the CREST variant of scleroderma. Most symptomatic patients with the CREST syndrome exhibit motility disturbances and acid reflux on esophageal testing. Esophageal motility abnormalities commonly seen in patients with scleroderma include body aperistalsis and decreased lower esophageal

sphincter pressure. An esophageal stricture must be ruled out in patients with dysphagia. Barrett esophagus with adenocarcinoma has been reported in patients with scleroderma and acid reflux. (Ch. 57; pg 1227)

25. b

Food impaction usually occurs in the setting of underlying esophageal disease, such as a Schatzki ring or a stricture. A history of prior food impaction is common. An overtube should be used in conjunction with endoscopy to prevent aspiration of the food bolus as it is removed. Once the esophagus has been cleared, the patient should be treated with acid-suppressive therapy and begin a liquid diet. The underlying esophageal stricture should not be dilated at this time. (Ch. 61; pg 1304)

26. b

Symptoms of chest pain induced by acid, distention, or cholinergic stimuli frequently overlap with symptoms of chest pain of cardiac origin. By ambulatory pH monitoring, acid reflux events are associated with pain less than 50% of the time. Left arm pain and exercise-induced pain are equally common in cardiac and esophageal pain. (Ch. 31; pg 695)

27. d

The results of diagnostic tests are usually normal in patients with noncardiac chest pain, particularly if there are no associated gastrointestinal symptoms. Only 20% of patients have abnormal baseline manometry. Empiric trials of high-dose H_2-receptor antagonists or proton pump inhibitors have been useful for diagnosis. Altered sensory perception and contractility have been implicated in the pathogenesis of noncardiac chest pain. (Ch. 31; pg 703)

28. a

Psychologic profiles of patients with noncardiac chest pain are similar to those with the irritable bowel syndrome and are more abnormal than the profiles of healthy subjects and hospitalized patients without chest pain. Psychologic stress increases pain perception but not acid reflux scores. (Ch. 31; pg 704)

29. b

Diagnostic yields are less than 50% even if all tests are used. A Bernstein test and balloon distention can predict an esophageal source but not the mechanism. Many patients do not have pain during elective testing. A positive result on any one test increases the likelihood that other tests will also be positive. (Ch. 31; pg 699)

30. b

Pain thresholds are lower in women, and pain is most common after balloon distention. Like patients with the irritable bowel syndrome, patients with noncardiac chest pain experience pain with lower levels of visceral balloon distention compared to healthy subjects. (Ch. 31; pg 698)

31. d

Cardiac mortality in this group of patients with noncardiac chest pain (NCCP) is similar to that of the general population. Endoscopically visualized esophagitis is seen in only 30% to 40% of patients with acid-induced NCCP. However, acid reflux is the most common esophageal cause of NCCP, and 24-hour pH monitoring is the most useful initial diagnostic test. Measurements of 24-hour pH levels and esophageal pressure may demonstrate both acid-induced and dysmotility-induced pain episodes, even if standard esophageal manometry detects nothing abnormal. Esophageal balloon distention and acid infusion may induce pain in patients with irritable bowel syndrome and cardiac disease as well. (Ch. 31; pg 702)

32. a

Infection with *Helicobacter pylori* may be inversely correlated with gastroesophageal reflux disease. (Ch. 58; pg 1238)

33. d

Odynophagia is uncommon in gastroesophageal reflux disease. (Ch. 58; pg 1244)

34. c

Fewer than 50% of patients with gastroesophageal reflux disease have esophagitis on upper endoscopy. Barium studies are even less sensitive than upper endoscopy. Radionuclide scintiscanning reportedly has a specificity of more than 90%; however, its sensitivity ranges from 14% to 90%. Empiric proton pump inhibitor trials have a sensitivity of more than 80% for gastroesophageal reflux disease. (Ch. 58; pg 1245)

35. c

Most patients with gastroesophageal reflux disease (GERD) do not have a hiatal hernia (<20%). In contrast, almost all patients with reflux esophagitis have a hiatal hernia. Acid clearance is poor in patients with a hiatal hernia and GERD. Transient lower esophageal sphincter relaxations occur more commonly in patients with a hiatal hernia and GERD. (Ch. 58; pg 1238)

36. c

Posterior laryngitis is the major finding with reflux laryngitis. Almost all patients have microaspiration. False negative results on ambulatory esophageal pH monitoring occur in up to 30% of cases. Poor acid neutralization in the pharynx, rather than poor acid clearance, has been associated with this disorder. (Ch. 46; pg 1008) (Ch. 58; pg 1244)

37. c

The perforation rate for the dilation of benign esophageal strictures is less than 1% when using polyvinyl dilators. Perforation of the cervical esophagus may occur with improper dilator introduction, although this is much more common with mercury dilators (e.g., Maloney) and metal olive dilators (e.g., Eder-Puestow). Perforations of the thoracic esophagus proximal to the stenosis result from dilator or guidewire kinking. Perforation of the stricture itself is unusual. Achalasia is one exception; the perforation rate is 1% to 5% and usually involves dilation of the lower esophageal sphincter. In this instance, dilation is much more aggressive with a large pneumatic balloon. (Ch. 126; pg 2819)

38. d

Barrett esophagus is the most common precursor lesion for esophageal adenocarcinoma. Infection with *Helicobacter pylori* decreases the risk for Barrett esophagus, possibly by decreasing acid secretion. Asymptomatic cases are 5 to 20 times more common than symptomatic cases and therefore, treatment of only those patients with endoscopically defined Barrett esophagus may not alter overall mortality. (Ch. 58; pg 1250)

39. c

Barrett esophagus occurs predominantly in white males. Up to one-third of patients report no symptoms at initial diagnosis. Esophageal cancer develops in approximately 1% of patients, and it predominantly affects the intestinal metaplasia of the esophagus. (Ch. 58; pg 1250)

40. d

A premalignant change in the distal esophagus requires specialized intestinal epithelium, not just columnar epithelium. Alcohol and smoking are risk factors for squamous cell cancer but not adenocarcinoma of the distal esophagus. Men are more commonly affected with Barrett esophagus. *Helicobacter pylori* infection is not increased in patients with Barrett esophagus; in fact, *H pylori* infection may be inversely related to the development of Barrett esophagus. (Ch. 60; pg 1287)

41. d

Positive celiac lymph nodes indicate metastatic disease. When found, a biopsy should be performed. The prognosis of esophageal cancer is related to the depth of tumor invasion. Only T4 lesions that involve stricture have been shown to respond similarly to surgical as opposed to medical therapy. Nodes in the chest away from the tumor are a poor prognostic sign. (Ch. 60; pg 1283) (Ch. 136; pg 3007)

42. e

Both esophageal cancer and benign esophageal strictures usually produce progressive dysphagia, which is predictable and reproducible. Both conditions can be associated with heartburn; thus, directed biopsy and cytology at the time of diagnostic endoscopy are required to exclude cancer. Barium radiographic studies may give an unacceptably high false-negative rate for the detection of esophageal malignancy. (Ch. 30; pg 687)

43. d

Computed tomography is superior to endoscopic ultrasonography for the detection of hepatic metastases in patients with esophageal carcinoma. Otherwise, endoscopic ultrasonography is superior for TNM staging, as well as for detecting local invasion of the surrounding vascular structures—a finding that precludes curative surgery. (Ch. 136; pg 3006)

44. c

Stent placement is critical, and most endoscopists use both fluoroscopy and endoscopy to aid in the positioning and deployment of stents. External markers or submucosal contrast injections are used for the fluoroscopic marking of the tumor length. Excess stent length of 3 to 4 cm allows for a margin of error and helps to lessen the risk of tumor overgrowth around the stent. Stents impair esophageal motility and should not be excessively long. Furthermore, although placement of the stent across the lower esophageal sphincter permits frank gastroesophageal reflux, this positioning is sometimes unavoidable. (Ch. 126; pg 2816)

45. d

Maloney dilators are not designed for passage over a guidewire and are therefore blindly placed. This is reasonably safe for "simple" lesions like webs, rings, and mild strictures. Long, angulated, or eccentric esophageal strictures require the use of a guidewire system (e.g., American or Savary-Gillard dilators). Similarly, tight (<7 mm) strictures or the presence of a hiatal hernia are best managed with a guidewire system. These "complicated" lesions may cause dilator coiling and increase the risk of perforation when Maloney dilators are blindly passed. (Ch. 126; pg 2816)

46. c

Diets high in vitamin C have been shown to be protective, likely because of their antioxidant effect. (Ch. 60; pg 1278)

47. c

Tylosis is an autosomal dominant disorder. (Ch. 60; pg 1279)

48. d

Barrett esophagus occurs in up to 90% of patients with adenocarcinoma of the esophagus. *Helicobacter pylori* infection is less common in these patients than in controls with gastroesophageal reflux disease (GERD). GERD is more common in patients with cancer of the gastroesophageal junction, and men have this cancer more commonly than women (3 to 5 times). (Ch. 60; pg 1278)

49. b

Although the intravenous photosensitizing agent is cleared from many tissues within 72 hours, the skin and other organs retain the drug for a longer period of time. Exposure to direct sunlight and bright indoor light should therefore be avoided for 1 month or more. (Ch. 130; pg 2885)

50. c

Damage consistently occurs with radiation doses of more than 60 Gy. Radiation does not increase the risk of perforation with stenting. Dysphagia can occur after 5 years, but it usually occurs in the first year. (Ch. 115; pg 2607)

51. b

The esophagus is the most radioresistant gastrointestinal organ, although damage may be potentiated by concomitant chemotherapy. Fibrosing esophagitis may develop, but not for months to years following radiation therapy. (Ch. 115; pg 2607)

52. d

Clinical symptoms usually occur hours after medication ingestion, although onset may be delayed for days or weeks. Most patients with drug-induced injury have normal esophageal anatomy and function. Oval tablets usually pass more easily through the esophagus than round ones. (Ch. 61; pg 1314) (Ch. 120; pg 2688)

53. a

Mucosal contact is the mechanism for most medication-induced esophagitis, with the exception of nonsteroidal antiinflammatory drugs. Dysmotility and strictures increase the risk. Tetracycline, doxycycline, erythromycin, and ampicillin are the most common medications to be implicated. Swallowing medications in the upright position and with adequate amounts of water decrease the likelihood of medication-induced esophagitis. (Ch. 61; pg 1314)

54. a

Varices develop when a threshold pressure of 12 mm Hg is achieved in the portal venous system. Once varices develop, the relative level of portal hypertension above this threshold value is less important and other factors become more important predictors for variceal hemorrhage. (Ch. 32; pg 721)

55. b

Variceal rebleeding occurs in 30% to 50% of patients before complete variceal obliteration can be accomplished with sclerotherapy. This process usually takes

1 to 3 months. Variceal rubber band ligation appears to achieve variceal obliteration more quickly than sclerotherapy. (Ch. 128; pg 2837)

56. e

The administration of pH-neutralizing substances is contraindicated after caustic ingestion because the ensuing exothermic reaction could extend the esophageal injury. The other therapies listed may be appropriate if burns are extensive or if there is a stricture, although none of the choices has been adequately validated by clinical trials. (Ch. 120; pg 2687)

57. c

Almost all esophageal ruptures occur at the gastroesophageal junction or above. Massive rupture is life-threatening with circulatory collapse and 80% mortality. Most patients do not develop the Mackler triad; these symptoms are observed in 30% of cases. Loss of compliance is a major factor. Other causes of major vascular collapse are identified in differential diagnoses, including aortic dissection, cardiac rupture, variceal bleeding, and abdominal perforation. (Ch. 61; pg 1313)

58. d

Mallory-Weiss tears are characterized by nonpenetrating mucosal lacerations in either the distal esophagus or the proximal stomach. Hiatal hernias occur in 42% to 80% of these patients. Not all patients have a history of retching or nonbloody emesis prior to the onset of hematemesis. The bleeding may vary from a self-limited episode to massive hemorrhage with melena and shock, occasionally requiring intensive care and blood transfusions. Most patients stop bleeding spontaneously and require no intervention other than hemodynamic support. Endoscopic electrocoagulation or epinephrine injection therapy are the preferred therapies for active bleeding. Balloon tamponade is dangerous, because it can extend the tear. (Ch. 61; pg 1311)

True/False

59. false

Botulinum toxin inhibits acetylcholine release. (Ch. 57; pg 1219)

60. false

Most patients with these features have primary achalasia. (Ch. 57; pg 1218)

61. false

Focal discrete ulcers are the primary endoscopic finding in patients with esophagitis caused by the herpes simplex virus. (Ch. 59; pg 1269)

62. false

Although ketoconazole is cheaper and acid secretion is not a problem in AIDS patients, fluconazole has

performed better in randomized trials. (Ch. 59; pg 1267)

63. false

Dysphagia is the predominant symptom, not fever and chest pain. (Ch. 59; pg 1264)

64. false

Regardless of whether a patient does or does not have oral thrush, an empiric antifungal trial is still the most appropriate course of action. Endoscopy should be reserved for the patient who does not respond to empiric treatment. The optimal treatment duration is 7 days. (Ch. 59; pg 1266)

65. false

Most of these patients have normal findings on endoscopy. (Ch. 58; pg 1247)

66. true

The correlation is almost linear. (Ch. 58; pg 1248 [Fig. 58.18], pg 1254)

67. false

Only endoscopy can diagnose reflux esophagitis. Empiric proton pump inhibitor therapy is the best test to diagnose all forms of reflux disease (i.e., erosive and nonerosive). (Ch. 58; pg 1247)

68. false

The prevalence of gastroesophageal reflux disease increases with gestational age. (Ch. 50; pg 1064)

69. false

Gastroesophageal reflux during pregnancy is mediated primarily by hormonal alterations, especially progesterone. (Ch. 50; pg 1065)

70. false

Progesterone levels are more important than estrogen levels in mediating gastroesophageal reflux during pregnancy. (Ch. 50; pg 1065)

71. false

Lifestyle modifications should be attempted prior to any medical therapies. (Ch. 50; pg 1065)

72. true

This action prevents bolus retropulsion into the pharynx. (Ch. 9; pg 165)

73. false

The lower esophageal sphincter is relaxed throughout the passage of the entire bolus through the esophagus. (Ch. 9; pg 179)

74. true

Both sphincters relax simultaneously. Relaxation of the upper esophageal sphincter is brief (<1 second), whereas the duration of the relaxation of the lower esophageal sphincter is long (>5 seconds). (Ch. 9; pg 179)

75. false

The lower esophageal sphincter does not open until bolus passage occurs. This is a major reason for the lack of acid regurgitation during normal swallowing. (Ch. 9; pg 175)

76. true

The UES has residual compliance, which is increased by a large or thick bolus. (Ch. 9; pg 167)

77. false

78. false

79. true

The rate of failure of lower esophageal sphincter (LES) relaxation increases with age but remains at less than 15% of all wet swallows. Dry swallows may produce simultaneous esophageal body contractions and are rarely used for the diagnosis of esophageal dysmotility. Maximal esophageal body and LES pressures are lower than 180 and 45 mm Hg, respectively, in healthy individuals. (Ch. 131; pg 2899)

80. true

The central control of esophageal and lower esophageal sphincter function arises from preganglionic parasympathetic neurons originating in the dorsal vagal complex located in the dorsomedial hindbrain medulla. The neurocircuitry that controls swallowing begins with sensory afferents from the esophagus projecting to the nucleus tractus solitarius (NTS) and terminating on the premotor neurons in the subnucleus centralis. Cell bodies from the subnucleus centralis project directly to somatic motor neurons within the nucleus ambiguus, which control the buccopharyngeal pattern generator for swallowing. This provides a direct transfer of information coming into the NTS from peripheral sensory endings in the esophagus to the motor neurons in the nucleus ambiguus that innervate the muscles involved with deglutition. (Ch. 9; pg 159)

81. true

Pain does not characterize most episodes (75%) of gastroesophageal reflux. If the refluxate pH is 1, 100% of reflux episodes produce pain, whereas at a pH of 3, only 60% of reflux episodes cause symptoms. (Ch. 31; pg 695)

82. false

Neither test has been shown to predict a satisfactory response to medical therapy. (Ch. 58; pg 1246)

83. false

Approximately 50% of patients with reflux symptoms have endoscopic evidence of mucosal injury in the distal esophagus. (Ch. 58; pg 1247)

84. true

The antidepressant agent trazodone decreases chest pain in some patients with esophageal dysmotility syndromes, but this does not correlate with improvement in manometric parameters. (Ch. 31; pg 710)

85. true

Acid ingestion represents 15% of all caustic ingestions. Commonly ingested agents include toilet bowel cleaners and antirust compounds. Acid ingestion most commonly leads to gastric injury; esophageal injury occurs in only 6% to 20% of cases. (Ch. 61; pg 1316)

86. false

A history of lye ingestion increases the risk of esophageal carcinoma. For this reason, the clinician should have a low threshold for evaluating a symptomatic patient with such a history. However, although it is increased, the risk for esophageal carcinoma is not high enough to warrant routine surveillance. (Ch. 60; pg 1280)

87. false

Direct microscopic examination of endoscopic brush cytology and biopsy specimens remain the most accurate means of diagnosing fungal infection of the esophagus. Cultures are not useful, because *Candida* organisms may be present in the mouth and esophagus in the absence of microscopic evidence of epithelial attachment or injury. (Ch. 59; pg 1264)

88. false

Graft-versus-host disease of the esophagus is uncommon and only occurs in the setting of multisystem involvement. (Ch. 112; pg 2558)

89. true

The 5-year survival of patients with squamous cell carcinoma of the esophagus is based on the depth of tumor invasion. In particular, the 5-year survival rate is 46% with invasion of the submucosa, 30% with invasion of the muscularis propria, and 20% with invasion of the adventitia. If there is extension to contiguous tissues and organs, the 5-year survival rate is 7%. (Ch. 60; pg 1283)

90. false

Cytology has a much higher false-negative rate when used to detect adenocarcinoma in patients with Barrett esophagus than it does when used to detect squamous cell carcinoma of the esophagus in patients without Barrett esophagus. Cytologic determinations of high-grade dysplasia or early carcinoma are usually reliable, but samples that show low-grade dysplasia or that are indeterminate for dysplasia are ambiguous because of high interobserver variation. Biopsy specimens are much more useful. (Ch. 60; pg 1290)

91. false

92. true

93. false

94. true

Esophageal rings and webs are predominantly congenital lesions. They can produce intermittent symptoms and are rarely progressive. Symptoms usually manifest when the lumenal diameter is less than 13 mm, but even then, the individual may remain asymptomatic. Symptomatic rings are best detected by solid bolus barium radiography, which is not part of the routine upper gastrointestinal radiographic examination. (Ch. 56; pg 1190)

95. true

96. true

97. false

Esophageal dysphagia can produce symptoms referable to the suprasternal notch, and thus, the diagnosis may be misinterpreted as pharyngeal dysphagia. Gastroesophageal reflux and collagen vascular diseases that produce skeletal muscle dysfunction (e.g., polymyositis, mixed collagen vascular disease) can produce pharyngeal dysphagia. Scleroderma, on the other hand, does not involve the upper esophagus, which is composed of striated muscle. Barium radiographic studies, usually cinefluoroscopy, are the best diagnostic tests, because the findings on manometry are often normal. (Ch. 30; pg 684)

98. false

99. false

100. false

101. false

102. false

Clinical symptoms are helpful but rarely can be used to reliably differentiate between chest pain from cardiac or esophageal sources. Radiation of pain to the jaw and hand, and rapid relief with nitroglycerin are more commonly associated with cardiac pain but may be reported with esophageal disease as well. Radiation of pain to the back and posterior neck are more commonly reported with esophageal pain but may be noted with heart conditions. Both types of chest pain are gradual in onset and gradual in relief, and both decrease with rest. (Ch. 31; pg 695)

Matching

103. c

104. a

105. b

106. d

Cowden's disease is associated with marked squamous cell and neural hypertrophy, and growths on the face and tongue called trichilemmomas. Patients with Peutz-Jegher syndrome may present with mucosal and cutaneous melanin spots. Supernumerary teeth, osteomas, sebaceous cysts, and fibromas characterize familial adenomatous polyposis. Hyperpigmentation, alopecia, and onchodystrophy are manifestations of Cronkhite-Canada syndrome. (Ch. 45; pg 992) (Ch. 46; pg 1008)

107. b

108. c

109. a

110. d

Telangiectasias of the lips and the extremities occur in patients with scleroderma. Lichen planus of the tongue is a manifestation of infection with the Epstein-Barr virus in AIDS patients. Severe mucositis throughout the gastrointestinal tract is the hallmark of graft-versus-host disease. A gingival "lead line" is a manifestation of lead poisoning. (Ch. 45; pg 992) (Ch. 46; pg 1008)

111. b

112. d

113. a

114. c

Bluish nodules (hamartomas) that bleed occur with blue rubber bleb nevus syndrome. Nasal bleeding is the predominant form of bleeding in Osler-Weber-Rendu disease. Pseudotumors that mimic leiomyomas can cause massive gastrointestinal hemorrhage in Ehler-Danlos syndrome. Angioid streaks of the retina are a sign of vascular weakness and thus indicate a predisposition to bleeding in pseudoxanthoma elasticum. (Ch. 45; pg 992) (Ch. 46; pg 1008)

115. a

116. b

117. d

118. c

Cheilosis is a manifestation of B vitamin deficiencies of all types, whereas gingival bleeding is a hallmark of scurvy (vitamin C deficiency). Lingual atrophy occurs with vitamin B_{12} and folate deficiency. Dysgeusia and night blindness can result from vitamin A deficiency. (Ch. 45; pg 992) (Ch. 46; pg 1008)

119. c

120. e

121. g

122. a

123. d

124. b

125. f

Intermittent solid or liquid food dysphagia is a hallmark of intermittent esophageal dysmotility, and characterizes diffuse esophageal spasm. Progressive heartburn with solid and liquid food dysphagia indicates decreased lower esophageal sphincter pressure and esophageal dysmotility, both of which occur with scleroderma. Intermittent solid food dysphagia suggests the presence of a ring in the distal esophagus, whereas progressive solid or liquid food dysphagia suggests achalasia. Progressive solid food dysphagia with or without reflux symptoms may be caused by an underlying stricture or cancer. (Ch. 30; pg 686)

126. c

127. a

128. b

129. a

130. c

Immunocompromised patients are at increased risk for viral esophagitis. Herpes simplex virus (HSV), and rarely varicella-zoster virus (VZV), may also infect the healthy esophagus. Cytomegalovirus infects subepithelial endothelial cells and fibroblasts. Observation of definitive biopsy specimens will reveal cytoplasmic inclusion bodies. In contrast, HSV typically causes intranuclear inclusions. Infection with VZV may produce necrotizing panesophagitis in severely immunodeficient patients. (Ch. 59; pg 1268)

131. c

132. b

133. d

134. a

135. e

Nutcracker esophagus is characterized by high-amplitude (>180 mm Hg) peristaltic contractions of the esophageal body. As the name implies, a hypertensive lower esophageal sphincter (LES) involves elevated LES pressures, but normal sphincter relaxation on swallowing. Nonspecific esophageal dysmotility refers to a group of disorders that includes frequent nonperistaltic contractions (20% of wet swallows), retrograde contractions, low-amplitude contractions (<30 mm Hg), prolonged peristaltic waves (6 seconds), and isolated incomplete LES relaxation. In diffuse esophageal spasm, manometry reveals frequent simultaneous contractions intermixed with normal peristaltic contractions of the esophageal body. The hallmark of achalasia is esophageal body aperistalsis. Other manometric findings of achalasia include incomplete LES relaxation, elevated resting LES pressure, and elevated intraesophageal pressures. (Ch. 57; pg 1221)

136. d

137. a

138. e

139. c

140. b

α-Fetoprotein (AFP) is a marker for hepatoma (75% sensitivity at best). CEA is the standard marker for colon cancer; however, it is elevated in only 25% of patients on initial evaluation. CA72.4 has been reported to be a tumor marker in patients with gastric cancer. Currently, there is no reliable marker for esophageal cancer, although mucosal p53 mutation may help predict risk. CA19-9 is the reliable marker for pancreatic cancer. (Ch. 60; pg 1281)

CHAPTER 2

Multiple Choice

1. c

Although the patient has hypergastrinemia and basal gastric hypersecretion, the maximal acid output and the trivial rise in serum gastrin in response to secretin injection are not typical of Zollinger-Ellison syndrome. Before pursuing additional diagnostic or therapeutic options, a standard meal study should be considered. Antral G-cell hyperplasia can produce hypergastrinemia and gastric acid hypersecretion, but gastrin levels will increase minimally after secretin injection. Ingestion of a standard meal will lead to a prominent rise (>200 pg/mL) in the serum gastrin level with antral G-cell hyperplasia. (Ch. 65; pg 1448)

2. b

In addition to gastrinomas, the differential diagnosis of hypergastrinemia includes hypochlorhydria or achlorhydria, retained gastric antrum, antral G-cell hyperplasia, renal insufficiency, massive small bowel resection, gastric outlet obstruction, rheumatoid arthritis, vitiligo, diabetes mellitus, and pheochromocytoma. (Ch. 65; pg 1449)

3. a

Hypergastrinemia may lead to active gastric and small bowel secretion, but it does not cause colonic hypersecretion. (Ch. 65; pg 1447)

4. a

The drugs of choice for the treatment of the clinical manifestations of gastrinoma (e.g., peptic ulcer, diarrhea) are the proton pump inhibitors. Although octreotide is the drug of choice for other secretory tumors such as carcinoid and VIPoma, it is considered to be a second-line therapy for Zollinger-Ellison syndrome. (Ch. 65; pg 1454)

5. b

The most common clinical manifestation of multiple endocrine neoplasia (MEN) type I is hypercalcemia secondary to hyperparathyroidism. (Ch. 65; pg 1447)

6. c

With the advent of potent antisecretory agents, there is no need to perform a gastrectomy for the initial treatment of gastrinoma. This procedure is currently used only in rare patients with unresectable gastrinomas who have not responded to medical therapy, or in individuals who are unable to take oral medications. Chemotherapy is used only for unresectable metastatic gastrinoma. (Ch. 65; pg 1454)

7. b

Cushing syndrome in a patient with gastrinoma is a poor prognostic indicator. (Ch. 65; pg 1456)

8. c

A noninvasive imaging study of the abdomen, such as computed tomography, magnetic resonance imaging, or somatostatin receptor scintigraphy to exclude metastasis should be performed prior to surgery. Endoscopic ultrasonography and selective arterial stimulation of secretin are adjunctive studies to consider once metastatic disease has been ruled out by more traditional imaging studies. (Ch. 65; pg 1450)

9. d

Transcutaneous ultrasonography is the least sensitive of the imaging studies used to evaluate gastrinoma, with a maximal sensitivity of 28% for the primary lesion and 14% for metastasis. Although computed tomography is a useful imaging modality, its maximum sensitivity is closer to 50% and 70% for detecting primary lesions and metastatic disease, respectively. Endoscopic ultrasonography is generally not useful for the detection of metastatic gastrinoma. (Ch. 65; pg 1451)

10. d

Cirrhosis does not cause marked elevations in serum gastrin. (Ch. 65; pg 1449)

11. c

Button batteries are sometimes ingested by children. These batteries can cause corrosive injury if they become lodged in the esophagus. Batteries that have passed through the esophagus to the stomach need not be removed unless the patient shows obvious signs or symptoms indicating injury of the gastrointestinal tract, such as hematochezia or abdominal pain. (Ch. 69; pg 1553)

12. c

Atropine delays gastric emptying and is counterproductive for bezoar eradication. Metoclopramide has been reported to be somewhat effective in treating bezoars. (Ch. 69; pg 1552)

13. b

Nonproductive retching, rather than vomiting of intragastric contents, is the characteristic clinical manifestation of acute gastric volvulus. (Ch. 69; pg 1557)

14. e

Hepatomegaly does not predispose patients to a gastric volvulus. The other conditions have been shown to be risk factors for gastric volvulus. (Ch. 69; pg 1556)

15. c

Gastric sympathetic efferents emerge at the level of T5 through T9. They are preganglionic fibers that eventually synapse at the celiac ganglion. (Ch. 14; pg 281)

16. d

The retained antrum syndrome is characterized by the presence of residual antral tissue within the duodenal stem after a Billroth II resection. This commonly leads to elevated serum gastrin levels, increased gastric acid secretion, and ultimately recurrent peptic ulcer disease. The take-up of technetium pertechnetate by the gastric mucosa of the duodenal stem can be of diagnostic utility. A negative result from a secretin stimulation test is necessary to exclude Zollinger-Ellison syndrome in patients with postoperative ulcer recurrence and hypergastrinemia. Modified sham feeding is used to rule out incomplete vagotomy and is not useful in the diagnosis of the retained antrum syndrome. (Ch. 14; pg 308)

17. d

All except pure alcohol stimulate acid secretion. However, red wine and beer stimulate acid secretion, which suggests that substances in alcoholic beverages other than the alcohol are responsible for acid secretion. Similarly, caffeine is a potent acid secretogogue. Decaffeinated coffee also stimulates acid secretion, suggesting the involvement of other substances, such as the amines or amino acids. (Ch. 14; pg 287)

18. a

Pepsinogen secretion is evoked by the same stimulants that increase gastric acid secretion. (Ch. 14; pg 302)

19. c

Pepsinogen II is produced by chief and mucous cells in the gastric body, as well as by pyloric, Brunner, and metaplastic glands. (Ch. 14; pg 302)

20. b

When parietal cells are activated, H^+,K^+-ATPase is translocated from vesicular membranes within the cells to the canalicular membranes at the apical cell surface, where it actively pumps hydrogen ions in exchange for potassium. (Ch. 14; pg 281)

21. c

Basal gastric acid secretion is highest at night and lowest in the early morning. Cholinergic vagal fibers are primarily responsible for the cephalic phase of gastric acid secretion. The primary stimulatory factors involved in the intestinal phase include distention, proteins, and products of protein digestion. (Ch.14; pg 285)

22. c

Occupancy of muscarinic receptors on parietal cells results in phospholipase C activation, which leads to the hydrolysis of phosphatidylinositol bisphosphate to diacylglycerol (DAG) and inositol triphosphate (IP$_3$). IP$_3$ promotes an increase in cytosolic calcium, and DAG leads to the translocation of protein kinase C. These events in turn lead to the stimulation of parietal cell secretory activity. (Ch. 14; pg 292)

23. b

Intrinsic factor (IF) secretion is stimulated by the same pharmacologic agents as acid secretion (i.e., pentagastrin, histamine, and cholinergic agonists); however, the secretory response is not linked to acid secretion. Therefore, proton pump inhibitors do not block IF secretion. (Ch. 14; pg 306)

24. c

Transforming growth factor–α, amphiregulin, betacellulin, heparin-binding epidermal growth factor (EGF), and neuregulins are members of the EGF family. (Ch. 3; pg 58)

25. c

Enterochromaffin-like (ECL) cells of the gastric mucosa release histamine by the action of the gastrin. (Ch. 3; pg 50, Fig. 3.13)

26. a

Most of the stomach is supplied by branches of the celiac artery (i.e., splenic, left gastric, and common hepatic arteries). The right, middle, and left hepatic arteries supply the liver and biliary tree. (Ch. 62; pg 1327)

27. c

Lung cancer has surpassed gastric cancer as the most common cancer world-wide. There has been a dramatic decrease in the incidence of gastric cancer over the past 30 to 50 years despite an increase in the use of outdoor charcoal grills in the United States. N-nitroso compounds are thought to be carcinogenic as a consequence of their ability to alkylate nucleic acids. The spontaneous formation of N-nitroso compounds from dietary components is enhanced by the relatively high gastric pH levels that occur in patients with pernicious anemia or in those who have undergone gastric surgery for ulcer disease. Gastric cancer has a predilection for men in virtually every population studied, and men have been reported to have significantly higher concentrations of N-nitroso compounds than women. (Ch. 67; pg 1502)

28. b

Cancers involving the upper one-third of the stomach have a worse prognosis than those involving the distal stomach. The diffuse variant of gastric cancer is not associated with chronic atrophic gastritis. Diffuse-type carcinomas are cytologically less well-differentiated than the intestinal type, and they make up a larger proportion of the stomach cancers in the low-risk populations of the world, such as in North America. (Ch. 67; pg 1515)

29. d

Patients with common variable hypogammaglobu-
linema are at an increased risk for gastric cancer.
Because of exposure of the stomach to bile in the setting of hypochlorhydria and hypergastrinemia, patients with a Billroth II gastrojejunostomy have an
increased cancer risk. Atrophic gastritis has a similar
premalignant potential. Long-term proton pump inhibitor therapy can produce enterochromaffin-like
cell hyperplasia and carcinoid tumors in rats but not in
humans. Lynch syndrome II is also known as the cancer family syndrome, a genetic disease with a propen-
sity for gastrointestinal and other tumors. (Ch. 67;
pg 1509)

30. b

Men have up to a 2-fold risk for the development of
gastric cancer compared with women in some populations. Gastric cancer is associated with *Helicobacter
pylori* seropositivity and with lower socioeconomic
status; it is likely that these two factors are at least
partially related to each other, because *H pylori* infection is more common in lower socioeconomic groups.
Gastric cancer affects first-generation emigrants at
rates comparable to those in their countries of origin.
Gastric cancer is more common in areas where there
are high nitrate levels in the water, such as Columbia.
(Ch. 67; pg 1500)

31. e

Tumor markers have been studied as prognostic markers for gastric cancer; however, they are not predictive
of survival. Depth of invasion (e.g., T stage) and
nodal involvement predict outcome. Proximal tumors
tend to have a worse prognosis, possibly because they
are frequently advanced at the time of diagnosis.
(Ch. 67; pg 1515)

32. d

Computed tomography is required to exclude distant
metastatic disease, particularly to the liver. Endoscopic ultrasonography is very accurate for TNM
staging and for the evaluation of tumor extent, but
cannot determine whether lymph node enlargement
is the result of tumor involvement or inflammation.
Enlarged nodes should be biopsied prior to pre-
cluding a curative resection. Laparoscopy is used
in some centers prior to resection for cure to investi-
gate for peritoneal lesions that may have been
missed by preoperative radiographic studies.
(Ch. 67; pg 1517)

33. c

Palliative resection is most appropriate in patients undergoing resection when preoperative staging has
failed to predict unresectability and survival is expected beyond a few months. (Ch. 67; pg 1518)

34. b

Gastric lymphomas arise from mucosa-associated
lymphoid tissue and are B cell in origin. (Ch. 67;
pg 1521)

35. c

Surgical therapy may be beneficial for patients with
gastric lymphoma, but its central role in management
is being challenged by advances in chemotherapy and
radiotherapy. The diffuse variant is the most common
subtype in the stomach. Mucosa-associated lymphoid
tissue lymphomas have a relatively good prognosis
and have been reported to regress with therapy to eradicate *Helicobacter pylori* infection. (Ch. 67; pg 1520)

36. a

Only 2% to 3% of carcinoid tumors are found in the
stomach. Carcinoid tumors are most commonly found
in the appendix (47%), ileum (28%), and rectum
(17%). (Ch. 67; pg 1522)

37. a

Benign hyperplastic polyps constitute about 80% of
all gastric polyps. They are usually less than 2 cm in
diameter, sessile, and often multiple. (Ch. 67; pg 1523)

38. b

The most important predictors of prognosis in patients
with gastric adenocarcinoma include depth of invasion and the distribution of lymph node metastasis.
The degree of histologic differentiation of the tumor is
not an independent predictor of prognosis. Proximal
tumors tend to have a worse prognosis than more distal lesions (Ch. 67; pg 1515). Increased p53 expression in cancers is associated with a reduced 5-year
survival rate. (Ch. 67; pg 1506)

39. c

Infection with *Helicobacter pylori* has been linked to
both histologic variants of gastric adenocarcinoma—the
intestinal type and the diffuse type. (Ch. 67; pg 1503)

40. b

The onset of dyspeptic symptoms in patients older
than 45 to 50, or the presence of "warning signs" such
as dysphagia, nausea, vomiting, bleeding, weight loss,
or a family history of gastric cancer support the need
for early diagnostic evaluation with endoscopy.
(Ch. 67; pg 1512)

41. c

The eradication of *Helicobacter pylori* leads to both
ulcer healing and decreased recurrence rates. The documentation of *H pylori* eradication is absolutely necessary only in patients with complicated peptic ulcer
disease, mucosa-associated lymphoid tissue lymphoma, and after the resection of early gastric cancer.
(Ch 64; pg 1417)

42. b

In patients with a gastric ulcer, biopsy specimens of the stomach should be obtained from the ulcer center and rim to rule out malignancy, and from uninvolved mucosa to rule out *Helicobacter pylori* infection. (Ch. 67; pg 1513)

43. c

Diet and stress do not appear to play a role in ulcer pathogenesis. In contrast, cigarette smoking appears to decrease ulcer healing and is associated with an increased risk for ulcer complications. (Ch 64; pg 1391)

44. a

Antibody tests may remain positive for years following successful eradication of *Helicobacter pylori*. This patient received empiric therapy, which may or may not have been directed toward active ulcer disease. Thus, the most appropriate approach would be for this patient to undergo endoscopy to definitively evaluate the cause of her symptoms. Biopsy specimens to assess *H pylori* status should be obtained at the time of endoscopy. (Ch. 64; pg 1397)

45. b

Mucosa-associated lymphoid tissue lymphoma is strongly associated with *Helicobacter pylori* infection and may be preceded by the development of lymphoid follicles. Lymphoid follicles are rare in normal gastric mucosa, except in children, and correlate with *H pylori* density and antibody titers. Lymphoid follicles decrease in number with antibiotic therapy. (Ch. 66; pg 1469) (Ch. 67; pg 1521)

46. b

Basal and gastrin-releasing peptide (GRP)-stimulated acid secretion levels are elevated in *Helicobacter pylori*–infected patients with a duodenal ulcer (DU). Cytokines may play a role in the secretory abnormalities seen in DU patients. The oral administration of urea does not increase gastrin release. (Ch. 64; pg 1384)

47. a

Zollinger-Ellison syndrome is a rare cause of refractory peptic ulcer disease. Poor compliance with medical therapy and the ingestion of nonsteroidal antiinflammatory drugs are important factors to exclude in patients with no evidence of *Helicobacter pylori*. Gastric acid hypersecretion may contribute to the failure of standard medical therapies in a subset of patients with peptic ulcer disease. (Ch. 64; pg 1427)

48. b

Fifty percent to 70% of ulcer recurrences are asymptomatic in patients on maintenance therapy with H_2 blockers. (Ch. 64; pg 1426)

49. e

Helicobacter pylori and nonsteroidal antiinflammatory drugs alter the integrity of the mucus barrier and reduce the surface hydrophobicity of the mucosa. Mucosal regeneration is impaired by *H pylori* toxins. Mucosal regeneration is prostaglandin-dependent, as is microvascular blood flow. Neutrophilic infiltration is seen only in *H pylori*–induced injury. (Ch. 66; pg 1471)

50. b

COX-1 expression occurs in response to physiologic stimuli and leads to the synthesis of thromboxane A_2, PGI_2, and PGE_2. (Ch. 64; pg 1374)

51. d

While there is some debate as to the relationship between *Helicobacter pylori* and nonsteroidal antiinflammatory drugs (NSAIDs) in causing ulcers, the weight of the evidence suggests they are independent risk factors for ulcer disease. Thus, the eradication of *H pylori* infection, as recommended by the NIH consensus conference, is recommended for all patients with ulcer disease. Patients who continue to use an NSAID remain at risk for recurrent ulcer disease and should be considered for co-therapy with a prophylactic agent. Either full-dose misoprostol or proton pump inhibitor (PPI) therapy (i.e., the equivalent of 20 mg of omeprazole) reduces the likelihood of NSAID-induced peptic ulcer disease. H_2 blockers are less effective than PPIs in decreasing ulcer recurrence; they are mainly effective at reducing damage in the duodenum if administered at low doses (150 mg twice daily). Switching to a COX-2–specific inhibitor fails to eradicate *H pylori* or heal the ulcer, and such agents may in fact impair ulcer healing. (Ch. 64; pg 1420)

52. d

Alcohol use has not been clearly identified as a risk factor for the development of peptic ulcer disease in people who use nonsteroidal antiinflammatory drugs, though it has been suggested to exacerbate acute damage. (Ch. 64; pg 1389)

53. b

Symptoms caused by nonsteroidal antiinflammatory drugs (NSAIDs) that persist in the setting of antisecretory therapy increase the likelihood of a peptic ulcer. The role of *Helicobacter pylori* in NSAID-induced ulcer disease is complex. It appears that both NSAIDs and *H pylori* are independent risk factors for peptic ulcer disease. Thus, simply testing the patient for *H pylori* and treating the infection if tests are positive ignores and inadequately treats the NSAID-associated ulcer risk. Treating the patient with a proton pump inhibitor (PPI) may prove effective, as PPIs can heal ulcers caused by NSAIDs; single daily doses are adequate for this purpose. However, the persistent symptoms in this patient are best evaluated with endoscopy to determine whether or not long-term therapy with a PPI will be required to treat active ulcer disease. Use of a safer antiinflammatory, such as a COX-2 inhibitor or Arthrotec, is potentially hazardous in this patient, who may have ulcer disease. It is therefore best to confirm the diagnosis with endoscopy. (Ch. 64; pgs 1390, 1394, 1419)

54. a

Switching to nonacetylated salicylates or reducing the analgesic dose, avoiding concomitant corticosteroid use, and co-therapy with misoprostol or a proton pump inhibitor have all been demonstrated to reduce the incidence of nonsteroidal antiinflammatory drug–induced ulcers. (Ch. 64; pg 1423)

55. c

There are differences in the ability of nonsteroidal antiinflammatory drugs (NSAIDs) to selectively block COX-1 and COX-2; the newer selective agents are associated with less gastrointestinal toxicity. The potency and duration of COX-1 inhibition is related to duodenal ulcer development. Nonacetylated NSAIDs do not significantly inhibit COX activity. (Ch. 64; pg 1374)

56. d

Nonsteroidal antiinflammatory drug–related complications occur most commonly in the elderly and in women and often are not accompanied by warning symptoms, such as dyspepsia or nausea. (Ch. 64; pg 1389)

57. d

Proton pump inhibitors, high-dose H_2 blockers, and misoprostol are reasonable options for the prophylaxis of nonsteroidal antiinflammatory drug–induced ulcer. However, these agents are not routinely recommended for patients taking corticosteroids. (Ch. 64; pgs 1389, 1420)

58. d

The nonsteroidal antiinflammatory drug should be discontinued given the size of the ulcer and the evidence of gastrointestinal bleeding. Proton pump inhibitors appear to have an advantage in treating large ulcers (i.e., 1.5 cm or larger), especially if there are related complications. (Ch. 64; pgs 1389, 1420)

59. b

Although nonsteroidal antiinflammatory drugs have likely played a significant role in this patient's clinical picture, *Helicobacter pylori* may have contributed to the ulcer development. Therefore, eradication therapy for *H pylori* would be appropriate. The presence of gastrointestinal bleeding places this patient at even higher risk if she were to have a recurrent ulcer.

Consequently, documentation of the *H pylori* eradication with a urea breath test or a stool antigen test 4 to 6 weeks after the completion of antibiotic therapy is appropriate. Serology is generally not useful for documenting *H pylori* eradication because test results can remain positive for years after successful cure of the infection. (Ch. 64; pg 1417)

60. c

Pain is a poor predictor of ulcer versus nonulcer causes of dyspepsia. (Ch. 64; pg 1395)

61. b

Surface active phospholipids are a component of mucosal defense at the pre-epithelial level. (Ch. 64; pg 1375)

62. b

A decreased rate of peptic ulcer disease is associated with diabetes mellitus. This may be the result of decreased acid and pepsin secretion. (Ch. 64; pg 1392)

63. c

Cigarette smokers are at increased risk for developing ulcer disease and related complications. In addition, ulcer healing rates are lower in smokers than in nonsmokers. Genetic factors appear to play an important role in the development of peptic ulcer disease. Neither ethanol nor diet appear to play a role in the pathogenesis of peptic ulcer disease. (Ch. 64; pg 1391)

64. d

Proton pump inhibitors (PPIs) inactivate the H^+,K^+-ATPase pump, which provides the final common pathway to gastric acid secretion. PPIs are transformed into active inhibitors in an acidic environment. Within 2 weeks of beginning PPI therapy, many patients have elevated fasting serum gastrin levels. PPIs have been associated with the development of enterochromaffin-like (ECL) cell hyperplasia and carcinoid tumors in rats. In humans, the available data do not support any substantial change in the ECL cell population with PPI use. (Ch. 64; pg 1407)

65. d

Proton pump inhibitor (PPI) regimens heal ulcers more rapidly than do H_2-receptor antagonist regimens after 2 and 4 weeks of therapy. (Ch. 64; pg 1409)

66. a

H_2-receptor antagonists are effective but are inferior to proton pump inhibitors for the treatment of nonsteroidal antiinflammatory drug (NSAID)–related ulcers when NSAID therapy is continued. (Ch. 64; pg 1421)

67. c

Omeprazole undergoes hepatic metabolism to three metabolites, 80% of which are excreted in the urine. Consequently, it is not necessary to reduce the dosage of omeprazole in patients with renal failure. (Ch. 64; pg 1409)

68. b

Annual ulcer recurrence rates may be as high as 60% to 100% if *Helicobacter pylori* is not eradicated. (Ch. 64; pg 1424)

69. b

Intestinal metaplasia most commonly occurs in the incisura angularis of patients with type B atrophic gastritis. (Ch. 66; pg 1473)

70. d

Patients with hemorrhagic gastritis usually present with painless bleeding. Pathologic findings are not specific for the inciting agent. Biopsy specimens exhibit sparse inflammation with extensive regenerative epithelia. (Ch. 66; pg 1469)

71. a

This is the classic presentation for Ménétrier disease. Gastric lymphoma can be excluded if multiple, deep mucosal biopsy specimens do not show signs of malignancy. Zollinger-Ellison syndrome is characterized by gastric acid hypersecretion and hypergastrinemia. (Ch. 66; pg 1487)

72. e

Although autoimmune metaplastic atrophic gastritis is associated with an increased risk of gastric cancer ranging from 3-fold to 18-fold higher than expected, no accepted surveillance protocol has been established. (Ch. 66; pg 1473)

73. b

Stress gastritis is very common among patients in the intensive care unit (ICU), even in those individuals who are not mechanically ventilated. Up to 3% of patients in the ICU develop overt gastrointestinal hemorrhage requiring blood transfusions. (Ch. 32; pg 720)

74. e

Gastroparesis is not a gastrointestinal manifestation of rheumatoid arthritis. (Ch. 63; pg 1344)

75. c

The effects of erythromycin on gastric emptying are mediated by way of its action as a motilin receptor agonist. Erythromycin induces strong antral contractions and appears to accelerate emptying in association with impaired gastric sieving, which results in the delivery of large, poorly dispersed food particles to the proximal intestine. (Ch. 63; pg 1350)

76. d

Patients with functional dyspepsia often have reduced symptomatic tolerance to balloon distention of the prox-

imal stomach. However, this alteration in visceral perception has not been associated with changes in fundic wall compliance. (Ch. 63; pg 1358)

77. b

Although its periodicity and regularity can be altered by sectioning of the extrinsic nerves, antral phase III activity is usually not interrupted by vagotomy. Unlike the heart, the stomach has no specialized electrical conduction system. The fed motor pattern in the antrum exhibits irregular phasic activity—contractions occur in about half of all slow-wave cycles. Indigestible residue is cleared by phase III of the fasting migrating motor complex. The migrating motor complex is not impaired in the elderly. (Ch. 10; pg 192)

78. c

Intraduodenal lipid perfusion inhibits antral motor activity but stimulates phasic and tonic motor activity of the pylorus, which further delays gastric emptying, presumably by producing a relative outlet obstruction of the pylorus. (Ch. 10; pg 195)

79. a

Gastric emptying of inert liquids follows the principles of first-order kinetics. The volume of liquid that is emptied into the duodenum is a constant fraction of the volume that remains in the stomach. Thus, a 500-mL bolus will empty twice as rapidly as a 250-mL bolus. (Ch. 10; pg 199)

80. e

Corticotropin-releasing factor is believed to be an important central mediator of the effects of stress on the gastrointestinal tract. Intestinal nutrients delay the gastric emptying of solids by prolonging the lag phase. Ileal lipid perfusion delays the emptying of both liquids and solids from the stomach. Exogenous cholecystokinin delays gastric emptying. Nonpainful rectal distention delays the gastric emptying of solids. (Ch. 10; pg 204)

81. b

Delays in gastric emptying in patients with diabetic gastroparesis correlate poorly with symptom severity. Many asymptomatic diabetics exhibit profoundly delayed gastric emptying, whereas severely nauseated patients may have normal emptying. Furthermore, relief of symptoms with prokinetic treatment is not necessarily associated with accelerated gastric emptying. (Ch. 63; pg 1341)

82. e

All of these statements concerning the treatment of diabetic gastroparesis are true. (Ch. 63; pg 1348)

83. b

Tachygastria is considered to be the result of ectopic pacemaker activity in the distal stomach that results in the propagation of depolarizations in a retrograde direction. Because tachygastric electrical activity is too low in amplitude to reach a contractile threshold for gastric smooth muscle, the stomach is usually atonic during tachygastria. (Ch. 63; pg 1353)

84. c

The symptom complex that this individual describes is most consistent with the early-dumping syndrome, which is believed to result from fluid shifts into the intestine, and from the supraphysiologic release of a number of vasoactive hormones such as vasoactive intestinal polypeptide, neurotensin, and enteroglucagon. The late-dumping syndrome, in which dumping occurs 90 to 240 minutes after a meal, is believed to result from hyperinsulinemia. Symptoms that accompany the late-dumping syndrome include palpitations, tremulousness, weakness, confusion, and syncope. (Ch. 68; pg 1543)

85. e

All of these statements concerning treatment of the early-dumping syndrome are correct. (Ch. 68; pg 1543)

86. a

After truncal vagotomy, both the receptive relaxation and accommodation reflexes are blunted in response to a meal, resulting in accelerated liquid emptying. Vagal denervation of the antrum reduces the force and frequency of contractions during the fasted and fed states. Conversely, reflex inhibition of antral contractions elicited by food passing into the small intestine is also impaired. Truncal vagotomy shortens the duration of fed motor activity after a meal. (Ch. 68; pg 1544)

87. c

In addition to decreasing the sensitivity of parietal cells to gastrin and histamine, truncal vagotomy reduces basal acid output by 85% and maximal acid output by 50%, decreases the influence of acetylcholine on parietal cells, and abolishes proximal gastric non-phasic motor activity. (Ch. 68; pg 1531)

88. d

In patients with anorexia nervosa, changes in gastrointestinal function underlie the common complaints of early satiety, bloating, belching, vomiting, and constipation. There is evidence for gastric electrical dysrhythmias, impaired antral contractions, and delayed emptying of a solid meal. Improvement in gastric emptying after the administration of domperidone suggests that dopaminergic pathways in the central and enteric nervous systems may be impaired. Many gastrointestinal symptoms associated with anorexia nervosa resolve with refeeding. (Ch. 63; pg 1345)

89. d

Although some patients with a visible vessel at the base of an ulcer crater require surgical intervention, many can be treated with endoscopic procedures such as heater probe therapy, injection therapy, or electrocautery. Dumping syndrome occurs in up to 15% of patients after vagotomy coupled with antrectomy. In contrast, dumping syndrome occurs in only 5% of patients after proximal gastric vagotomy. Preoperative gastric acid analysis does not identify those patients at highest risk for postoperative ulcer recurrence. Ulcer recurrence after truncal vagotomy and antrectomy is lower than after proximal gastric vagotomy. Unfortunately, truncal vagotomy and antrectomy is associated with a higher mortality rate and incidence of postoperative complications than is proximal gastric vagotomy. (Ch. 68; pg 1530)

90. b

When perforation of an anterior duodenal bulb ulcer is associated with a bleeding posterior "kissing" ulcer, it is necessary to perform a definitive surgical procedure. (Ch. 68; pg 1538)

91. d

Although rapid transit can occur after vagotomy and antrectomy with resultant malabsorption of nutrients, hypocalcemia as a result of malabsorption is not common. (Ch. 68; pg 1543)

92. a

Iron deficiency is a common cause of anemia in post-gastrectomy patients. This condition is related to reduced postoperative acid secretion and a decreased ability to dissociate ferric iron from food. Folate and vitamin B_{12} deficiencies can also develop in these patients, but these deficiencies are much less common. (Ch. 68; pg 1543)

93. d

Poor surgical candidates and patients with a negative result from a Gastrografin swallow can be managed conservatively if there are no signs of generalized peritonitis. There is no evidence suggesting that octreotide is of any benefit in the management of these cases. (Ch. 68; pg 1540)

94. c

During the act of vomiting, there typically is involuntary contraction of the abdominal musculature, which in turn increases intraabdominal pressure and facilitates the retropulsion of gastric contents through the mouth. (Ch. 35; pg 778)

95. b

In most patients, 5-fluorouracil does not induce nausea and vomiting. (Ch. 35; pg 781, Table 35.1)

96. c

Prior use of oral contraceptives does not alter the incidence of nausea and vomiting during pregnancy. However, nausea during the first trimester of pregnancy is more common in nonsmokers, primigravidas, obese women, and women with lower levels of education. (Ch. 35; pg 783)

97. b

Hyperemesis gravidarum usually starts at 4 weeks of gestation and resolves by the end of the first trimester. Although serum human chorionic gonadotropin levels are increased in patients with hyperemesis gravidarum, these levels do not correlate with the severity of symptoms. One percent to 5% of women with pregnancy-associated nausea and vomiting develop hyperemesis gravidarum, which is characterized by volume depletion and electrolyte abnormalities. (Ch. 35; pg 783)

98. b

Unlike the other metabolic abnormalities listed, acidosis is not a consequence of vomiting. (Ch. 35; pg 785)

99. a

In a patient with an obvious upper gastrointestinal source of bleeding (indicated by a history of hematemesis), a nasogastric tube allows the assessment of ongoing acute hemorrhage. (Ch. 32; pg 715)

100. c

Maintenance of tissue perfusion with adequate intravascular volume is more important than replacement of blood cells in the initial management of the patient with acute gastrointestinal hemorrhage. (Ch. 32; pg 715)

101. a

Urgent endoscopy is warranted in patients with continued bleeding. Diagnostic endoscopy alone has not been shown to significantly alter the outcome of acutely bleeding patients. (Ch. 32; pgs 715)

102. a

Gastric varices usually accompany esophageal varices and are most often the result of underlying liver disease. They most commonly span the gastroesophageal junction along the wall of the lesser curve and often disappear spontaneously with the obliteration of esophageal varices. Splenic vein thrombosis complicating pancreatitis can lead to isolated gastric variceal formation, which is best treated by splenectomy. (Ch. 32; pg 726)

103. d

Pancreatitis can be complicated by splenic vein thrombosis, which can be successfully managed by splenectomy. (Ch. 32; pg 726)

104. b

Angiodysplasias cause 5% to 7% of upper gastrointestinal hemorrhages. High rates of rebleeding occur after endoscopic therapy for gastrointestinal angiodysplasia because most patients will have multiple lesions, especially those with hereditary hemorrhagic telangiectasia. (Ch. 32; pg 727)

105. a

Most studies have shown that patients with a clean ulcer base at endoscopy have a 0% to 3% risk of rebleeding. The identification of a visible vessel or adherent clot at endoscopy is associated with a significantly increased risk of ulcer rebleeding. Visible vessels are identified in 20% to 50% of endoscopies performed within 6 to 24 hours of hospital admission. Other stigmata, such as the flat pigmented spot or white clot, confer a lower risk of rebleeding. (Ch. 32; pg 716)

106. c

In general, prompt follow-up endoscopy in patients with hemorrhage from peptic ulcer disease is reserved for those with recurrent bleeding. (Ch. 129; pg 2861)

107. b

Thermal methods have been reported to be superior, inferior, and equal to injection techniques for bleeding ulcers; in general, their efficacy rates are comparable. The ulcer patients who seem to benefit most from therapeutic endoscopy, in terms of need for surgery, transfusion requirements, and length of hospitalization, are those with major stigmata (e.g., arterial spurting, visible vessels). The joules per tamponade station vary from 60 to 150, and a mean of 40 seconds of electrocoagulation per ulcer has been used safely. (Ch. 32; pg 718) (Ch. 129; pg 2870)

108. a

Gastric varices have not been shown to benefit from epinephrine injection or thermal therapy. (Ch. 32; pg 726)

109. b

Duodenogastric reflux is not more common in patients with nonulcer dyspepsia than in control subjects. (Ch. 29; pgs 661, 666)

110. c

An aberrant localization of pancreatic tissue, also known as a pancreatic rest or heterotopic pancreas, is usually an asymptomatic condition. Although 70% of pancreatic rests are found in the upper gastrointestinal tract, other sites include the gallbladder, liver, small intestine, colon, appendix, omentum, and Meckel diverticula. Pancreatitis, biliary obstruction with jaundice, intestinal obstruction, and intussusception have all been associated with heterotopic pancreas. These lesions can be confused with leiomyomas, lymphomas, or adenomatous polyps and can be distinguished only by an examination of endoscopic biopsy specimens. Asymptomatic individuals in whom heterotopic pancreas is discovered incidentally do not require any specific treatment. (Ch. 92; pg 2116)

111. b

Upper endoscopy identifies structural disease in about 50% of previously unevaluated dyspeptic patients. An extended functional workup can identify abnormalities in about 50% of the remaining patients. (Ch. 29; pgs 661, 671)

112. b

A single intravenous dose of antibiotics can be given periprocedurely to decrease the risk of infection with *Staphylococcus aureus* and β-hemolytic streptococci. (Ch. 127; pg 2825)

113. a

Prophylactic shunt surgery reduces rebleeding rates (vs. sclerotherapy) but does not improve long-term mortality in patients with cirrhosis. β-Adrenergic antagonists have a beneficial effect for large (i.e., grade II or III) varices only. The Child-Pugh score correlates better with mortality than with variceal size. (Ch. 128; pg 2841)

114. a

A Dieulafoy lesion is a condition in which a histologically normal artery running within the submucosa fails to reduce in caliber near the mucosal surface, thus causing pressure erosion of the overlying epithelium, and possible rupture and hemorrhage. The optimal surgical treatment is a wide wedge resection. Endoscopic coagulation is often successful and precludes the need for surgical management. (Ch. 32; pg 727)

115. d

In patients with retained antrum syndrome, little or no gastrin is released after a meal, although the basal gastrin level is increased. Unlike the results in patients with gastrinoma, secretin stimulation tests in patients with retained antrum syndrome do not produce significant increases in the serum gastrin concentration. Acid secretion in these individuals is significantly elevated, compared to the levels expected after antrectomy and gastrojejunostomy. (Ch. 14; pg 308)

116. b

Pernicious anemia is caused by circulating intrinsic factor or parietal cell antibodies that lead to a decrease in cobalamin absorption in the terminal ileum and consequent megaloblastic anemia. (Ch. 14; pg 308)

True/False

117. false

Similar to benign peptic ulcers, ulcers associated with Zollinger-Ellison syndrome occur most commonly in the first portion of the duodenum (75%). (Ch. 64; pg 1447)

118. true

Endoscopic biopsy of all gastric ulcers diagnosed radiographically is required to exclude malignancy, because their radiographic appearance does not definitively exclude malignancy. (Ch. 64; pg 1396)

119. false

Only 5% of H^+,K^+-ATPase pumps are active in the resting or basal state. (Ch. 64; pg 1374)

120. false

In patients with duodenal ulcer, mucosal bicarbonate output in the proximal duodenum is decreased; it is normal in the distal duodenum. (Ch. 64; pg 1380)

121. true

Neutrophil endothelial adherence and their extravasation into submucosal tissue with the release of cytotoxines and the generation of oxygen-derived free radicals are important factors in experimental mucosal injury. (Ch. 64; pg 1375)

122. false

Both type A and type B gastritis are risk factors for the development of gastric cancer. (Ch. 66; pg 1473)

123. false

Recent use of a proton pump inhibitor, antibiotics, or bismuth-containing compounds decreases the accuracy of both rapid urease tests and histologic evaluations for *Helicobacter pylori*. Diagnostic yield can be maximized by obtaining multiple biopsies from the gastric body and antrum. (Ch. 64; pg 1397)

124. false

Proton pump inhibitors effect the accuracy of both rapid urease tests at endoscopy and the urea breath test. These drugs should be withheld for 7 to 14 days prior to testing. (Ch. 64; pg 1400)

125. false

The urea breath test and the stool antigen test are reliable means of establishing a cure of *Helicobacter pylori* infection. Serologic tests for antibodies can remain positive for years after the successful cure of infection, and therefore are not recommended as a reliable or practical means of testing for eradication. (Ch. 64; pg 1401)

126. false

In both developing and developed countries, the acquisition of *Helicobacter pylori* infection occurs in childhood. The age-dependent increase in *H pylori* prevalence seen in the United States is a consequence of the cohort effect rather than an acquisition of infection in adulthood (Ch. 64; pg 1382)

127. false

In the United States, the reinfection rate after successful eradication of *Helicobacter pylori* is less than 1% per year. (Ch. 64; pg 1419)

128. false

A follow-up of research subjects with gastritis (and therefore presumptively with *Helicobacter pylori* infection) for up to 10 years revealed that 11% developed peptic ulcers. (Ch. 64; pg 1382)

129. false

Metronidazole resistance can be found in up to 60% of persons infected with *Helicobacter pylori* in developed countries. (Ch. 64; pg 1418)

130. true

Unlike proton pump inhibitors, the absorption of H_2-receptor antagonists is not affected by ingesting food. (Ch. 64; pg 1405)

131. true

N-nitroso compounds are powerful carcinogens for upper gastrointestinal malignancy because of their ability to alkylate nucleic acids, and because they are spontaneously synthesized from dietary components. Nitrosamides are a subset of the *N*-nitroso compounds formed in the stomach from nitrates and amides. There is a high degree of correlation between per capita intake of nitrate and age-adjusted mortality from gastric cancer. (Ch. 67; pg 1503, Fig. 67.2)

132. false

Healing rates of duodenal ulcers approach 85% to 99% after 8 weeks of therapy with sucralfate. (Ch. 64; pg 1416)

133. false

Long-term regimens of omeprazole and lansoprazole have been shown to be safe in humans, with no increased risk for dysplasia or carcinoid tumors. (Ch. 64; pg 1411)

134. false

Currently, ulcer prophylaxis is recommended only for patients simultaneously taking nonsteroidal anti-inflammatory drugs and corticosteroids or those with a history of ulcer disease. Although early studies indicated a risk of increased ulcer disease in patients taking large doses of steroids over long periods, subsequent randomized trials have failed to confirm this association. (Ch. 64; pg 1389)

135. false

Normal gut mucosa is insensitive to pH extremes as well as to pinching, stabbing, cutting, and electrical and thermal stimulation. The gut generally responds to distention, contraction, traction, compression, torsion, stretch, and inflammation. (Ch. 36; pg 795)

136. false

Bezoars composed of insoluble material such as hair must be removed mechanically or surgically. (Ch. 69; pg 1549)

137. true

Gastric bezoars can cause a host of nonspecific symptoms including anorexia, bloating, early satiety, dyspepsia, malaise, weakness, weight loss, headache, nausea, vomiting, and abdominal pain. If a bezoar is discovered incidentally on radiography or endoscopy in a patient without clear-cut symptoms, no therapy (e.g., a prokinetic agent or a trial of enzymes) may be appropriate. (Ch. 69; pg 1550)

138. true

Unless associated with gastric volvulus, gastric outlet obstruction rarely produces abdominal pain. The predominant complaints in the setting of gastric outlet obstruction are nausea and vomiting. (Ch. 69; pg 1556)

139. true

The incidence and mortality of gastric adenocarcinoma are up to 3 times higher in lower socioeconomic groups. Men are affected 1.4 to 1.7 times more often than women. (Ch. 67; pg 1500)

140. false

The Borrmann classification is based solely on morphology and provides little insight into the biology or clinical behavior of the tumor. (Ch. 67; pg 1507)

141. false

The risk of gastric adenocarcinoma does not increase for at least 15 years after surgery for peptic ulcer disease. (Ch. 67; pg 1511)

142. false

Apparent healing as documented by upper gastrointestinal radiography with a barium swallow has been reported for some malignant gastric ulcers. (Ch. 67; pg 1512) (Ch. 64; pg 1396)

143. true

The yield of biopsy for the diagnosis of gastric malignancy is 74% to 86%; for cytology, it is 77% to 85%. The combination produces a diagnostic yield of 88% to 91%. (Ch. 67; pg 1512)

144. false

No tumor marker has sufficient sensitivity or specificity to allow an early diagnosis of gastric malignancy. (Ch. 67; pg 1515)

145. false

Local lymph node metastases do not universally adversely affect prognosis in patients with gastric adenocarcinoma. (Ch. 67; pg 1515)

146. true

Gastric cancer in young people is more likely to be the diffuse type, which is associated with a poorer prognosis. (Ch. 67; pgs 1507, 1516)

147. true

The TMN stage is the most significant prognostic factor in gastric cancer. The exception to this is in the case of early gastric cancer, in which local lymph node metastases do not significantly adversely affect the prognosis. (Ch. 67; pg 1515)

148. true

Endoscopic ultrasonography (EUS) provides the best preoperative local staging of gastric cancer. EUS has an overall accuracy of 80% for T stage and 70% for N stage for gastric adenocarcinoma. EUS has an accuracy of 96% in predicting tumor resectability. (Ch. 67; pg 1517)

149. true

Mucosa-associated lymphoid tissue (MALT) lymphoma is a low-grade primary B-cell lymphoma that affects the stomach. Antibiotic eradication of *Helicobacter pylori* can lead to the regression of MALT lymphoma. (Ch. 67; pg 1521)

150. true

The overall 5-year survival rate in patients with gastric cancer is 7.4% to 16.5%. In patients resected for cure, the 5-year survival rate is 20.5% to 42.8%. (Ch. 67; pg 1518)

151. false

In general, adjuvant chemotherapy following a curative resection of gastric cancer has yielded disappointing results. (Ch. 67; pg 1519)

152. false

Familial genetic mechanisms play only a minor role in the pathogenesis of gastric cancer. (Ch 67; pg 1504)

153. true

The molecular mechanisms involved in the pathogenesis of cancer are largely those of genetic lesions in the tumor cells. Although there is not yet a comprehensive hypothesis for the development of gastric cancer, several genetic alterations have been reported, including mutation of the *APC* gene, microsatellite instability, overexpression of p53, and loss of heterozygosity. (Ch. 67; pg 1505)

154. true

Most gastrointestinal stromal tumors occur in the stomach. (Ch. 67; pg 1522)

155. false

Histologic factors that increase the risk of a malignant gastric stomach tumor include size larger than 5 cm, more than 5 mitoses per 50 high-power microscopic fields, tumor necrosis, nuclear pleomorphism, dense cellularity, and microscopic invasion of the lamina propria or blood vessels. Endosonography cannot reliably distinguish between benign and malignant lesions. (Ch. 67; pg 1523)

156. false

Carbohydrates do not stimulate cholecystokinin release. (Ch. 3; pg 52)

157. true

Pepsins are maximally active at a pH of 1 to 3 and rapidly inactivated at pH levels above 4.5. (Ch. 14; pg 303)

158. true

Normal stomach acidity causes aspirin, a weak acid, to associate with a hydrogen ion and thus become uncharged. The uncharged molecule is more readily absorbed than is the charged molecule, which predominates in a less acidic stomach. (Ch. 26; pg 613)

159. true

Even when test conditions are standardized, the percent of a solid meal emptied from the stomach at 2 hours can vary in the same patient from day to day by up to 30%. This marked variation may explain why up to one-half of patients with chronic nausea and vomiting have normal results on gastric emptying studies. (Ch. 10; pg 201)

160. true

Digestible solids are triturated to particles less than 1 mm in diameter in the antrum and pylorus. (Ch. 10; pg 202)

161. false

Hyperosmolar solutions in the duodenum delay gastric emptying. (Ch. 10; pg 199)

162. true

Entry of food into the stomach relaxes the gastric fundus by two vagally mediated reflexes: receptive relaxation and accommodation. (Ch. 10; pg 190)

163. false

Ingestion of liquid nutrients inhibits the activity of the migrating motor complex. Liquid nutrients are emptied by tonic effects produced by the fundus, with contributing motor effects produced by the antrum, pylorus, and duodenum. (Ch. 10; pg 199)

164. true

Vagal denervation of the stomach eliminates both the gastric accommodation and receptive relaxation reflexes. This results in a rapid rise of intragastric pressure after ingestion of a meal. The end result is rapid emptying of liquids soon after completion of a meal. This effect is seen with truncal, selective gastric, and proximal gastric vagotomies. The addition of an antrectomy or pyloroplasty compounds the problem by removing a secondary control of gastric outflow to liquids. (Ch. 68; pg 1531)

165. false

Chronic idiopathic intestinal pseudoobstruction is characterized clinically by nausea, vomiting, diffuse abdominal pain, constipation or diarrhea, and bladder dysfunction. Small bowel dysmotility is the predominant finding in these patients, and delayed gastric emptying is often demonstrable. (Ch. 63; pg 1345) (Ch. 85; pg 1920)

166. false

Gastric motility abnormalities have been demonstrated in patients with viral gastroenteritis. However, as with other disorders of gastric emptying, symptoms do not universally correlate with the presence or absence of a motility disorder on diagnostic testing. (Ch. 63; pgs 1342, 1345)

167. true

The frequency of the gastric slow wave is 3 cycles per minute (cpm) in humans and 5 cpm in dogs, whereas the frequency of the duodenal slow wave is 11 cpm in humans and 18 cpm in dogs. (Ch. 10; pg 191)

168. false

The fasting pattern of the interdigestive migrating motor complex is comprised of four phases. In phase I, a few weak gastric contractions occur. In phase II, contractions become more frequent, building to phase III, in which each gastric slow wave is followed by a forceful contraction. These contractions are propagated well into the small intestine. Phase IV serves as a transition period to the next phase I. The entire cycle typically lasts 90 to 120 minutes in humans. (Ch. 10; pgs 191, 198)

169. true

Radioimmunoassays indicate that blood levels of motilin peak when phase III activity starts in the esophagus and stomach. When motilin is removed by neutralizing antibodies, antral contractions become intermittent and weak. In addition to motilin, input from the vagus nerve may also contribute to the generation of phasic activity. (Ch. 10; pg 193)

170. false

Sensors involved in the feedback regulation of gastric emptying are located throughout the small bowel as well as the colon. They respond to a variety of nutrients and other stimuli. (Ch. 10; pg 204)

171. true

Breakdown products of protein (e.g., dipeptides, amino acids, amines), rather than the proteins themselves, appear to be responsible for stimulating acid secretion. (Ch. 14; pg 287)

172. true

Antral resection coupled with truncal or selective vagotomy is associated with the lowest risk of ulcer recurrence for chronic duodenal ulcer (0% to 2%). (Ch. 68; pg 1535, Table 68.4)

173. true

The characteristics of the fed pattern are determined by the type, composition, and amount of nutrients consumed. For example, solid foods lead to higheramplitude contractions in the antrum than do liquid foods. Fats lead to a more prolonged fed pattern than do carbohydrates. The duration of the fed pattern is dependent on calorie ingestion. (Ch. 10; pg 194)

174. true

Distal antral receptors respond mainly to gastric contractions, whereas receptors in the fundus and proximal gastric body respond to distention. Mechanoreceptors in the middle portions of the stomach are activated by both contractile activity and passive distention. (Ch. 10; pg 189, Fig. 10.1)

175. true

Diagnostic endoscopy with biopsy can usually be performed safely in patients who are taking oral anticoagulation medication. However, a patient who is to be treated with electrocoagulation for polypectomy or for hemostasis should stop taking anticoagulants for as long as 2 weeks after the procedure, if possible. (Ch. 120; pg 2680)

176. false

Negative nasogastric aspirates are not uncommon and are the result of either the lack of duodenogastric reflux of blood in the patient with a duodenal source of bleeding or the cessation of bleeding. (Ch. 32; pg 716)

177. true

Hematochezia from upper gastrointestinal hemorrhage occurs as a result of rapid gastrointestinal transit and usually is a manifestation in patients who are bleeding rapidly. (Ch. 32; pg 716)

178. true

Effective coagulation begins by applying firm pressure with a contact probe that in turn applies sufficient heat to weld the artery walls together. (Ch. 129; pg 2860)

179. false

Duodenal varices are found deeper in the gut wall and are less likely to rupture than are esophageal varices. (Ch. 128; pg 2841)

180. false

Manifestations related to pituitary adenoma are the least common clinical presentation in multiple endocrine neoplasia type 1. (Ch. 65; pg 1447)

181. true

Gastric acid is the primary inhibitor of gastrin release; therefore, its absence leads to enhanced gastrin secretion and potentially to G-cell hyperplasia. (Ch. 65; pg 1449)

182. false

Large clinical trials have failed to demonstrate improved survival using either of these agents to manage acute upper gastrointestinal hemorrhage. (Ch. 32; pg 718) (Ch. 64; pg 1415)

183. true

Variceal size is the most important predictor of hemorrhage. (Ch. 32; pg 721)

184. true

Blood loss from portal gastropathy that necessitates transfusion is uncommon; however, when it occurs, it appears to respond to either portosystemic shunt or propranolol. (Ch. 32; pg 725)

185. true

Rebleeding and liver failure account for most deaths in the first week after an index hemmorhage. (Ch. 128; pg 2842)

186. false

The Child classification is more closely associated with mortality rates. (Ch. 128; pg 2836)

187. false

Endoscopic band ligation is associated with a complication rate of 5%, which is significantly lower than the 26% reported with sclerotherapy. (Ch.128; pg 2847)

188. true

The average rebleeding rate after transjugular portosystemic shunt surgery is 20% compared to 40% after sclerotherapy. (Ch. 128; pg 2844)

189. false

Patients with onset of bleeding prior to a hospital admission have a lower mortality rate than patients who suffer the onset of bleeding during a hospital admission. (Ch. 32; pg 716)

Matching

190. c

191. d

192. a

193. b

Scopolamine is an anticholinergic agent useful in treating motion sickness. Domperidone acts on dopamine receptors in the gut and the chemoreceptor trigger zone, but does not penetrate the blood-brain barrier. Among its many actions, cisapride stimulates enteric cholinergic neurons. Because of central anti-dopaminergic activity, dystonia is a complication of metoclopramide therapy. (Ch. 35; pg 788)

194. c

195. d

196. a

Gastric acid analysis should be the first test for patients with elevated serum gastrin levels that are below 1000 pg/mL. Gastric acid hypersecretion that is near maximal in the basal state (i.e., the ratio of basal to maximal acid output is >0.6) and associated with a rise in serum gastrin of more than 200 pg/mL after a secretin infusion confirms the diagnosis of Zollinger-Ellison syndrome. Retained gastric antrum after Billroth II surgery, antral G-cell hyperfunction, and rarely, duodenal ulcer disease can all give similarly high baseline gastrin levels, but the result from the secretin stimulation test is usually negative in patients with these entities. Patients with pernicious anemia have profound hypochlorhydria or achlorhydria and do not need secretin stimulation testing. (Ch. 65; pg 1448)

197. a

198. a

199. a

200. c

201. a

202. c

Benzamides, antiparkinsonian drugs, opiates, and butyrophenones induce nausea and vomiting through the activation of the area postrema. Erythromycin and nonsteroidal antiinflammatory drugs can cause nausea and vomiting by activation of peripheral afferent pathways. (Ch. 35; pg 780)

203. b

204. a

205. a

206. b

The dumping syndrome is a complication of surgical procedures used to treat peptic ulcer disease. It can be divided into early-dumping syndrome and late-dumping syndrome. In early-dumping syndrome, large quantities of hyperosmolar chyme are dumped into the upper small intestine. The consequent distention and osmotic load lead to a number of consequences, including increased motility, shift of fluid from the intracellular compartment to the gut lumen, and a release of vasoactive substances that may cause peripheral vasodilation and flushing. In addition, patients often experience abdominal discomfort, borborygmi, and diarrhea. Systemic manifestations include weakness, sweating, flushing, tachycardia, and palpitations. In early dumping, glucose is rapidly absorbed from the gut and leads to hyperglycemia. This in turn causes hyperinsulinemia. This hyperinsulinemia outlasts the hyperglycemia and eventually causes hypoglycemia. This set of circumstances defines late-dumping syndrome. (Ch. 68; pg 1543)

207. b

208. b

209. a

210. a

Gastrin increases gastric acid secretion via the phosphoinositide signaling system. Acetylcholine binds to cholinergic M_3 receptors, which in turn activates the phosphoinositide signaling system. Activation of the parietal cell H_2 receptors leads to an increase in cAMP. The simultaneous activation of the H_2 and M_3 receptors on the parietal cell leads to an additive response in acid secretion (Ch. 64; pg 1373). Somatostatin is produced in antral D cells and has an inhibitory effect on gastric acid secretion and gastric emptying. Somatostatin receptors are in the rhodopsin/β-adrenergic receptor family and couple predominantly to adenylate cyclase. (Ch. 3; pg 54)

211. c

212. a

213. b

Ulcers recur after vagotomy and antrectomy in only 0% to 2% of patients. Ulcer recurrence is 10% to 17% after vagotomy and drainage and after parietal cell vagotomy. Subtotal gastrectomy can be complicated by abnormalities in calcium absorption, and by iron and B_{12} deficiencies. The likelihood of developing postoperative gastroparesis is lowest after highly selective vagotomy. (Ch. 68; pg 1542)

214. b

215. d

216. a

217. c

Gastric carcinoids tend to be slow growing. If confined to the submucosa and smaller than 1 cm in diameter, these tumors can be resected endoscopically. Gastric lipomas account for 50% of all gastrointestinal lipomas and are usually found incidentally at endoscopy. Endoscopic biopsy specimens of gastric leiomyomas usually reveal normal mucosa. Gastric leiomyomas are sometimes difficult to differentiate from leiomyosarcoma. The risk of carcinoma in gastric adenomas may be 10% or higher; the risk correlates with the size of the lesion. (Ch. 67; pg 1522)

CHAPTER 3

Multiple Choice

1. c

    Tropical sprue is a chronic diarrheal illness associated with malabsorption that often leads to severe nutritional deficiencies. The etiology is presumed to be bacterial overgrowth of the small bowel by toxigenic strains of coliform bacteria. The diagnosis is made by small bowel biopsy. Histologic examination reveals partial villous atrophy. Ileal involvement is common. Megaloblastic anemia caused by vitamin B_{12} and folate deficiencies is the hallmark of tropical sprue. Treatment involves a regimen of folic acid and tetracycline for 6 months. (Ch. 73; pg 1647)

2. d

    Gastrointestinal tuberculosis is caused by *Mycobacterium tuberculosis* and *Mycobacterium bovis*. Persons at increased risk for tuberculosis infection include those infected with human immunodeficiency virus, older people, persons from endemic areas, persons taking long-term steroids, alcoholics, and persons who abuse intravenous drugs. The most common presenting symptom is abdominal pain. The differential diagnosis includes Crohn's disease, lymphoma, and infections including *Mycobacterium avium* complex enteritis, histoplasmosis, and cryptosporidiosis. (Ch. 73; pg 1650)

3. d

    Gastrointestinal tuberculosis involves areas of high lymphoid density, especially the distal small bowel, the cecum, and the appendix. The diagnostic procedure of choice is colonoscopy with biopsies of the terminal ileum and cecum. The organism can frequently be identified on intestinal biopsy specimens using an acid-fast stain. (Ch. 73; pg 1651)

4. a

    Mycotic infections of the gastrointestinal tract can result from the dissemination of pulmonary infections. Histoplasmosis can disseminate in immunocompetent as well as immunocompromised persons. Intestinal aspergillosis, candidiasis, and mucormycosis affect only severely immunocompromised persons. (Ch. 73, pg 1653)

5. c

    Viral ulcerations are the most common cause of bleeding in patients who have undergone bone marrow transplant. Peptic-appearing gastroduodenal ulcers that are resistant to standard ulcer therapy may be caused by cytomegalovirus. Epstein-Barr virus does not cause direct mucosal ulcerations but often presents with large small intestine mucosal nodules and diffuse mucosal immunoblast infiltration. In acute graft-versus-host disease, the most common sources of bleeding are esophagitis and gastric erosions. (Ch. 48; pg 1037)

6. a

    Acid-peptic disease is the most common cause of occult-gastrointestinal bleeding in western countries. Hookworm infection is the most common cause worldwide, but it is rare in the industrialized countries of the western world. (Ch. 33; pg 745) (Ch. 109; pg 2448)

7. a

    Although *Giardia lamblia* is a common cause of enteric infection worldwide, it is not considered a particularly important pathogen in acquired immunodeficiency syndrome. In the United States, *G lamblia* is the most commonly identified intestinal parasite, with prevalence rates as high as 16% in some communities. Diagnosis of *Giardia* infection can be made by examining fresh stool for trophozoites or preserved stool for cysts, which provide diagnostic yields of approximately 50%. (Ch. 107; pg 2429)

8. c

    Diarrhea resulting from colonic disease commonly presents with 3 to 30 bowel movements per day, whereas diarrhea from small intestine pathology usually presents with only about 3 to 8 bowel movements per day. Stool volumes are variable but are often large in small intestine disease and small in colonic disorders. Diarrhea from small intestine disease commonly occurs at irregular intervals, especially at night and in the early morning, and does not commonly contain blood. Diarrhea from colonic disease occurs at more regular intervals throughout the day and night and is often associated with an inflammatory colitis, which results in occult or gross blood loss. (Ch. 40; pg 859)

9. c

    Pinworm (*Enterobius vermicularis*) is the most prevalent small intestine helminth, followed by *Ascaris lumbricoides*. (Ch. 109; pg 2443)

10. c

    Visceral larva migrans is a syndrome that produces the clinical triad of eosinophilia, hepatomegaly, and hypergammaglobulinemia that results from infection by *Toxocara* ova found in dog or cat feces. It is most commonly seen in children with a history of pica, but it is occasionally seen in adults. (Ch. 109; pg 2450)

11. c

    Evidence of increased intestinal permeability or inflammation is found in up to 70% of patients taking nonsteroidal antiinflammatory drugs (NSAIDs). Nonspecific small intestine ulcers have been observed in 8.4% of patients prescribed NSAIDs in the 6 months prior to their death. NSAID-associated intestinal injury primarily occurs in the distal small intestine.

Stricture formation occurs in 5% of patients on chronic NSAID therapy and can mimic the presentation of Crohn's disease in the small intestine. NSAIDs have been associated with several other small intestine disorders, including collagenous colitis, celiac sprue, and nonceliac flattening of the small intestine mucosa. (Ch. 79; pg 1741)

12. c

The basic mechanism of action of cocaine-induced ischemia is inhibition of the presynaptic reuptake of norepinephrine, dopamine, and serotonin as well as an increased synthesis of norepinephrine and dopamine. Therefore, this drug may lead to arterial vasoconstriction and subsequent intestinal ischemia. There have been several reports of intestinal ischemia secondary to the administration of ergot alkaloids with subsequent splanchnic vasoconstriction. Oral contraceptives can cause mesenteric thrombosis leading to small bowel infarction. Angiotensin-converting enzyme inhibitors do not cause intestinal ischemia. (Ch. 79; pg 1747)

13. c

A high index of suspicion is necessary to make the diagnosis of an aortoenteric fistula as a source of gastrointestinal hemorrhage, because the fistula is difficult to discern by endoscopy or angiography. Aortoenteric fistulas almost always involve the third portion of the duodenum. In patients with Dacron grafts, the fistula usually arises from the proximal portion of the graft. (Ch. 32; pg 727)

14. a

Necrotizing enterocolitis is seen in premature, low-birth-weight babies and is believed to be caused by the entry of bacteria into damaged intestinal mucosa. Breast feeding may be protective by providing additional antibody protection not afforded by cow's milk or formula feeding. Pneumatosis intestinalis secondary to bacterial gas formation can be seen on abdominal radiography and is characteristic of necrotizing enterocolitis. The condition may occur anywhere in the small bowel but is most common in the ileocecal region. (Ch. 79; pg 1751)

15. a

Radiation enteritis is uncommon when the total radiation dose is less than 45 Gy. A dose of 60 Gy increases the risk of intestinal damage to 25% to 50%. In the early stages of radiation enteritis, the most common symptom is diarrhea. Later, the patient may present with obstructive symptoms. The radiographic evaluation may be normal or reveal dilated, edematous loops of small bowel. (Ch. 40; pg 883)

16. a

This patient has acute jejunitis secondary to infection with *Clostridium perfringens*. Epidemics of this type

of infection have been described in New Guinea. Patients are typically observed with a 3- to 10-day history of upper abdominal cramps, vomiting, and often bloody diarrhea. Stool cultures are usually positive for *C perfringens* and leukocytosis is often present. Patients often require surgical intervention, although medical management, including antibiotics, is frequently successful in patients who have not developed fulminant toxemia. (Ch. 72; pg 1618)

17. a

In the absence of nephrotic syndrome or significant liver disease, hypoalbuminemia associated with lower extremity edema suggests protein-losing enteropathy (PLE). Although lower extremity deep vein thrombosis may cause edema, this would not explain the hypoalbuminemia noted in this patient. PLE may be secondary to lymphatic obstruction (e.g., lymphoma, tuberculosis, right-sided heart failure) or enterocyte barrier breakdown (e.g., Crohn's disease, celiac sprue). The diagnostic evaluation should focus on these considerations. The fecal α_1-antitrypsin concentration may confirm the diagnosis of PLE, because α_1-antitrypsin is highly resistant to proteolytic digestion and therefore is elevated in conditions that lead to intestinal protein loss. Significant steatorrhea is commonly associated with many of the disorders that cause PLE. (Ch. 79; pg 1752)

18. c

Hereditary hemorrhagic telangiectasia is an autosomal dominant disease characterized by vascular ectasias of the skin and mucous membranes. Other connective tissue disorders are seen in association with this syndrome. Patients often present with epistaxis or gastrointestinal hemorrhage from either upper or lower sources. (Ch. 113; pg 2572)

19. b

Giardia lamblia, Isospora belli, and diverticulitis would be unlikely causes for melena and guaiac-positive stools in a patient with acquired immunodeficiency syndrome. The most likely diagnosis is Kaposi sarcoma, which may present with gastrointestinal tract bleeding. (Ch. 107; pg 2413)

20. e

Pneumatosis intestinalis is often benign, occurring in association with hematologic cancer or acquired immunodeficiency syndrome and following chemotherapy or organ transplantation. This diagnosis does not necessarily represent a severe form of enteritis. It can also be associated with scleroderma, in which gas accumulations assume a cystic pattern, and in some cases, the rupture of the cysts may lead to pneumoperitoneum. In the setting of intestinal ischemia, gas may accumulate in the bowel wall in a linear pattern.

This may be associated with gas in the portal system and likely represents intestinal infarction. (Ch. 83; pg 1877)

21. b

Ischemic injury to the gut wall may largely occur at the time of tissue reperfusion. The breakdown of ATP leads to the production of free radicals by xanthine oxidase. Reperfusion supplies the oxygen needed to catalyze this reaction. The already damaged mucosa may be further injured by lumenal toxins such as hydrochloric acid in the stomach, proteases, and bacterial toxins. Superoxide dismutase does not exacerbate ischemic injury. (Ch. 23; pg 537) (Ch. 114; pg 2588)

22. b

The sympathetic rather than the parasympathetic nervous system contributes to the modulation of gastrointestinal blood flow. (Ch. 23; pg 529)

23. c

Most small intestine tumors are benign and remain asymptomatic, whereas at least 80% of malignant small intestine tumors produce symptoms. Small intestine tumors account for approximately 1% of all gastrointestinal malignancies and are more common in western industrialized nations than in other parts of the world. Japanese persons who migrate to Hawaii acquire the higher incidence of malignant small intestine tumors found in the Hawaiian white population. (Ch. 78; pg 1723)

24. d

Familial adenomatous polyposis coli, celiac sprue, Crohn's disease, an ileal conduit, and neurofibromatosis are associated with an increased risk of developing small intestine adenocarcinoma. Acquired immunodeficiency syndrome is associated with an increased risk of developing non-Hodgkin lymphoma and Kaposi sarcoma, but not adenocarcinoma. (Ch. 78; pg 1728)

25. a

Symptoms of carcinoid syndrome are improved or abolished in more than 90% of patients during treatment with octreotide. Although plasma serotonin levels are not altered, octreotide reduces the urinary excretion of 5-hydroxyindoleacetic acid (5-HIAA) in 66% of patients. Claims that long-term octreotide therapy retards or reverses tumor growth have not been substantiated. (Ch. 78; pg 1731)

26. e

Although some small intestine carcinoids produce peptide and steroid hormones leading to the development of carcinoid syndrome, most are completely asymptomatic. (Ch. 78; pg 1731)

27. c

The prevalence of prior infection with adenovirus serotype 12 is higher in patients with celiac sprue compared with healthy controls. In addition, there is significant amino acid homology between A-gliadin and E16 protein of adenovirus serotype 12. The D region of the HLA genes (i.e., HLA-DR and HLA-DQ) has the highest association with celiac sprue. These genes are necessary, but not sufficient, for the development of celiac sprue. (Ch. 74; pg 1665)

28. c

There are multiple underlying causes for adynamic ileus, including inflammatory disorders, metabolic abnormalities, and vascular insufficiency. The intralumenal pressures generated with an ileus are not great enough to compromise the mucosal blood flow. Focal pain, borborygmi, and multiple air fluid levels are more characteristic of mechanical obstruction than of adynamic ileus. (Ch. 71; pg 1603)

29. c

Esophageal involvement is common in patients with chronic intestinal pseudoobstruction. Myopathic causes of pseudoobstruction may involve the urinary tract. A manometric evaluation of a patient who has pseudoobstruction usually reveals a loss of normal migrating motor complex activity in the small intestine. (Ch. 71; pg 1602)

30. e

Chronic intestinal pseudoobstruction occasionally can be focal in nature, causing megaduodenum, and it can also be caused by drugs that affect gastrointestinal motility. Scleroderma and amyloidosis typically cause a myopathy, but in their earliest stages, they can produce neuropathies. Familial myopathies have been described with urinary tract involvement. Idiopathic forms are more likely to be neuropathic than myopathic. (Ch. 71; pg 1585)

31. a

Anorectal manometry is likely to be nonspecific or normal and is of limited value in arriving at a diagnosis of chronic intestinal pseudoobstruction. Colonic manometry may be useful, but stereotyped patterns have not been well described, and normal patterns are not well established. Pupillary pharmacologic testing may be useful in selected patients suspected of having idiopathic forms of visceral neuropathy. The most specific test is full-thickness biopsy of the small bowel obtained at laparotomy. Unfortunately, mucosal biopsy specimens obtained at the time of endoscopy are not helpful. Of the nonsurgical studies available, small intestine manometry is likely to be the most useful in the diagnosis of chronic intestinal pseudoobstruction. (Ch. 71; pg 1601)

32. d

Type I familial visceral myopathy is inherited in an autosomal dominant fashion and commonly leads to esophageal dilation, megaduodenum, redundant colon, and megacystis. In some patients, the proximal jejunum may also be slightly dilated. Mydriasis occurs in more than 50% of patients. Esophageal manometry is abnormal in 75%, and the most common abnormalities encountered are reduced lower esophageal sphincter pressure and low-amplitude contractions in the smooth muscle portion of the esophagus. Gastroparesis has not been observed in any patients with type I familial visceral myopathy. (Ch. 71; pg 1585)

33. d

The small intestine is the second most frequently involved gastrointestinal organ in scleroderma after the esophagus. Small intestine dysmotility is presumably caused by degeneration of smooth muscle with replacement by collagen and is characterized by dilation of the small intestine, delayed intestine transit, and occasionally an accordion appearance of the small intestine mucosa on radiographic evaluation. The circular muscle layer is more often involved than is the longitudinal muscle layer. (Ch. 71; pg 1592)

34. e

A dilated, atonic small intestine predisposes to the development of bacterial overgrowth, which in turn can result in diarrhea and steatorrhea. Diarrhea can also be caused by the intestinal dysmotility itself. Malnutrition secondary to poor intake is frequent, because symptoms discourage patients from eating. Pneumatosis cystoides intestinalis is a relatively rare condition, but it occasionally can occur in patients with small intestine dysmotility. It is usually an incidental finding on radiographic evaluation. Ascites is not a typical complication of small intestine dysmotility. (Ch. 71; pg 1600)

35. d

Dihydroxy bile salts that escape absorption in the terminal ileum can evoke an osmotic and secretory diarrhea in the colon. When a larger segment of terminal ileum is removed or diseased, the hepatic synthesis of bile acids cannot keep pace with the bile salt loss, and depletion of the bile salt pool occurs, followed by steatorrhea. This distinction is sometimes referred to as the "100-cm rule." When less than 100 cm of terminal ileum is removed or diseased, the ensuing diarrhea is probably the result of the effects of bile acid in the colon. When more than 100 cm of terminal ileum is removed, the diarrhea is the result of depletion of the bile salt pool, followed by steatorrhea. The former is more likely to respond to bile salt–binding agents, and the latter to a low-fat diet. (Ch. 40; pg 878)

36. e

Most extraintestinal manifestations occur more commonly with ulcerative colitis or Crohn's colitis than with Crohn's disease confined to the small intestine. (Ch. 81; pg 1782)

37. d

Celiac sprue typically causes a reduction or loss of the valvulae conniventes rather than thickening. (Ch. 74; pg 1671)

38. c

Enterocytes from patients with abetalipoproteinemia contain numerous small, clear vacuoles that are visible under light microscopy and reflect lipid accumulation within the enterocyte. (Ch. 75; pg 1684)

39. d

Microfold (M) cells transport but do not process antigens. M cells lack class II antigens on their surface but express MHC class II molecules in lysosomal organelles, suggesting that under certain circumstances, they may serve as antigen-presenting cells. (Ch. 6; pg 115)

40. d

A few intraepithelial lymphocytes (IELs) are CD4$^+$ T cells, but most express the CD8 $\alpha\beta$ heterodimer, the CD45RO isoform. They have suppressor and cytolytic activities; however, their exact roles are unknown. (Ch. 6; pg 118)

41. d

Secretory IgA inhibits the adherence of bacteria to epithelial cells, interfering with bacterial colonization and replication. (Ch. 6; pg 118)

42. b

IgD is not involved in mucosal defense against parasitic infection. (Ch. 7; pg 137)

43. a

Vasoactive intestinal polypeptide, substance P, and somatostatin can trigger histamine secretion by both connective tissue and intestinal mucosal mast cells. (Ch. 7; pg 137)

44. d

IgA deficiency is the most common primary immune deficiency. Biopsy specimens from the jejunum in IgA-deficient subjects are morphologically normal, whereas immunofluorescence studies show a paucity of IgA-producing cells and an increase in IgM-secreting cells. (Ch. 112; pg 2548)

45. b

Gastrointestinal infection with *Giardia lamblia* occurs in approximately 30% of X-linked hypogammaglobulinemia patients. Severe combined immunodeficiency syndromes show a markedly increased risk of viral infections in early childhood, but *Giardia* infections do not predominate. Giardiasis is a common cause of steatorrhea and malabsorption in common variable hypogammaglobulinemia. Giardiasis has been reported with IgA deficiency, but the incidence is probably the same or only slightly increased in comparison with the general population. (Ch. 112; pg 2548)

46. c

Secretory component is released into external secretions bound to IgA, although it may also occur in a free form. (Ch. 6; pg 117)

47. b

Under most conditions, the apical intercellular tight junctions are the rate-limiting barrier restricting the passive movement of hydrophobic solutes through the paracellular space. The plasma membrane and transmembrane proteins are the rate-limiting barriers to transcellular absorption. (Ch. 8; pg 147)

48. b

Tight junctions are selective pores that allow the passage of water and small molecules of molecular weight less than 300 d. Tight junctions are the route for the net movement of those substances that are not actively transported to maintain the osmotic and electrical balance of the cell. (Ch. 8; pgs 146, 152)

49. a

Gap junctions assist in coordinating the activities of adjacent cells within the epithelial sheet by allowing them to behave as syncytia with respect to the transfer of small molecules. (Ch. 8; pg 146)

50. b

In the small intestine, the most important chloride channel is the cAMP-activated low-conductance channel, which participates in hormone-stimulated chloride secretion. This channel is defective in cystic fibrosis. A separate calcium-activated chloride channel has been isolated in airway epithelial cells and in colon cancer cell lines. This appears to be regulated by calcium-calmodulin. The role of the calcium-activated chloride channel in intestinal chloride secretion is unclear. (Ch. 15; pg 336)

51. c

In contrast to patients with selective IgA deficiency, up to 60% of patients with common variable hypogammaglobulinemia have chronic recurrent diarrhea, and two-thirds of these have malabsorption. Nodular lymphoid hyperplasia is frequently found in common variable hypogammaglobulinemia, does not occur in X-linked hypogammaglobulinemia, and is rare in selective IgA deficiency. Selective IgA deficiency is the most common primary immunodeficiency syndrome in adults. (Ch. 112; pg 2549)

52. d

Every organ is vulnerable to infection, but hepatic and gastrointestinal disorders are a prominent feature of chronic granulomatous disease. Hepatomegaly is very common, and liver abscess formation occurs in more than 30% of patients. (Ch. 112; pg 2551)

53. a

Abdominal pain, vomiting, and watery diarrhea are common features of hereditary angioedema. Pitting edema, pruritus, and leukocytosis are notably absent. Anabolic steroids can be effective in treating some cases of hereditary angioedema. (Ch. 112; pg 2552)

54. b

Patients with intestinal lymphangiectasia most commonly exhibit lymphopenia, resulting in anergy, and increased excretion of α_1-antitrypsin in the stool. (Ch. 112; pg 2552)

55. b

Skin tests or oral challenges with peanuts should not be performed in those with a suspected allergy to peanuts because of the risk of anaphylaxis. (Ch. 112; pg 2555)

56. b

Eosinophilic gastroenteritis can involve the mucosa, muscularis, or serosa in any region of the gastrointestinal tract. The condition commonly results in the release of Charcot-Leyden crystals into the stool. (Ch. 112; pg 2557)

57. a

Eosinophilic gastroenteritis may, to some degree, mimic Crohn's disease or lymphoma, with barium radiography showing cobblestoning of the stomach in some patients. The stomach and small intestine are most frequently involved, and prednisone is effective in most patients. Although some parasites can produce increases in circulating eosinophils similar to that seen in eosinophilic gastroenteritis, neither amebiasis nor giardiasis is associated with eosinophilia. (Ch. 112; pg 2557)

58. b

Most cases of travelers' diarrhea develop within the first week of travel. Antibiotic prophylaxis reduces the incidence of travelers' diarrhea by about 90%. Bismuth is an effective prophylaxis and has been effective in the treatment of mild to moderate cases of traveler's diarrhea. Because of increasing drug resistance and the high incidence of illness caused by *Campylobacter jejuni*, the quinolones are now the treatment of choice for adults. (Ch. 72; pg 1615)

59. a

Bacillus cereus is also associated with a diarrheal illness following ingestion of a preformed toxin. The emetic illness associated with this toxin is confined to the ingestion of contaminated fried rice; the ingestion of the toxin in other foodstuffs is associated with a diarrheal illness. Botulinum toxin blocks acetylcholine at the neuromuscular junction and produces skeletal muscle weakness with a 15% case-fatality rate. There is also a mild associated disturbance of gastrointestinal function. The clinical features of ingestion of *Staphylococcus aureus* enterotoxin include profuse vomiting and nausea, typically beginning within 6 to 24 hours of ingestion. *S aureus* is the most common ingested food-borne pathogen in the United States. (Ch. 72; pg 1612)

60. c

The glucose–amino acid–sodium cotransport mechanism is not affected by cholera toxin, and in mild to moderate disease, can provide adequate rehydration of patients. *Vibrio parahaemolyticus* is halophilic, or salt-loving, and is usually found in salt water fish or shellfish. *Aeromonas* infections can be associated with a chronic diarrheal illness that can last as long as a year. (Ch. 72; pg 1624)

61. b

Fever is not characteristic of *Staphylococcus aureus* food poisoning. (Ch. 72; pg 1612)

62. c

Primary infection does confer long-term immunity to the development of recurrent illness from *Vibrio cholerae* infection. Person-to-person contact is not thought to play a role in the transmission of this disease. (Ch. 72; pg 1625)

63. c

With the exception of metronidazole, all of the listed agents decrease the incidence of travelers' diarrhea. However, prophylaxis for travelers' diarrhea is not currently recommended because of the risk of adverse side effects (e.g., photosensitivity, rash, hematologic disorders, antibiotic-associated colitis), and because of the development of antibiotic resistance in bacterial strains. Bismuth subsalicylate has been shown to impart protection rates of 62% to 65% against travelers' diarrhea. (Ch. 72; pg 1615)

64. b

Clostridium botulinum is a ubiquitous anaerobe that can form spores in foods that have undergone improper canning techniques. The heat-labile neurotoxin produced by *C botulinum* is capable of blocking acetylcholine action at the neuromuscular junction. Symptoms can include all of those listed except urinary incontinence. (Ch. 72; pg 1613)

65. b

This clinical presentation, which can be mistaken for acute appendicitis, is classic for *Yersinia enterocolit-*

ica infection. Subsequent to gastrointestinal infection, this patient's course was complicated by the development of erythema nodosum. (Ch. 72; pg 1623)

66. d

This is the typical presentation of tropical sprue. Many patients with tropical sprue can trace the onset of their disease to an episode of acute watery diarrhea. It usually occurs in visitors or natives who have lived in an endemic area for more than 1 year; however, it can occur within weeks of arriving in an endemic area. It is not associated with any underlying immunodeficiency of the host and it is rare among children. Tropical sprue is believed to result from the persistent colonization of the intestine with toxigenic coliform bacteria (not anaerobes), although no specific microorganism has yet been implicated. Folate deficiency, vitamin B_{12} deficiency, and associated megaloblastic anemia can occur after 6 months of disease. (Ch. 73; pg 1647)

67. a

Although no test is diagnostic for tropical sprue, small intestine biopsy specimens show shortening of the villi and lengthening of the crypts along with infiltration of the lamina propria with chronic inflammatory cells. A completely flat mucosa, similar to that observed with celiac sprue, is seen in less than 10% of cases. Demonstration of lipid droplets adjacent to the surface epithelium with oil red O stain is a more specific finding. (Ch. 73; pg 1648)

68. c

Tropical sprue results from damage to the small intestine wall from coliform bacterial toxins, leading to malabsorption and megaloblastic anemia resulting from folate and vitamin B_{12} deficiency. (Ch. 73; pg 1649)

69. d

Ascariasis may present with any of the clinical manifestations listed with the exception of hepatic granulomas, which are more typical of schistosomiasis. (Ch. 109; pg 2447)

70. a

Trichuris trichiura (whipworm) infections are often asymptomatic and result from the ingestion of embryonated ova. The other helminths listed have a component of their life-cycle that includes migration of larvae to the lung, which can be associated with pulmonary hypersensitivity reactions. (Ch. 109; pg 2443)

71. c

Hookworm disease (*Necator americanus* infection) was once prevalent in the southeastern United States but is now unusual. Persons from an endemic region who present with abdominal pain, flatulence, iron deficiency, or pulmonary hypersensitivity reactions should undergo direct fecal examination for ova, which is adequate to detect clinically significant infections. (Ch. 109; pg 2448)

72. b

Stem cells located near the base of the crypt-villus axis give rise to four major epithelial cell types in the small intestine. The enterocyte is the main functional cell of the crypt-villus axis. Enteroendocrine cells are distributed throughout the intestinal mucosa but are found predominantly in the crypts. Goblet cells secrete an acidic mucus and are located along the crypts and villi. Paneth cells are serous and zymogenic cells located at the base of the crypt; their exact physiologic function has not been determined. Intraepithelial lymphocytes are also present in a ratio of about 1 lymphocyte for every 5 epithelial cells; however, these lymphocytes are predominantly T-suppressor cells. (Ch. 70; pg 1567)

73. d

Congenital atresias and stenoses can occur anywhere in the small intestine, but 40% of atresias and 70% of stenoses occur in the duodenum. The overall mortality rate for atresias has been reduced to about 20%, but the prognosis worsens with proximal or multiple atresias. A number of cases are associated with other birth defects such as malrotation, annular pancreas, and cardiac anomalies. Thirty percent of duodenal atresias or stenoses are associated with Down syndrome. (Ch. 70; pg 1573)

74. d

Malrotation can produce small intestine volvulus with associated obstruction and ischemia. Ladd bands from cecal peritonealization can also obstruct the duodenum. Malrotation has been associated with other anomalies, including small bowel atresia, Hirschsprung disease, and abdominal wall defects, but not arteriovenous malformations. (Ch. 70; pg 1575)

75. b

This is the classic presentation of intussusception, one of the most common causes of abdominal pain in infancy. In addition to confirming the diagnosis, a gentle barium enema will frequently reduce the idiopathic intussusception in patients in the pediatric age group. (Ch. 70; pg 1577)

76. d

A Meckel diverticulum results from a failure of the vitelline duct—the structure that connects the fetal yolk sac to the primitive gut—to be completely resorbed. In adults, gastrointestinal hemorrhage is by far the most frequent presentation, and intestinal obstruction is relatively uncommon. Crohn's disease and other inflammatory diseases of the bowel can lead to

false-positive readings on a Meckel scan. (Ch. 70; pg 1571)

77. a

Patients with congenital lymphangiectasia (Milroy disease) usually present with asymmetric edema of the extremities as a result of peripheral lymphatic obstruction, or in a manner similar to secondary lymphangiectasia, with diffuse symmetric edema exacerbated by hypoalbuminemia. Despite lymphocytopenia and delayed hypersensitivity reactions, opportunistic infections resulting in the development of diarrhea are rare. (Ch. 70; pg 1578)

78. c

Volvulus of the small intestine occurs in newborns and is rare in adults, unlike the more common colonic volvulus and sigmoid volvulus, which occur in persons of a broad age range, including older persons. Small intestine volvulus is often associated with an underlying defect, such as an inadequate mesenteric attachment in malrotation, a fibrous band, or an adhesion. Treatment is surgical, and is often performed emergently if evidence of intestinal ischemia is present. (Ch. 70; pg 1576)

79. c

The plicae circulares increase the surface area of the small intestine and have no role in small intestine propulsion. The plicae circulares are invaginations of the submucosa and mucosa only, and are most prominent in the duodenum and jejunum. (Ch. 70; pg 1561)

80. b

Most evidence, collected using selective antisera and relatively selective receptor antagonists, suggests that vasoactive intestinal polypeptide contributes to the descending relaxation component of peristalsis. Other data support the participation of nitric oxide in smooth muscle relaxation as well. (Ch. 5; pg 97)

81. b

Studies using selective antagonists and relatively selective receptor antagonists suggest that tachykinins such as substance P participate in the ascending contraction component of peristalsis. Acetylcholine may also contribute to this contractile event. (Ch. 5; pg 98)

82. c

Stimulation of sympathetic pathways in the gastrointestinal tract tends to inhibit gastrointestinal motility, except in sphincteric regions, where sympathetic innervation may be excitatory. Secretomotor neurons stimulate the epithelial cells to pump chloride ions into the lumen, in association with cations and water. Sympathetic neurons tonically inhibit this process. Vagal afferent neurons terminate centrally in the nucleus tractus solitarii. The dorsal motor nucleus of the vagus provides motor neurons that supply the gastrointestinal tract. The perception of visceral pain is mediated by visceral afferents traveling in the thoracolumbar splanchnic and pelvic nerves, and not in the vagal sensory neurons. (Ch. 11; pg 219)

83. b

A diagnosis of lactose intolerance should always be considered in patients with bloating, abdominal pain, and diarrhea. Symptoms do not always correspond to the intake of lactose; thus, lactose intolerance should not be excluded on the basis of a negative dietary history. A mucosal assay for lactase is the definitive diagnostic tool to evaluate lactose tolerance, but it requires invasive measures to perform. Lactose tolerance testing involves the ingestion of 50 g of oral lactose followed by serial measurements of glucose levels. If lactase deficiency is not present, the serum glucose should rise by more than 20 mg/dL within 2 hours. Unfortunately, this test lacks sensitivity, and therefore does not definitively rule out lactase deficiency. Hydrogen breath testing should produce a rise of 20 ppm in breath hydrogen after the ingestion of oral lactose if the patient is lactase-deficient. However, hydrogen breath testing can also give false-negative results if the colonic bacterial flora do not metabolize the ingested lactose or produce hydrogen gas. (Ch. 40; pg 893) (Ch. 75; pg 1690)

84. e

All of the choices listed are risk factors for the development of bacterial overgrowth except pancreatic insufficiency. Other factors that confer an increased risk for developing bacterial overgrowth include enterocolic fistulas, small intestine dysmotility syndromes, immunodeficiency syndromes, gastric achlorhydria, and very young age. (Ch. 76; pg 1698)

85. c

Patients with long-term diabetes mellitus and autonomic neuropathy are at increased risk for bacterial overgrowth. The diagnosis can be made definitively by performing microbiologic cultures of small intestine aspirates. The growth of more than 10^5 colony-forming units/mL in duodenal or jejunal fluids is diagnostic of bacterial overgrowth. $^{14}CO_2$, or hydrogen breath testing, provides a noninvasive means for making the diagnosis of bacterial overgrowth. Successful treatment of bacterial overgrowth can be achieved with a number of antibiotics, including tetracycline, ampicillin, and metronidazole. Celiac sprue has been associated with diabetes mellitus but is only a rare cause of diarrhea in these patients. Anal sphincter dysfunction is quite common in the setting of chronic diabetes mellitus, particularly in those with autonomic neuropathy. (Ch. 76; pg 1698)

86. d

Risk factors for primary small bowel lymphoma include immunodeficiency syndromes, celiac sprue, and the human immunodeficiency virus. The gastrointestinal tract is the most common location for primary extranodal lymphoma. Primary small bowel lymphomas are typically of the non-Hodgkin variety; two-thirds are B-cell and one-third are T-cell derived. (Ch. 78; pg 1733)

87. c

Tropheryma whippelii is a gram-positive bacillus. It is not acid-fast, which distinguishes it from *Microbacterium avium* complex bacilli, which are acid-fast. The source of the infection is unknown. *T whippelii* is closely related to aerobic organisms present in soil; transmission by direct person-to-person contact has not been documented. Small bowel biopsy specimens are usually diagnostic, revealing lamina propria infiltration with large foamy macrophages filled with periodic acid–Schiff (PAS)-positive glycogen granules. (Ch. 73; pg 1645)

88. c

The incidence of gallstones is increased in patients 2 to 3 times with extensive ileal resection. However, the explanation that the bile salt pool is depleted leading to supersaturation of bile with cholesterol may be too simplistic. Forty percent of patients with ileostomies have radiopaque calcium-containing stones. In addition, interruption of the enterohepatic circulation may predispose to pigment stones. (Ch. 77; pg 1711)

89. c

Calcium oxalate stones are formed in the setting of fat malabsorption when terminal ileal disease or resection inhibits bile-salt resorption. Fatty acids bind calcium in the lumen, which leaves oxalate, normally bound to calcium, free to enter the colon where it is absorbed and precipitated in the kidney. The colon is required to absorb the oxalate. (Ch. 81; pg 1789)

90. b

Neutrophils do not secrete immunoglobulin. (Ch. 81; pg 1781)

91. c

Olsalazine is composed of two 5-ASA moieties linked by an azo bond. This drug can elicit a secretory response from small bowel epithelium, resulting in watery diarrhea in 5% to 10% of treated patients. (Ch. 81; pg 1807)

92. b

Diarrhea is a clinical feature in nearly all patients with Crohn's disease. Perianal disease and bleeding occur more commonly in patients with Crohn's colitis and ileocolitis than in patients with isolated ileal disease.

Abdominal pain occurs in more than 50% of patients with disease at any site. (Ch. 81; pg 1785)

93. d

94. e

This is a case of Behçet syndrome, the clinical features of which have significant overlap with other disorders, particularly Crohn's disease. If the patient develops genital ulcers, hypopyon, and superficial thrombophlebitis, the possibility of Behçet syndrome should be considered. Involvement of the intestinal tract occurs in up to 10% of cases, and usually manifests as discrete ulcerations in the terminal ileum or the esophagus. Turkey and Japan have much higher incidences of this disorder than most western countries. In Turkey, this syndrome is associated with HLA-B51. A positive pathergy test is useful to establish this diagnosis. Small bowel biopsy may reveal granulomatous inflammation, and therefore is not particularly helpful in distinguishing Behçet syndrome from Crohn's disease. Histoplasmosis involving the gastrointestinal tract causes ulcers in the terminal ileum; the constellation of other symptoms that this patient develops renders this diagnosis less likely. Nonsteroidal antiinflammatory drug–induced small bowel ulcers manifest as diaphragm-like strictures and ulcers that can affect any part of the small bowel; the extraintestinal manifestations reduce the likelihood of this diagnosis. Whipple disease does not cause terminal ileal ulcerations. (Ch. 45; pg 997) (Ch. 79; pg 1744)

95. b

The most common cause of bacterial overgrowth is stasis, resulting from abnormal motility as occurs with scleroderma and amyloidosis, or prior surgery. Achlorhydria and immunodeficiency may be associated with bacterial overgrowth as a result of decreased bacterial clearance. Vitamin B_{12} deficiency may ensue due to competitive bacterial utilization. Malabsorption of vitamins A, D, and E may accompany steatorrhea, but gastrointestinal bacterial synthesis prevents vitamin K deficiency. All noninvasive tests for bacterial overgrowth suffer from variable sensitivity. Several tests can be used depending on the expertise of the institution. The only breath analysis test recommended by the Clinical Efficacy Committee of the American College of Physicians for the diagnosis of bacterial overgrowth is the ^{14}C-D-xylose breath test. A high level of breath glucose after oral ingestion of ^{14}C-D-xylose is consistent with the diagnosis. (Ch. 76; pg 1700)

96. b

Short bowel syndrome is the result of extensive small bowel resection. With the exception of celiac sprue, all the entities listed may be complicated by extensive small intestine resection. (Ch. 77; pg 1705)

97. a

This patient meets the Rome criteria for the diagnosis of irritable bowel syndrome: abdominal pain that is relieved with defecation and associated with altered bowel habits. The initial evaluation should focus on the patient's predominant symptoms. To evaluate for possible pain-predominant irritable bowel syndrome, plain abdominal radiography during a pain episode has been recommended to exclude intermittent bowel obstruction. When determining the aggressiveness of the diagnostic evaluation, the clinician should also consider the duration of symptoms, the change in symptoms over time, the age and sex of the patient, prior diagnostic studies, a family history of colorectal malignancy, and the degree of psychosocial dysfunction. Thus, a younger person with mild symptoms requires a minimal diagnostic evaluation, while an older person or an individual with rapidly progressive symptoms should undergo a more thorough evaluation to exclude organic disease. (Ch. 84; pg 1894)

98. b

For the treatment of irritable bowel syndrome (IBS), prokinetic agents have proven to be of limited benefit, even for those patients with constipation-predominant IBS. A high-fiber diet, antispasmotic and anticholinergic agents, as well as tricyclic antidepressant drugs are all reasonable therapeutic alternatives. (Ch. 84; pg 1896)

99. c

Irritable bowel syndrome (IBS) is not associated with an increased mortality rate. Symptoms usually persist over a long period. The quality of life for many patients with IBS can be enhanced by appropriate physician intervention. Male patients who exhibit an acute onset but short history of symptoms, a predominant symptom of constipation, and a good initial response to treatment are most likely to achieve long-term improvement. Also, patients who are included in detailed discussions about their diagnoses, psychological issues, precipitating factors, and treatments return fewer times to physicians. Education, counseling, and a judicious use of medications improve the outcomes for many patients with IBS. (Ch. 84; pg 1902)

100. b

Extraintestinal symptoms of irritable bowel syndrome (IBS) include chronic pelvic pain, symptoms of genitourinary dysfunction, impaired sexual function, and primary fibromyalgia. Hypertension and peptic ulcer disease also occur at a higher rate in patients with IBS. (Ch. 84; pg 1886)

101. c

Although the pathophysiology of irritable bowel syndrome (IBS) is poorly understood, abnormal colonic motor activity and heightened sensitivity to normal intestinal stimulation have been implicated. Small intestine motor patterns observed in IBS do not consistently correlate with abdominal symptoms and are not diagnostic. (Ch. 84; pg 1886)

102. d

Glucose and galactose influx occurs through the apical Na⁺-coupled glucose transporter SGLT1. SGLT1 is the only known Na⁺-coupled glucose transporter expressed in enterocytes. Data suggest that there is a differential expression of this transporter along the crypt-villus axis. (Ch. 75; pg 1677)

103. c

Infants expressing the glucose-galactose malabsorption (GGM) phenotype typically present with profuse watery diarrhea and hyperosmolar dehydration in the first week of life. The defect was initially thought to be caused by a single missense mutation in *SGLT1* resulting in asparagine rather than aspartate at position 28. However, genetic studies have demonstrated that there is more than one missense mutation responsible for this disorder. Glycosuria is often detected in these patients and may be present without hyperglycemia. (Ch. 75; pg 1678)

104. c

Menkes syndrome is a primary defect in copper transport. Infants may present with vomiting, diarrhea, and failure to thrive. The prognosis of Menkes syndrome is poor, secondary to cerebral degeneration that persists despite copper supplementation. (Ch. 75; pg 1680)

105. b

Omeprazole is reportedly of benefit in the treatment of congenital chloride diarrhea. Investigators have proposed that the inhibition of gastric chloride secretion reduces exposure of the distal bowel to unabsorbed chloride. In contrast, neither NaCl nor glucose can ameloriate the metabolic abnormalities seen in congenital chloride diarrhea, nor is there any evidence that histamine H₂ receptor blockade is of any benefit. (Ch. 75; pg 1682)

106. d

Both the mRNA for apolipoprotein B (apoB) and the apoB protein are expressed in the intestinal mucosa and liver of persons affected with abetalipoproteinemia. The defect resides in the protein complex, microsomal triglyceride transfer protein (MTP). Studies of patients with abetalipoproteinemia have shown that the assembly of apoB-containing lipoproteins is defective as a result of nonfunctional MTP. (Ch. 75; pg 1685)

107. a

The most likely cause of this man's discomfort is lactose intolerance. The disorder is very common in persons from Asia and Africa. It is characterized by intermittent symptoms that are exacerbated by the ingestion of lactose-containing food. The absence of bloody diarrhea, weight loss, fever, and metabolic abnormalities render the diagnosis of irritable bowel syndrome, amebiasis, or sprue less likely. (Ch. 75; pg 1689)

108. c

109. b

110. b

111. c

Clostridium botulinum, a gram-positive anaerobic bacterium, produces a neural toxin that blocks the release of acetylcholine at the neuromuscular junction. This bacterium produces heat-resistant spores that require anaerobic conditions and a pH higher than 4. The most common source of infection is home-canned foods of any kind. Symptoms of infection, including nausea, vomiting, abdominal pain, and diarrhea usually manifest 12 to 36 hours after ingestion of the preformed toxin. Neurologic symptoms include diplopia, dysphasia, dysarthria, dysphonia, ophthalmoplegia, descending bilateral weakness, and respiratory muscle weakness. *C botulinum* produces seven types of toxins (types A to G). Wound botulism is similar, without the gastrointestinal complications. Diagnosis is confirmed by symptoms and by the clinical assay of the vomitus, stool, or suspected food for the toxin. Treatment is supportive along with the administration of antitoxin. (Ch. 72; pg 1613)

112. a

Host factors associated with an increased risk of developing travelers' diarrhea include travel in an underdeveloped country, hypochlorhydria secondary to surgery or medication use, immunosuppression, and young age. (Ch. 72; pg 1614)

113. c

Nontyphoid salmonellosis is a foodborne infection that is caused by *Salmonella enteritidis* or *Salmonella typhimurium*. Risk of infection correlates with the number of ingested organisms and depends on predisposing host factors. The most important risk factor for this illness is a high gastric pH. In the intestine, the organisms interact with enterocytes and M cells and are transported to the submucosal lymphoid tissue by a process termed bacteria-mediated endocytosis. Infection does not cause epithelial damage. For the treatment of severe infections, a combination of two antibiotics from different classes is recommended until sensitivities are known. Possible agents include ampicillin, amoxicillin, trimethoprim-sulfamethoxazole, a cephalosporin, chloramphenicol, or a fluoroquinolone. (Ch. 72; pg 1621)

114. b

115. b

116. c

117. b

Whipple disease is caused by the bacterium *Tropheryma whippelii*. It occurs most often in the fifth and sixth decades of life and exhibits a male predominance (male:female, 8:1). Diarrhea affects 75% of patients. Weight loss is a common presenting symptom. Extraintestinal symptoms may precede the gastrointestinal symptoms by years. Migratory arthritis involving the large and small joints is the most common extraintestinal symptom; fever is second most common. Tropical sprue is associated with chronic diarrhea and malabsorption in patients from an endemic area; extraintestinal manifestations are not common. The diagnosis of Whipple disease is best made by small bowel biopsy, which demonstrates infiltration of the lamina propria with large foamy macrophages that grossly distort the normal villous architecture, giving the villi a blunted clublike appearance. Treatment is with one of several antibiotic regimens, including trimethoprim-sulfamethoxazole, penicillin, amoxicillin, or chloramphenicol for 1 year. (Ch. 73; pg 1641)

118. a

119. c

120. c

Celiac disease occurs as a consequence of sensitivity of the small bowel mucosa to gluten. There is a strong association with HLA-DQ2 antigen and high circulating levels of antigluten, antireticulum, and antiendomysial antibodies in untreated patients. Persons with celiac disease are at risk for lactose and sucrose intolerance and hyposplenism. Gluten-sensitive enteropathy is closely associated with dermatitis herpetiformis; 100% of patients with dermatitis herpetiformis have abnormal jejunal biopsies. Celiac disease is associated with an increased risk of small bowel lymphoma; the risk is significantly decreased if the patient adheres to a gluten-free diet. Persons with celiac disease are at increased risk for several other skin disorders including psoriasis, eczema, pustular dermatitis, cutaneous amyloid, cutaneous vasculitis, nodular prurigo, acquired ichthyosis, epidermal necrolysis, pityriasis rubra pilaris, and mycosis fungoides. (Ch. 74; pg 1660)

121. b

The histologic characteristics of celiac sprue include flattening of intestinal villi, loss of normal villous architecture, and a reduction in the normal ratio of villous height to crypt depth. The total thickness of the mucosa is increased because of crypt hyperplasia and cellular infiltration of the lamina propria with plasma cells and lymphocytes. The crypt mitotic activity is no longer confined to the base of the crypt, and the migration time of cells from the base of the crypt to the villus tip is shortened to 12 to 24 hours from a normal rate of 3 to 5 days. The ratio of intraepithelial lymphocytes to epithelial cells is also increased. (Ch. 74; pg 1661)

122. d

While a small bowel biopsy is mandatory to confirm or exclude a diagnosis of celiac sprue, the presence of antigliadin and antiendomysial antibodies has both positive and negative predictive values approaching 99%. There is a 15% prevalence of celiac sprue among first-degree relatives, and 10% of patients with celiac sprue have IgA deficiency. Complement deficiency is not associated with celiac sprue. (Ch. 74; pg 1665)

123. b

Hypoalbuminemia in a compliant patient with celiac sprue should heighten suspicion for a complication such as small bowel lymphoma or ulcerative jejunitis. Other possible causes of hypoalbuminemia in this include disaccharide deficiency, bacterial overgrowth, or the ingestion of foods thought to be gluten-free that in fact contain gluten. (Ch. 74; pg 1669)

124. b

Gluten shock is a rare event and occurs in patients who are rechallenged with gluten-containing foods. These patients develop nausea, vomiting, tachycardia, and cardiovascular collapse. Systemic corticosteroids are used in the treatment of this condition. Steroids can be used to treat moderate to severe celiac sprue, but they should not be a part of routine management. (Ch. 74; pg 1674)

True/False

125. false

126. false

127. true

128. true

Patients with deficiencies of immunoglobulins are susceptible to infections caused by encapsulated bacteria, enteric organisms, protozoa, and *Mycoplasma*. Common variable hypogammaglobulinemia most commonly presents with recurrent sinopulmonary infections, but may also be associated with giardiasis, jejunal villous atrophy, nodular lymphoid hyperplasia, and bacterial overgrowth. Achlorhydria is a common manifestation of most immunoglobulin deficiency syndromes. Achlorhydria and reductions in lumenal immunoglobulin secretion increase the risks of acquiring chronic *Salmonella, Shigella,* and *Campylobacter* infections. One-third of patients with common variable hypogammaglobulinemia develop atrophic gastritis and pernicious anemia, which confers an increased risk of gastric adenocarcinoma. In addition, there is an increased incidence of lymphomas in patients with common variable hypogammaglobulinemia. (Ch. 112; pg 2549)

129. true

130. false

131. true

132. false

Schistosoma mansoni primarily migrates within the superior mesenteric vein, and *Schistosoma japonicum* primarily migrates within the inferior mesenteric veins. Pipestem hepatic fibrosis is the classic histopathologic finding with schistosomiasis. Praziquantel is the drug of choice for the treatment of infection with all species of *Schistosoma*. (Ch. 109; pg 2455)

133. false

Perforation is a well-recognized risk of chemotherapy for lymphoma of the gastrointestinal tract. This risk can be minimized by resection of significant transmural disease prior to instituting chemotherapy. (Ch. 78; pg 1734)

134. true

For patients with mesenteric arterial occlusion, a second-look operation is rarely required. With venous occlusion however, the progression of thrombosis postoperatively is insidious and often can only be detected by a second-look procedure. (Ch. 114; pg 2600)

135. true

Malrotation usually presents within the first month of life as proximal small bowel obstruction. (Ch. 80; pg 1770)

136. false

137. false

138. true

139. true

Arterial mesenteric emboli most frequently originate from the heart and are associated with a 50% to 90% mortality rate. Mesenteric arterial thrombosis often occurs at the site of atherosclerotic lesions and may first present during a low-flow state. Typically, at least 2 of the 3 major vessels (i.e., inferior mesenteric artery, superior mesenteric artery, celiac artery) must be involved for mesenteric ischemia to occur. (Ch. 114; pg 2593)

140. false

141. true

142. true

143. false

Patients with intestinal angina or chronic mesenteric ischemia classically present with the triad of intermittent postprandial pain, weight loss, and sitophobia. Physical examination of the abdomen during an attack typically reveals hyperperistalsis with increased bowel sounds. Most patients do not develop acute small bowel infarction, but surgical management may be necessary to alleviate pain. In general, this condition does not respond well to anticoagulant therapy. (Ch. 114; pg 2599)

144. false

In patients with unexplained weight loss for which an etiology cannot be found despite an extensive evaluation, the long-term prognosis is good with little risk of development of an unsuspected disease. (Ch. 34; pg 765)

145. false

The appendix is the most common site for the development of carcinoid tumors (approximately 70%); however, appendiceal carcinoid tumors very rarely metastasize. The ileum is the most common site of metastatic carcinoid tumors. (Ch. 78; pg 1731)

146. true

Most small intestine adenomas are located in the second part of the duodenum. This applies to sporadic adenomas as well as those in patients with familial adenomatous polyposis coli. (Ch. 78; pg 1728)

147. false

Patients with celiac sprue are at increased risk primarily for lymphoma, but they also develop adenocarcinoma of the esophagus, mouth, pharynx, and small intestine at increased rates compared to the general population. (Ch. 74; pg 1672)

148. false

This is a typical presentation of ulcerative jejunoileitis, a serious complication of celiac sprue that is characterized by small bowel ulcerations and strictures. Strictures are uncommon in celiac sprue, refractory sprue, and lymphoma. Ulcerative jejunoileitis is often refractory to a gluten-free diet as well as to corticosteroids and has a high mortality rate. (Ch. 74; pg 1672)

149. true

This lesion is consistent with collagenous sprue. This condition may complicate celiac sprue and typically presents as a flare of symptoms despite compliance with a gluten-free diet. Patients with this complication often do not respond to a gluten-free diet or to corticosteroids. (Ch. 74; pg 1673)

150. true

151. true

152. true

Mechanisms for intestinal adaptation after extensive small intestine resection include stimulatory and trophic effects of dietary nutrients, polyamines, pancreatic and biliary secretions, hormones, neural factors, and increased blood flow. (Ch. 77; pg 1707)

153. true

The small intestine mucosa possesses great metabolic requirements and is very susceptible to ischemic damage. Loss of mucosal integrity can rapidly lead to hemorrhage and translocation of gut bacteria. (Ch. 114; pg 2587)

154. true

Mucosal disease is often caused by an inflammatory process with a release of inflammatory mediators, particularly cytokines, which contribute to the systemic symptoms mentioned. In contrast, these factors are often not increased by pancreatic disease. (Ch. 40; pg 885)

155. false

Myosin light chain is phosphorylated by myosin light chain kinase. The phosphorylation of myosin light chain induces a conformational change in the myosin head that enhances actin-stimulated ATP hydrolysis. Myosin light chain phosphatase catalyzes the dephosphorylation of the myosin light chains. (Ch. 5; pg 84)

156. true

Calcium is needed for the contraction of gastrointestinal smooth muscle. One mechanism involves the interaction of a contractile agonist with a plasma membrane receptor that initiates the opening of agonist- or voltage-gated calcium channels. The other major mechanism involves interaction with a plasma membrane receptor that generates inositol trisphosphate from the hydrolysis of membrane phospholipids. Inositol trisphosphate then evokes the release of calcium from intracellular stores. (Ch. 5; pg 90)

157. true

The membrane potential is largely determined by the Na^+,K^+-ATPase pump, which sets up diffusion gradients for Na^+ and K^+ across the membrane. The permeability of the membrane to K^+ is greater than that to Na^+, and the flow of K^+ ions down their electrochemical gradient creates a diffusion potential that is the major contributor to the resting membrane potential. (Ch. 5; pg 91)

158. false

The human intestinal slow wave frequency decreases from 11 to 12 cpm in the duodenum to 7 to 8 cpm in the distal ileum. (Ch. 11; pg 217)

159. true

The interstitial cells of Cajal are a distinctive population of fibroblast-like stellate cells that make contact with muscle cells and nerve terminals. The interstitial cells of Cajal generate wave-like depolarizations analogous to the slow wave in gastrointestinal smooth muscle. (Ch. 2; pg 27)

160. false

The gap junction provides a pathway for close electrical coupling of adjacent gastrointestinal smooth muscle cells. However, the nexus is a characteristic of circular smooth muscle. Few or no nexuses are found in the longitudinal layer. (Ch. 5; pg 83)

161. true

Motilin is synthesized in the duodenal and jejunal mucosa. Peak plasma motilin levels occur immediately before the initiation of endogenous phase III activity. An exogenous motilin infusion induces premature phase III activity beginning in the stomach. The administration of motilin antiserum interrupts phase III cycling in the proximal gut. (Ch. 11; pg 222)

162. true

The ileocecal sphincter maintains a region of high pressure to delay the passage of ileal contents into the colon. Nonadrenergic noncholinergic inhibitory neurons mediate relaxation of the sphincter. Distention of the ileum relaxes and distention of the proximal colon increases the ileocecal sphincter pressure. (Ch. 11; pg 235)

163. true

Chronic intestinal pseudoobstruction from paraneoplastic visceral neuropathy has been most commonly reported in oat cell carcinoma of the lung. Epidermoid carcinoma of the lip has also been reported. Histologic examination of the myenteric plexus shows widespread neuronal and axonal degeneration. (Ch. 71; pg 1596)

164. false

Constipation is the most common reported symptom in diabetes mellitus–related gastrointestinal dysmotility, occurring in 60% of patients. Diarrhea (22%) and steatorrhea (10%) occur less commonly. (Ch. 41; pg 911) (Ch. 111; pg 2513)

165. true

Gastrointestinal symptoms, including abdominal distention, pain, diarrhea, constipation, nausea, and bloating may precede the development of sclerodactyly, the Raynaud phenomenon, or arthritis in patients with scleroderma. (Ch. 111; pg 2509)

166. false

Intestinal pseudoobstruction in the setting of hypoparathyroidism is thought to be related to hypocalcemia. The administration of calcium improves gastrointestinal symptoms in these patients. (Ch. 71; pg 1598)

167. true

The ability of B cells to alter their immunoglobulin production from IgM to IgA is a relatively unique mechanism in the immune system and is mediated by "switch" T lymphocytes within Peyer patches. (Ch. 6; pg 116)

168. true

Lymphoblasts recirculate or home to the sites of original antigenic stimulation as well as other mucosal secretory sites (e.g., breast, lung, eye) and mature into plasma cells that produce IgA. (Ch. 6; pg 115)

169. false

The removal of IgA-antigen complexes from the bloodstream by the liver may provide a protective mechanism against absorbed substances, including dietary antigens and bacterial products. (Ch. 6; pg 117)

170. false

Intestinal lamina propria lymphocytes, which are predominantly CD4 helper T lymphocytes, do not play a significant role in cell-mediated cytotoxicity. (Ch. 6; pg 117)

171. true

Enterovirus, reovirus, human immunodeficiency virus, and some bacteria (e.g., *Salmonella* species) gain access to the host after transport of the organism by M cells to Peyer patches. (Ch. 6; pg 115)

172. false

Although small amounts of submucosal tissue may occasionally be obtained, endoscopic biopsy rarely collects tissues deeper than the muscularis mucosa. (Ch. 120; pg 2672)

173. true

In addition to differentiation, the basement membrane can exert significant effects on the proliferation, adhesion, and migration of epithelial cells and may contribute to the barrier function of the gut as well. (Ch. 8; pg 146)

174. true

Although protein loss from the gut is nonselective, the synthetic rate of IgG is slower than that of IgA or IgM; thus, serum IgG levels will be reduced to a greater extent than the other immunoglobulin subtypes. It should also be noted that hypogammaglobulinemia attributed to protein-losing enteropathy is always associated with hypoalbuminemia. (Ch. 79; pg 1752)

175. false

The duodenum and jejunum are often sterile but can contain up to 100 colony-forming units per milliliter in healthy individuals. *Streptococci, Lactobacilli, Staphylococci*, and yeast are the predominant organisms. (Ch. 27; pg 625)

176. false

Gram-positive aerobic organisms resembling oropharyngeal flora are found in the proximal intestine, presumably delivered by the swallowing of salivary secretions and food. When bacterial overgrowth occurs, this flora is replaced by gram-negative bacteria, including facultative anaerobes such as *Escherichia coli*. In addition, there often is a predominance of strictly anaerobic bacteria such as *Clostridium* and *Bacteroides* species. (Ch. 27; pg 625)

177. true

A cutoff value of 10^5 colony-forming units per milliliter is used by many investigators for the diagnosis of small bowel bacterial overgrowth. The types of organisms are also important, with the presence of strict anaerobes, such as *Bacteroides fragilis*, confirming the diagnosis of bacterial overgrowth. (Ch. 76; pg 1701)

178. false

The Auerbach plexus, also known as the myenteric plexus, resides between the circular and longitudinal muscle layers in the small intestine. (Ch. 2; pg 14)

179. true

The vast majority of neuronal fibers carried within the vagus are afferent, rather than efferent. (Ch. 10; pg 189)

180. true

The pH at the surface microvillus border of the enterocyte is less than that of the intralumenal contents. Weak acids usually must be in their nonpolar (i.e., associated) form in order to traverse the enterocyte apical membrane and be absorbed. The acid microclimate promotes this process by increasing the fraction of the weak acid in the associated state. Thus, if this acid microclimate were abolished, weak acids such as folic acid would be less efficiently absorbed. (Ch. 26; pg 613)

181. false

In most cases, endogenous regulatory peptide hormones or neurotransmitters bind to and activate receptors on the basolateral membrane. (Ch. 3; pg 44)

182. true

Multiple biopsies and appropriate biopsy orientation aid in the histologic evaluation of tissue from persons with suspected celiac sprue. (Ch. 74; pg 1670) (Ch. 124; pg 2772)

183. false

Vibrio cholerae contaminates brackish water. Water and food are the major vehicles of transmission. Patients who recover from infection have long-lasting immunity. (Ch. 72; pg 1625)

184. true

Vibrio parahaemolyticus is a salt-loving vibrio that contaminates raw or improperly stored (after cooking) fish, shellfish and crustaceans. It is a common cause of bacterial diarrhea in Japan. It causes a spectrum of diarrheal illnesses, ranging from a mild diarrhea to a dysentery-like syndrome. (Ch. 72; pg 1626)

Matching

185. a

186. b

187. c

188. b

Small intestine obstruction is characterized by periodic crampy midabdominal pain, progressive nausea and emesis, and obstipation. A perforated duodenal ulcer, on the other hand, is usually marked by the sudden and severe onset of epigastric pain followed by more diffuse pain as peritonitis develops. A perforated duodenal ulcer may be associated with pneumoperitoneum. If this is absent, the diagnosis can be made by water-soluble contrast radiography. Pneumoperitoneum only occurs with small intestine obstruction if infarction has occurred. Both of these conditions are usually treated surgically, although a perforated duodenal ulcer may be managed medically in unusual circumstances. (Ch. 38; pg 832)

189. c

190. d

191. a

192. b

Cryptosporidiosis primarily involves the small intestine, with or without mild colonic involvement, and is associated with prolonged diarrhea and wasting in AIDS patients. Infection can extend to the bile ducts and gallbladder, causing cholecystitis and cholangitis. Treatment to date has been disappointing. Microsporida infections resemble cryptosporidiosis both clinically and microscopically. A diagnostic clue is the presence of a globular inclusion, the meront inclusion, in the supranuclear region of the epithelial cells, which produces a characteristic "cat's-eye" appearance on histologic examination. Isosporiasis is sensitive to antimicrobial therapy with pyrimethamine and

sulfadiazine or trimethoprim-sulfamethoxazole. Intestinal infections with *Salmonella* in AIDS patients are associated with bacteremia and a chronic relapsing course. (Ch. 107; pg 2406)

193. c

194. a

195. b

196. d

Histologically, cytomegalovirus infection is characterized by intranuclear inclusions, often surrounded by halos. Herpes simplex virus produces painful, chronic, shallow perineal ulcers. Latent Epstein-Barr virus (EBV) found in lymphomas of patients with AIDS suggests that the tumor may result from an outgrowth of EBV-transformed mucosal B cells. *Mycobacterium avium* complex (MAC) infection may cause massive thickening of the proximal small intestine, which is readily identified on a small bowel radiographic study. The pathophysiology of MAC is similar to Whipple disease in that intestinal thickening results from an infiltration of the lamina propria with macrophages and intramucosal blockage to lymphatic outflow. These abnormalities may lead to malabsorption and an exudative enteropathy. (Ch. 107; pgs 2408, 2411, 2414)

197. b

198. c

199. a

Achalasia with megaesophagus is a characteristic feature of *Trypanosoma cruzi* infection (i.e., Chagas disease), which can also cause megaduodenum, megacolon, megarectum, and megaureter. *Giardia lamblia* prefers to colonize the upper small intestine and is typically noninvasive. *Isospora belli* can be identified intracellularly on small intestine biopsy specimens. *I belli* oocysts can be identified in stool samples by using Kinyoun acid-fast stain. (Ch. 108; pgs 2429, 2436)

200. c

201. d

202. e

203. a

204. b

An ameboma from infection with *Entamoeba histolytica* may present as a manifestation of amebic colitis. This segmented collection of granulation tissue in the cecum or ascending colon may present as a tender, palpable abdominal mass. No effective medical therapy is available to treat cryptosporidiosis. In contrast, *Isospora belli* infection is responsive to trimethoprim-sulfamethoxazole, although prolonged or repeated courses of therapy may be required in patients with acquired immunodeficiency syndrome. *Endolimax nana* is a nonpathogenic enteric ameba. Trophozoite forms can be distinguished from *E histolytica* on the basis of size and motility. Although an examination of stool by microscopy is often diagnostic, duodenal aspiration and biopsy may be required for the diagnosis of giardiasis. (Ch. 108; pgs 2423, 2429, 2436)

205. d

206. a

207. b

208. c

Anisakiasis is caused by members of the family Anisakidae, which are pathogens of fish, including cod, herring, salmon, mackerel, Pacific pollock, Pacific red snapper, and squid. Anisakiasis occurs after eating raw or inadequately cooked fish and is relatively common in Japan and Europe. *Taenia saginata* (beef tapeworm) infection produces cysticercosis, which develops when the larvae invade the intestinal wall and disseminate, forming cysticerci in the brain and subcutaneous tissues. *Diphyllobothrium latum* (fish tapeworm) infection produces macrocytic anemia as a result of its successful competition with the human host for vitamin B_{12}. Echinococcosis is associated with production of hydatid cysts, most of which (about 66%) develop in the liver. Other locations of echinococcal cysts include the lung (20%), bone, brain, muscle, eye, and heart. Leakage of cyst contents can produce anaphylaxis or peritoneal seeding of the infection. (Ch. 109; pgs 2451, 2453)

209. c

210. e

211. d

212. b

213. a

Rotavirus is a common cause of diarrheal illness in young children. *Yersinia enterocolitica* infection of the ileum and cecum may produce a clinical picture indistinguishable from appendicitis. *Vibrio cholerae* produces cholera toxin, a potent diarrheogenic toxin that activates enterocyte adenylate cyclase. Certain shellfish contain a toxin that induces paralytic complications when ingested. *Campylobacter* infections can be complicated by the development of pseudomembranous colitis. (Ch. 72; pgs 1614, 1619, 1622, 1625) (Ch. 84; pgs 1894, 1897)

214. e

215. b

216. a

The stool osmotic gap is quantitated by subtracting $2 \times [Na^+ + K^+]$ from the measured stool osmolality. A

secretory diarrhea results from the excretion of electrolytes into the bowel; thus, most of the osmotic activity should be accounted for in the measured stool electrolytes, and the gap should be small. In an osmotic diarrhea, the diarrhea is the result of osmotically active particles other than secreted electrolytes and the calculated osmotic gap will therefore be large. Osmotic gaps between 40 and 100 mOsm have been used to distinguish an osmotic diarrhea from a secretory diarrhea. The measured stool osmolality should always be approximately equivalent to the serum osmolarity (280–330 mOsm). If a measured stool osmolality is significantly less than serum osmolality, contamination of the stool with water or dilute urine should be suspected. If the osmolality of fresh stool is significantly elevated, contamination of the specimen with concentrated urine should be suspected. (Ch. 40; pg 895)

217. a

218. c

219. b

220. b

Laxatives work by inducing either a secretory or an osmotic diarrhea. Castor oil induces a secretory diarrhea, whereas magnesium sulfate causes an osmotic diarrhea. Often diarrheas do not fit neatly into either category, because pathophysiologic mechanisms of each are operative. Diarrhea with celiac sprue is the result of the osmotic effects caused by the maldigestion of fats and the malabsorption of carbohydrates. In addition, there is net secretion in the small intestine as a result of the loss of villi, secretion in the colon resulting from malabsorption of fat, and production of hydroxylated fatty acids, which stimulate secretion by colonic epithelial cells. The fact that 90% of Asians are lactase-deficient must be a consideration in individuals with new-onset diarrhea who may have recently altered their diet. (Ch. 40; pg 864)

221. a

222. a

223. b

224. c

225. b

Intestinal secretion can be regulated by a number of endogenous and exogenous substances, each by different intracellular mediators. Cholera toxin causes an irreversible activation of the Gs protein by ADP ribosylation, resulting in the prolonged activation of adenylate cyclase and elevated cAMP levels. Vasoactive intestinal polypeptide also uses cAMP as its second messenger. Acetylcholine and histamine act through inositol trisphosphate–induced increases in intracellular calcium levels. The receptor for the

Escherichia coli heat-stable enterotoxin (ST$_a$) is a membrane-bound guanylyl cyclase. Upon binding, increased cGMP levels produce a secretory response. (Ch. 15; pg 340)

226. a
227. b
228. a
229. b
230. a
231. b

Dopamine, somatostatin, and glucocorticoids stimulate small intestine absorption, whereas calcitonin, substance P, and motilin cause secretion by the small intestine. (Ch. 15; pg 340)

232. c
233. d
234. a
235. b

Scleroderma is a connective tissue disease of unknown etiology. The most common gastrointestinal motor abnormalities encountered in scleroderma are dysmotility of the lower two-thirds of the esophagus and reduction of the lower esophageal sphincter pressure. This is consistent with the preferential involvement of gastrointestinal smooth muscle with scleroderma. In contrast, dermatomyositis preferentially affects skeletal muscle. For this reason, it typically causes dilation and/or dysmotility involving the proximal esophagus. Vasculitis associated with systemic lupus erythematosus can lead to small intestine ischemia. The gastrointestinal sequelae of diabetes mellitus are thought to be the consequence of autonomic neuropathy. The most common gastrointestinal manifestation of diabetes is constipation, but other problems include gastroparesis, small intestine dysmotility, low resting internal anal sphincter tone, and external anal sphincter incompetence. (Ch. 111; pg 2509)

236. b
237. c
238. d
239. a

Fat-soluble vitamin deficiency is sometimes seen in conjunction with bacterial overgrowth, most likely resulting from bile-salt deconjugation by intestinal bacteria. Lactase activity as well as the activities of other brush-border disaccharidases are decreased in the setting of bacterial overgrowth. There is evidence that anaerobic organisms produce proteases and glycosidases that release or destroy hydrolases on the brush border. Vitamin B$_{12}$ deficiency is most likely attribut-

able to the presence of intestinal anaerobes, which utilize vitamin B$_{12}$, either in the free form or when complexed with intrinsic factor. Not only do bacteria compete for the utilization of vitamin B$_{12}$, but they also produce inactive metabolites, which compete with vitamin B$_{12}$ for absorption. A rare complication of prolonged bacterial overgrowth is hepatobiliary injury. The pathogenesis of this problem remains obscure, but possible explanations include a toxin effect of bacterial cell wall polymers or other bacterial toxins in the setting of a genetically susceptible individual. Excessive flatus is a common complaint in patients with bacterial overgrowth and results from bacterial fermentation of ingested carbohydrates. (Ch. 76; pg 1700)

240. b
241. a
242. c

Some small intestine tumors exhibit characteristic arteriographic features. Leiomyomas are hypervascular and have a dense, well-circumscribed blush. Arterial tortuosity and narrowing draw carcinoid tumors into a stellate pattern. Adenocarcinomas are usually seen as hypovascular masses with arteries that are occluded or encased. (Ch. 141; pg 3111)

243. b
244. c
245. a

Salmonella species can be treated with ceftriaxone or ciprofloxacin. As for nonimmunocompromised patients, *Clostridium difficile* can be treated with metronidazole or vancomycin. A combination of rifabutin, ethambutol and clarithromycin was shown to decrease symptoms and increase survival in HIV-infected patients with *Mycobacterium avium* infection. (Ch. 107, pg 2403)

246. b

Immunoproliferative small bowel disease is more common in developing parts of the world such as South America and the Middle East. It is characterized by diffuse tumor infiltration involving long segments of the proximal small bowel. Its manifestations improve with the administration of antibiotics such as tetracycline, particularly if the regimen is started early in the prelymphomatous stage. (Ch. 78, pg 1733)

247. d

Persons with common variable immunodeficiency may develop diffuse nodular hyperplasia, infection with *Giardia lamblia*, and occasionally, small bowel lymphomas. Other conditions that predispose to small bowel lymphoma include celiac sprue and HIV infection. (Ch. 78; pg 1734)

248. c

Patients with familial adenomatous polyposis have an increased incidence of proximal small intestine adenomas and adenocarcinomas; these tumors can be peri-ampullary and present with obstructive jaundice. (Ch. 78; pg 1728)

249. a

250. c

251. b

252. d

253. c

Familial visceral neuropathies are a group of diseases characterized by degeneration of the myenteric plexus. Specific abnormalities include a reduced number of argyrophilic neurons and nerve fibers. (Ch. 71; pg 1589, Table 71.3)

254. c

255. b

256. d

257. a

Budesonide is a potent corticosteroid that undergoes first-pass hepatic metabolism, limiting its systemic toxicity. Budesonide is formulated in such a way as to allow delivery of the active drug to the terminal ileum and proximal colon. Azathioprine and 6-mercaptopurine are immunomodulators that are useful in treating steroid-resistant patients or as an alternative treatment for steroid-dependent patients. Leukopenia, pancreatitis, and a possible increase in lymphoma with long-term use are the most serious side effects with azathioprine and 6-mercaptopurine. Recent studies suggest that methotrexate is of limited value in the treatment of Crohn's disease. Infliximab is a chimeric anti–tumor necrosis factor-α antibody that has proven to be effective in treating patients with Crohn's disease who are steroid-resistant or who have refractory fistulous disease. (Ch. 81; pg 1811)

CHAPTER 4

Multiple Choice

1. c

   Although colonic transit can be measured by newer scintigraphic methods, standard colonic transit testing is performed using inert radiopaque markers and routine abdominal radiographs. When the test reveals slow transit, it generally allows division into two groups: one with diffuse slowing throughout the colon consistent with colonic inertia and one with slowing predominantly in the rectosigmoid colon consistent with a functional outlet obstruction. When the colonic transit test shows normal transit in a patient who complains of constipation, there may be significant psychologic or behavorial dysfunction. The study should be performed during ingestion of a 20- to 30-g/day high-fiber diet with discontinuation of all laxatives, enemas, or medications that can affect bowel function. Patients with mild to moderate symptoms and daily stools are less likely to benefit from the results of colonic transit testing than those with complaints of infrequent stools. (Ch. 41; pg 916)

2. a

   Rheumatoid arthritis and systemic lupus erythematosus are less likely to be associated with constipation than the other choices. (Ch. 41; pg 911)

3. a

   This patient has evidence of a functional outlet obstruction on colonic transit testing and a moderately large rectocele on defecography. In this case, the rectocele is large, and the patient clearly has an improvement in rectal expulsion when the rectocele is manually reduced. Surgery is indicated because medical therapy has not proven beneficial. Constipation biofeedback would not be helpful because there has been no evidence of paradoxical contraction of the puborectalis muscle during defecation. A subtotal colectomy would be indicated in a patient with severe colonic inertia, not functional outlet obstruction. Limited resection of the colon usually produces unsatisfactory results with high rates of anastomotic leaks. Division of the puborectalis muscle is usually not useful, and fecal incontinence may result. (Ch. 41; pg 922)

4. b

   It is important that a structural lesion of the colon such as colon cancer or diverticular stricture be excluded in any elderly patient complaining of new-onset constipation, even in the absence of occult bleeding or weight loss. Colonic transit testing, defecography, and anorectal manometry can be performed after structural lesions and other causes of constipation have been ruled out if symptoms persist despite a reasonable trial of medical therapy. (Ch. 41; pg 916)

5. e

   The interdigestive migrating motor complex is a stereotypical pattern that propagates from the stomach to the terminal ileum and is not present in the human colon. Short-duration contractions are associated with colonic slow waves, whereas long-duration contractions are believed to represent contractions resulting from periodic bursts of fast electrical oscillations. (Ch. 11; pg 226) (Ch. 85; pg 1911)

6. b

   The gastrocolonic response is defined as a feeding-induced increase in motor activity of the colon. Although the mechanism for the gastrocolonic response is uncertain, it appears to be cholinergically mediated, because it is markedly reduced by atropine. Although cholecystokinin (CCK) can induce colonic motility, the gastrocolonic response observed after a meal is not prevented by CCK receptor antagonism; therefore, this hormone probably does not play a physiologic role in the response. Colonic motor responses to eating can persist following a gastrectomy. (Ch. 85; pg 1911)

7. b

   The predominant direction of contraction in the right colon is antiperistaltic and in the left colon is peristaltic. The internal anal sphincter is tonically contracted most of the time, relaxing just before and during defecation. Although haustral markings were once considered to be fixed structures, they are now known to be transient and presumably represent tonic circular contractions in the colon. (Ch. 11; pgs 216, 235)

8. c

   The largest component of resting anal canal tone is determined by the tonically contracted internal anal sphincter muscle. However, when the continence mechanisms are stressed during periods of increased abdominal pressure, the external sphincter contracts and plays the key role in maintaining continence. The acuity of the anorectal angle, which is determined by puborectalis muscular contraction, helps to maintain fecal continence. Chronic constipation can cause fecal incontinence as a result of chronic stretch injury to nerves that control the sphincter musculature. Even during fecal impaction, loose stool can seep around the distended rectum, resulting in over-flow fecal incontinence. (Ch. 91; pg 2094)

9. a

   The symptoms described are typical for proctalgia fugax. Coccygodynia refers to pain in the coccyx, which can be reproduced by manipulation of the coccyx. The pain of anal fissure disease usually occurs during defecation, and the fissure should be visible during anorectal examination. The levator ani syndrome refers to an aching rectal pain that is more chronic in nature than proctalgia fugax, lasts longer, and is more typically seen in middle-aged women. (Ch. 91; pg 2101)

10. c

This is a presentation of complete rectal prolapse. It can be distinguished from prolapsing internal hemorrhoids by appearance alone. All layers of the rectum are palpable and visibly protrude through the anus as concentric mucosal folds. Solitary rectal ulcer syndrome is characterized by internal intussusception of rectal tissue, and may be present in a patient with complete rectal prolapse. Definitive surgical management involves replacement of the rectum into the sacral hollow with or without resection of the redundant rectosigmoid colon. (Ch. 91; pg 2091)

11. d

This patient has the classic signs of an anorectal abscess. Antecedent history may reveal a bout of constipation, diarrhea, or minor anal trauma. Anorectal abscesses are commonly caused by infection of the anal glands. The most common bacterial isolates are gram-negative enteric organisms. Crohn's disease is a possibility, but the vast majority of patients with anorectal abscess do not have inflammatory bowel disease. (Ch. 91; pg 2088)

12. e

This patient has suffered a traumatic sphincter injury at the time of episiotomy. Because symptoms clearly occurred immediately after the injury and there is no reason to suspect inflammatory or other bowel diseases, there is no reason to perform a flexible sigmoidoscopy. Anal sensory testing is a research tool and is not likely to be helpful in this case. Anorectal manometry with biofeedback therapy would give marginal if any benefit, given the anatomic defect present. This patient clearly needs surgical repair of the injured sphincter muscle. (Ch. 91; pg 2096)

13. b

This is a typical presentation of the levator ani syndrome. The pain is more of a chronic ache compared with the pain of proctalgia fugax. The key diagnostic finding is palpable tenderness and spasm of the levator ani muscle during digital rectal examination. Treatment includes local heat, smooth muscle relaxants, and digital rectal massage. Electrogalvanic stimulation is sometimes helpful. Antiinflammatory drugs and surgery have no proven efficacy. (Ch. 91; pg 2101)

14. e

Anal carcinoma is discovered late in more than 60% of cases because of the mild and nonspecific nature of the presenting symptoms. (Ch. 91; pg 2100)

15. a

Most anal fissures are in the midline; thus, a laterally located fissure should prompt a search for underlying diseases such as Crohn's disease. Patients with anal fissures exhibit an exaggerated overshoot contraction component of the rectoanal inhibitory reflex. Posterior midline sphincterotomy and manual anal dilation are associated with high incidences of postoperative complications. Primary fissures are located in the posterior midline more than 90% of the time. (Ch. 91; pg 2092)

16. c

The most common bacterial isolates from anorectal abscesses are *Escherichia coli, Enterococcus* species, and *Bacteroides fragilis.* (Ch. 91; pg 2089)

17. d

Acute appendicitis is a clinical diagnosis supported by carefully selected laboratory and radiographic studies. Abdominal ultrasonography may be helpful in ambiguous cases. Perforation should be suspected if symptoms have been present for more than 24 hours, if the temperature exceeds 38°C, or if the leukocyte count exceeds 15,000/mm^3. The prognosis is related to age; mortality rates are higher in patients older than 50 years. Appendiceal abscesses can be treated either operatively or nonoperatively, depending on the clinical setting. Some surgeons favor a nonsurgical approach initially, draining the fluid percutaneously and treating the patient with parenteral antibiotics. (Ch. 38; pg 831)

18. a

The most common gastrointestinal symptoms resulting from endometriosis include rectal pain, constipation, and painful defecation. Gastrointestinal involvement occurs in as many as 37% of women with documented pelvic endometriosis. Colonoscopy may be useful in excluding malignancy and in diagnosing the rare instance of mucosal endometriosis resulting in hematochezia, but in general, an evaluation for intestinal tract endometriosis is usually nondiagnostic. (Ch. 83; pg 1862)

19. b

By definition, acute colonic pseudoobstruction is never caused by a mechanical obstruction. The condition is usually precipitated by metabolic disturbances, medications, or other stresses in a patient with serious underlying medical illness. High mortality rates in these patients result from the underlying medical illnesses, not colonic perforation. An urgent decompressive colonoscopy should be performed if conservative measures such as nasogastric suction and correction of metabolic disturbances fail. A cecal size of 9 cm or larger is thought to be associated with an increased risk of cecal ischemia, and decompressive colonoscopy should be considered. If other measures fail, surgical decompression can be achieved by tube cecostomy. (Ch. 85; pg 1919)

20. d

This patient probably has sigmoid volvulus, given the association with Parkinson disease and a classic abdominal radiograph. In patients without peritoneal signs, flexible sigmoidoscopy with detorsion can be curative. However, because of the suggestion of peritonitis in this patient, emergent surgery is indicated. Barium studies are usually not therapeutic as they can be with intussusception and are contraindicated because of the peritoneal signs. (Ch. 80; pg 1772)

21. d

Colonoscopy and barium enema radiography are contraindicated in severe ulcerative colitis, because colonic distention can further limit blood supply and force lumenal contents and bacteria into the thin, ulcerated colonic wall. Antidiarrheals, opiates, and anticholinergics are all risk factors for the development of toxic megacolon. (Ch. 81; pg 1821)

22. c

This clinical presentation is most consistent with sclerosing cholangitis. Only 1% to 4% of patients with ulcerative colitis develop sclerosing cholangitis, but the majority of patients with sclerosing cholangitis have chronic ulcerative colitis. Colonoscopy should be performed despite the absence of intestinal symptoms. (Ch. 81; pg 1788)

23. c

Distal ulcerative colitis can recur following the discontinuation of 5-aminosalicylic acid enemas. To prevent recurrent disease, enemas should be gradually tapered. The administration of an oral 5-aminosalicylic acid preparation instead of enemas may also be appropriate. (Ch. 81; pg 1814)

24. b

Obliterative endarteritis with chronic radiation injury to the colon leads to tissue ischemia with fibrosis and possible ulceration and fissure formation. Acute symptomatic radiation injury does not appear to predispose to chronic injury. (Ch. 115; pg 2611)

25. a

There is little evidence of fertility problems with ulcerative colitis; however, studies suggest that women with Crohn's disease have a slightly increased rate of infertility that may be closely related to disease activity and nutritional status. Total parenteral nutrition by itself has not been shown to be detrimental to the fetus. Steroids have been widely used for many diseases during pregnancy and have not been shown to increase the risk of fetal abnormalities. (Ch. 81; pg 1830)

26. e

Although chronic watery diarrhea is characteristic, nocturnal symptoms and fecal incontinence can also occur with collagenous colitis. The normal intraepithelial lymphocyte ratio of 1:20 lymphocytes to epithelial cells is increased to 1:5 in lymphocytic colitis. The subepithelial collagen band, which is normally 4 μm in thickness, increases to greater than 10 to 15 μm in a patchy distribution. The collagen bands are most prevalent in the cecum and transverse colon and are less likely to be found in the rectum. (Ch. 83; pg 1857)

27. d

Both diseases commonly exhibit inflammatory cell infiltration of the lamina propria. The prominence of intraepithelial lymphocytes has led to use of the term lymphocytic rather than microscopic colitis. A prominent subepithelial collagen band larger than 10 to 15 μm in diameter is abnormal and is responsible for the term collagenous colitis. (Ch. 83; pg 1858)

28. a

This is a characteristic presentation of collagenous colitis. In some patients, the disease will spontaneously resolve or respond to antidiarrheals. Case reports describe responses to a variety of therapies, but sulfasalazine or 5-aminosalicylic acid or bismuth are the drugs of choice. In refractory cases, oral corticosteroids are the next line of therapy. (Ch. 83; pg 1860)

29. c

Fifteen percent of patients with inflammatory bowel disease (IBD) have a first-degree relative with IBD. The risk of developing ulcerative colitis (UC) is decreased among smokers, and the incidence of smoking among patients with Crohn's disease is as high or higher than the general population. Patients with IBD have an increased incidence of antibodies to cow's milk protein. A person with a first-degree relative with Crohn's disease has a higher risk of developing UC compared with the general population. Although the antineutrophil cytoplasmic antibody is present in 70% of patients with UC, there is no correlation with disease extent or activity. (Ch. 81; pg 1776)

30. a

Older patients are more likely than younger ones to experience prolonged periods without a relapse of symptoms. For patients younger than 50 years, the median time for relapse after the first attack is 2 to 3 years. Patients in the oldest age group are the least likely to suffer a relapse and the least likely to require bowel resection. (Ch. 81; pg 1784)

31. c

Backwash ileitis occurs in 15% to 20% of patients with ulcerative pancolitis. Terminal ileal involvement in Crohn's disease, in contrast, is characterized by lumenal narrowing, wall thickening, ulceration, and fistula formation. (Ch. 81; pg 1794)

32. c

Ulcerative proctitis and ulcerative colitis are thought to be part of a continuum. Most patients present initially with limited disease rather than pancolitis. Only 7% of patients with proctitis followed-up for 10 years have disease progression to the hepatic flexure. Depending on the severity of the first attack, the disease will go into remission in approximately 80% to 90% of patients with ulcerative colitis. Periodic colonoscopic evaluations demonstrating therapeutic responsiveness are not thought to provide any additional information beyond that obtained by a thorough history. (Ch. 81; pg 1783)

33. e

Omega-3 fatty acids treat inflammatory diseases such as inflammatory bowel disease (IBD) by reducing levels of leukotriene B_4 (LTB_4). Although prostaglandin levels are elevated in the mucosa and sera of IBD patients, studies using nonsteroidal antiinflammatory drugs show no improvement in disease, arguing against prostaglandins as the primary mediator of inflammation in IBD. LTB_4 is thought to be a major chemotactic agent in IBD. (Ch. 81; pg 1781)

34. d

The extraintestinal manifestations of inflammatory bowel disease are often categorized into those that correlate with disease activity and those that progress independently of intestinal disease activity. Ocular, dermatologic, and peripheral arthritic manifestations generally correlate with disease activity and usually resolve with colectomy. Sclerosing cholangitis and ankylosing spondylitis progress independently of intestinal disease and are not altered by colectomy. (Ch. 81; pg 1787)

35. c

Immunosuppressive agents are indicated in refractory inflammatory bowel disease for therapeutic benefit and as corticosteroid-sparing therapy. A disadvantage to the use of immunosuppressive agents is the incidence of adverse effects, including leukopenia and severe pancreatitis. In addition, these agents usually do not impact the disease for 2 to 4 months after beginning therapy. Colectomy is often preferable to long-term immunosuppressive therapy for ulcerative colitis, but many patients are willing to accept the potential side effects of immunosuppressive therapy to avoid colectomy. (Ch. 81; pg 1811)

36. b

Desmoid tumors, also referred to as mesenteric fibromatosis, may result in substantial morbidity and mortality. Bowel obstruction and ureteral obstruction are not uncommon, nor are complications related to the multiple surgeries needed to manage desmoid tumors in patients with Gardner syndrome. (Ch. 89; pg 2005)

37. c

Cronkhite-Canada syndrome is a noninherited condition of unknown etiology characterized by generalized hamartomatous gastrointestinal polyposis, mucocutaneous hyperpigmentation, nail atrophy, and hair loss. (Ch. 89; pg 2013)

38. a

Peutz-Jeghers syndrome has been associated with gastrointestinal malignancies as a result of adenomatous change in some polyps. Mucocutaneous pigmentation often begins during the first or second year of life. Polyps in Peutz-Jeghers syndrome are hamartomas and lack cellular atypia. The arborization of the epithelium leads to the unique microscopic picture of benign glands surrounded by smooth muscle extending well into the submucosa. This characteristic is called pseudoinvasion and is not indicative of malignancy. The most common location of polyps is the small intestine, followed in frequency by the colon and stomach. (Ch. 89; pg 2007)

39. e

Renal cell carcinoma has not been associated with familial adenomatous polyposis coli or Gardner syndrome. (Ch. 89; pg 2000)

40. c

Although fecal leukocytes are often seen with bacterial infections of the colon, they are also a common finding in ulcerative colitis and in other chronic inflammatory diseases of the colon. (Ch. 87; pg 1946)

41. d

This is a characteristic presentation of acute colonic pseudoobstruction. Appropriate management strategies include the elimination of medications that can adversely affect gastrointestinal motility and the correction of underlying metabolic abnormalities. The patient should not be fed, and a nasogastric tube should be placed to decompress the upper gut. A trial of a prokinetic agent such as erythromycin may be useful. These patients often have a cecal diameter of 9 to 10 cm—an arbitrary value of 11 cm can be considered as a criterion for decompressive colonoscopy or cecostomy if medical therapy is unsuccessful. However, the acuteness of colonic distention and the severity of symptoms are better determinants of the need for decompression than an absolute size criteria. It may be necessary to perform a partial colectomy if there is clinical evidence of perforation, but this procedure should otherwise be avoided. (Ch. 85; pg 1919)

42. c

In general, markers ingested over a 2- to 3-day period are mixed together in the stool and passed in a random manner. No significant differences in marker transit have been found when given either before or with a meal. Segmental colonic transit can be measured only if abdominal radiographs are taken to count markers. In normal volunteers, 80% of markers are passed by the fifth day after ingestion. (Ch. 41; pg 916)

43. e

Colonic diverticula should not be considered a source of occult bleeding. (Ch. 86; pg 1939)

44. a

Recurrence of diverticulitis is relatively common, occurring in 27% to 45% of patients. (Ch. 86; pg 1930)

45. c

Angiodysplasia from the stomach and right colon are histologically indistinguishable. (Ch. 113; pg 2565)

46. c

Symptoms of acute radiation proctitis occur in 75% of patients receiving greater than 40 Gy. Acute radiation injury almost always heals after the discontinuation of therapy and is not clearly related to chronic injury. The chance of developing chronic radiation proctitis is related to the total effective dose of radiation and the volume of bowel irradiated. Chronic radiation proctitis is related to vascular ischemic changes within the bowel wall, but acute proctitis is related to direct toxicity of the actively proliferating cell compartment. (Ch. 115; pg 2611)

47. c

Giardia lamblia typically infects the small bowel and does not result in dysentery. (Ch. 87; pg 1946) (Ch. 108; pg 2431)

48. b

Shigella species invade the colonic epithelium and produce enterotoxins, although the toxin is not essential for the development of colitis. Endoscopically, the severity of disease diminishes in more proximal regions of the colon. The entire colon is involved in 15% of patients. *Shigella* infection is highly contagious; the ingestion of even small numbers of organisms causes disease. (Ch. 87; pg 1947)

49. d

Enterohemorrhagic *Escherichia coli*, also known as serotype O157:H7, produces at least two toxins with properties similar to the toxin elaborated by *Shigella dysenteriae* type 1 (Shiga toxin), which causes severe abdominal cramps and watery diarrhea followed by the passage of grossly bloody stools. Enterohemorrhagic *E coli* infection may, in rare instances,

lead to the development of hemolytic uremic syndrome or thrombotic thrombocytopenic purpura. Enterotoxigenic *E coli* produces a heat-labile toxin remarkably similar to cholera toxin, which activates adenylate cyclase leading to a self-limited watery diarrhea syndrome. Enteropathogenic *E coli,* which lacks invasive properties, produces watery diarrhea primarily in children under age 2 years by its entero-adherence properties. Enteroinvasive *E coli* produces an illness indistinguishable from the dysentery-like disease caused by *Shigella* species and is the only *E coli* enteritis syndrome for which antibiotic treatment (i.e., trimethoprim-sulfamethoxazole or a quinolone) is clearly indicated. (Ch. 87; pg 1958)

50. d

Campylobacter jejuni infections are usually self-limited and frequently resolve by the time culture results are positive. Therapy is usually conservative and includes replacement of fluid and electrolytes. Weak evidence suggests that antibiotics (e.g., erythromycin, ciprofloxacin) may decrease the duration of symptoms if instituted within 3 days of the onset of diarrhea; however, most patients do not benefit from antibiotic administration. (Ch. 87; pg 1950)

51. c

Hirschsprung disease is diagnosed by a deep mucosal biopsy performed in the distal rectal region. If the aganglionic segment is relatively short, a biopsy in the proximal rectum or sigmoid colon will miss the area of abnormality. If the rectoanal inhibitory reflex is present during anorectal manometry, the disease can be ruled out without a rectal biopsy. Symptoms usually present in infants and not during toilet training. Surgery is required to treat this condition, but the majority of the colon is left in place. (Ch. 80; pg 1769)

52. d

Patients with acquired immunodeficiency syndrome may present with painful anorectal lesions caused by typical venereal organisms. Other etiologies include tuberculosis, Kaposi sarcoma, cloacogenic carcinoma, squamous cell carcinoma, and lymphoma, but not *Yersinia enterocolitica*. (Ch. 107; pg 2414)

53. d

The gut microflora synthesizes vitamin K and plays an essential role in the metabolism of drugs such as sulfasalazine and metronidazole. Probably the most important function of the colonic microflora is to suppress populations of other bacteria that are more pathogenic. (Ch. 27; pg 630)

54. b

Each of the listed mechanisms may play an etiologic role in the diarrhea associated with antibiotic therapy, with the exception of the osmotic effects of intralume-nal antibiotics. (Ch. 27; pg 631)

55. b

The toxin produced by *Shigella* species inhibits colonocyte protein synthesis and leads to diarrhea through the secondary failure of fluid absorption. The clinical course of adult infection begins with the onset of fever within 1 to 3 days of ingestion, followed by diarrhea within an additional day. The typical duration of the illness is 5 to 7 days. *Shigella* infections are associated with the hemolytic-uremic syndrome and with Reiter syndrome. Most patients with sympto-matic *Shigella* infections should be treated, except for selected patients with mild disease. Tetracycline ther-apy is effective for most infections acquired in North America, whereas ciprofloxacin will also treat cases acquired outside the United States, which may be caused by tetracycline-resistant organisms. (Ch. 87; pg 1947)

56. c

Campylobacter organisms are only found in 20% of stool cultures in patients with identifiable cases of acute bacillary diarrhea. The infection is most often acquired by eating infected foodstuffs, particularly poultry, eggs, and milk, although it can be spread by the fecal-oral route. The absence of fecal leukocytes makes *Campylobacter* infection unlikely. Clinically, there may be abdominal tenderness and pain that may mimic a surgical abdomen. Treatment of a *Campylobacter* infection with antibiotics shortens the duration of bacterial shedding, but does not affect the duration of clinical illness. (Ch. 87; pg 1951)

57. b

Diarrhea develops in only about one-third of patients with *Clostridium difficile* identified in their stool. The presence of confluent membranes in patients with pseudomembranous colitis is more unusual than scat-tered plaques. *C difficile* is associated with a spectrum of colonic disease including antibiotic-associated diar-rhea, antibiotic-associated colitis, and pseudomembra-nous colitis. The rate of isolation of *C difficile* and the detection of toxin in the stool increases with the sever-ity of disease. (Ch. 87; pg 1953)

58. b

The most frequent symptoms of gonorrheal proctitis are constipation and obstipation, although asympto-matic rectal carriage occurs in up to 53% of patients. *Chlamydia trachomatis* is responsible for up to 20% of proctitis in gay men. The condition may become chronic with fistula formation and clinically mimic Crohn's proctitis. The perianal warts of secondary syphilis are known as condyloma lata, while those caused by human papillomavirus are known as condy-loma acuminata. (Ch. 87; pg 1960)

59. e

Neuroleptic antidepressants have been reported to cause ischemic colitis. Nonsteroidal antiinflammatory drugs, gold, and isoretinoin have been known to pro-duce symptoms and signs of acute colitis. Marijuana has not been reported to cause features of acute coli-tis. (Ch. 83; pg 1869)

60. e

Recent reports suggest an equal male-female ratio for the occurrence of pneumatosis cystoides intestinalis. Secondary cases typically involve the small intestine and ascending colon, whereas idiopathic or primary cases usually involve the left colon. Radiographs show characteristic linear or curvilinear lucencies, and colonoscopy shows polypoid masses filled with air con-taining a high content of hydrogen. In asymptomatic patients, treatment is rarely indicated because the cysts usually resolve spontaneously. (Ch. 83; pg 1877)

61. b

Condyloma lata are the warty lesions of secondary syphilis, which can be confirmed by a dark-field micro-scopic examination for spirochetes. (Ch. 87; pg 1961)

62. b

The most common causes of acute diarrhea are infec-tious agents. In the United States, most cases of infec-tious diarrhea are self-limited and are not causes of significant morbidity. Attempting to determine the eti-ologic agent in all cases is not warranted for numerous reasons, including cost, the inability to make a defini-tive diagnosis in a large number of cases, and results that will not influence patient care. A thorough evalu-ation is warranted for patients who are likely to bene-fit from a specific diagnosis, such as for those with fever higher than 39°C, systemic illness, bloody diarrhea, dehydration, or a prolonged course (i.e., 2 weeks). (Ch. 40; pg 871)

63. e

64. d

Reiter syndrome, often presenting with the triad of arthritis, urethritis, and conjunctivitis, is a spondylo-arthropathy that usually develops 2 to 4 weeks after an enteric infection. All of the listed organisms can cause Reiter syndrome except enterohemorrhagic *Escherichia coli*. Incomplete presentations of Reiter syndrome are common. Other manifestations include painless oral ulcers on the tongue or palate, papulo-vesiculosquamous lesions on the palms and soles (i.e., keratoderma blennorrhagicum), carditis, and dystrophic nails. (Ch. 87; pg 1949)

65. d

About 50% of patients with pseudomembranous coli-tis (PMC) or antibiotic-associated colitis (AAC) do not have fecal leukocytes on stool examination. In cases of antibiotic-associated diarrhea, 15% to 25% have *Clostridium difficile* cytotoxin in their stool, and up to 40% are culture-positive. In about 30% of PMC cases, pseudomembranes are not seen in the rectum but are found more proximal in the colon. Pseudomembranes are not necessary for the diagnosis of AAC, which is confirmed by evidence of systemic illness or by evidence of colitis on flexible sigmoidoscopy. (Ch. 87; pg 1955)

66. c

Outbreaks of enterohemorrhagic *Escherichia coli* O157:H7 have been associated with ground beef served at fast-food restaurants, unpasteurized dairy products, and fecal contamination of municipal water. Children younger than 5 years are at greatest risk for developing hemolytic uremic syndrome as a complication of infection with *E coli* O157:H7. Strains of *E coli* O157:H7 produce at least two potent Shiga-like toxins: verotoxins I and II. In very rare cases, an intestinal uptake of these toxins may lead to severe systemic complications of *E coli* O157:H7 infection, including hemolytic-uremic syndrome and thrombotic thrombocytopenic purpura. The effectiveness of antibiotics has not been documented, and some strains may develop increased toxin production when exposed to antibiotics, raising theoretical concerns about their use. (Ch. 87; pg 1958)

67. d

IgA-deficient individuals are not at increased risk for infection with *Entamoeba histolytica*. (Ch. 108; pg 2424)

68. c

Acute amebic proctocolitis is commonly characterized by 1 to 3 weeks of increasingly frequent bloody diarrhea associated with abdominal pain and tenderness. Fever is present in about 33% of patients. Weight loss is common. (Ch. 108; pg 2426)

69. c

Atelectasis, elevation of the right hemidiaphragm, serous pleural effusion, and peritonitis are all common manifestations of amebic liver abscess. Pericarditis is an unusual complication that results from the direct spread of the liver abscess. Pulmonary embolism is not known to be specifically associated with amebic liver abscess formation. (Ch. 108; pg 2426)

70. c

With lumenal balloon distention, patients with irritable bowel syndrome (IBS) often experience pain in distant, ectopic, or even multiple sites. In contrast to healthy persons, patients with IBS and visceral hypersensitivity have normal or reduced perception of cutaneous stimulation, indicating that diffuse sensory

abnormalities are not present. Approximately 60% of patients with IBS exhibit enhanced perception of lumenal distention, indicating a lack of sensitivity for this maneuver as a diagnostic test for this disorder. (Ch. 84; pg 1888)

71. d

The presence of blood or sigmoidoscopic abnormalities is suggestive of inflammatory bowel disease. The presence of hypoalbuminemia with an increased stool volume may be seen with a protein-losing enteropathy. A stool volume of more than 1 L/day is consistent with a secretory diarrhea. Patients with irritable bowel syndrome classically present with normal laboratory studies, a lack of occult fecal blood, and normal stool volumes. Pain on sigmoidoscopy, which is not a consistent finding, results from visceral hypersensitivity in this condition. (Ch. 84; pg 1894)

72. c

There is only convincing evidence of the efficacy of fiber in treating constipation-predominant irritable bowel syndrome. (Ch. 84; pg 1895)

73. a

Flatulence is largely the result of dietary intake and the metabolic activity of the colonic flora. Passage of flatus up to 25 times per day is normal, but frequent flatulence may indicate an underlying disorder of intestinal motility or carbohydrate malabsorption. Dietary discretion is more likely to be effective than simethicone. (Ch. 37; pg 818)

74. b

Surveillance for dysplastic changes in chronic ulcerative pancolitis should begin 8 to 10 years after symptom onset. (Ch. 81; pg 1829)

75. b

Physiologic losses of blood from the gastrointestinal tract in normal subjects range from 0.5 to 1.0 mL/day. (Ch. 33; pg 744)

76. a

Streptococcus bovis infections have been associated with the presence of colonic adenomas and colon cancer but not gastric neoplasia. There is no association between telangiectasias and *S bovis* infection. (Ch. 90; pg 2044)

77. b

Endoscopic strip biopsy uses submucosal injection, usually of physiologic saline through an endoscopic needle. The horizontal separation of the lesion from the underlying tissues minimizes the extent of tissue required to resect the specimen and allows removal of a large area of mucosa while minimizing serious complications such as bleeding or perforation. Photodynamic therapy involves administering a photosensitizing drug that is then activated at close proximity by a laser. A problem associated with this form of therapy is significant photosensitivity. Endoscopic ultrasonography has been shown to complement computed tomography in the staging of tumors. Laser therapy is useful to ablate or recanalize malignant tumors. (Ch. 129; pg 2865) (Ch. 130; pgs 2882, 2885, 2895)

78. b

The lifetime risk for the development of colon cancer is approximately 5% for the average American. (Ch. 90; pg 2038)

79. c

Occult fecal bleeding and hematochezia do not necessarily indicate the presence of advanced colonic malignancy, and may instead be found in some individuals with early colorectal cancer. (Ch. 90; pg 2038)

80. c

Extensive disease extending proximal to the splenic flexure is usually treated the same as pancolitis involving the entire colon. This patient has had disease for 15 years and even if just isolated to the left side, a colonoscopy is indicated. Despite the mild, well-controlled nature of the disease, he is at substantial risk for the development of cancer because of the duration and extent of the disease. A barium enema radiographic study is not sufficiently sensitive for the detection of dysplasia or cancer, and sigmoidoscopy is an incomplete examination. The finding of high-grade dysplasia, when reviewed by an expert pathologist, is an indication for colectomy, whereas low-grade dysplasia requires careful follow-up but not necessarily resection. (Ch. 81; pg 1828)

81. a

A confirmed pathologic diagnosis of high-grade dysplasia is the equivalent of carcinoma in situ and must be removed. Often, a deeply infiltrating cancer may be found beneath the high-grade dysplasia. A hemicolectomy is inappropriate in this setting because of the risk of continued colitis and neoplasia in the residual colon. Although rectal sparing is typically associated with Crohn's disease, it may be the result of topical steroid 5-aminosalicylic acid therapy for rectal inflammation in ulcerative colitis and is not relevant in the face of high-grade dysplasia. (Ch. 81; pg 1829)

82. b

An increased incidence of colorectal cancer in patients with familial juvenile polyposis coli is apparently the result of adenomatous tissue contained within the juvenile polyps. It may be possible to manage this case with surveillance colonoscopy and the removal of the juvenile polyps. It is not necessary to perform a colectomy. This disease does not appear to be related to familial adenomatous polyposis. (Ch. 90; pg 2044)

83. b

Patients with Dukes stage C colon cancer can improve their 3- to 5-year disease-free survival from 37% to 49% by completing a 1-year course of adjuvant chemotherapy using levamisole and 5-fluorouracil. Radiotherapy is appropriate adjuvant therapy for rectal cancers but not for colon cancers above the level of the rectum. Adjuvant chemotherapy is associated with considerable side effects, but the improvement in survival is substantial enough that patients should be offered this treatment option. (Ch. 90; pg 2066)

84. a

The presence of cancer in the head of a pedunculated adenomatous polyp may be adequately treated by colonoscopic polypectomy. Invasion of the cancer into the stalk does not require additional surgical therapy as long as the pathologist and endoscopist agree that the polyp has been completely removed and that no adverse pathologic findings are present in the cancer (e.g., poor degree of differentiation, vascular invasion). The patient should undergo subsequent surveillance colonoscopy for metachronous tumors, but it is not necessary to do so every 6 months. (Ch. 88; pg 1984)

85. c

The presence of a solitary metastasis after prior surgical resection of a colonic adenocarcinoma is an indication for surgical resection in some clinical settings. It is not unreasonable to offer this patient surgery, acknowledging that he may have residual malignancy that is not apparent. Because he is symptomatic, he may benefit from intraarterial chemotherapy, although there is little evidence that this will prolong his life. However, it is a reasonable alternative to surgery. Although the patient may refuse both of these therapies, they should be offered unless the patient is not a surgical candidate or has previously expressed an unwillingness to undertake additional aggressive treatment. (Ch. 90; pg 2070)

86. d

Asymptomatic carcinoid tumors are frequently found when removing rectal lesions. These are very unlikely to produce the carcinoid syndrome. In a series of 38 rectal carcinoid tumors, 23 (61%) were less than 2 cm in diameter, and only one was malignant. Distant metastases were not observed. Among the 15 tumors that were larger than 2 cm in diameter, 14 were malignant, but only 1 metastasized. Thus, a small carcinoid tumor in the rectum may be considered an incidental finding that does not require aggressive surgical treatment. (Ch. 90; pg 2072)

87. a

The overwhelming majority of colonic bacteria are anaerobic. Facultative gram-negative organisms account for only 0.1% to 0.5% of the fecal flora. (Ch. 27; pg 624)

88. c

Colonic ischemia is the most common form of ischemic injury to the gut. The colon has relatively poor collateral arterial supply. As with ischemic events in the small intestine, colonic ischemia can occur as a result of either occlusive or nonocclusive disease, or generalized hypoperfusion. Digoxin and danazol can cause nonocclusive damage. Dehydration results in inadequate gut perfusion, and diabetes mellitus is one of several small vessel diseases of the colon, others being vasculitis and radiation injury, that promote ischemia. Doxycycline is not associated with vascular disease of the colon. (Ch. 114; pg 2594)

89. c.

Colonic ischemia is often difficult to diagnose. While it should always be a consideration in elderly patients with heart disease, the diagnosis should be entertained in all patients with moderate hematochezia, whether or not diarrhea or serious underlying disease is present. It may occur in young adults using cocaine or amphetamines, in pregnant women, and in women taking birth control pills. Patients with chronic renal disease, especially those requiring hemodialysis, are also susceptible. A patient undergoing peritoneal dialysis whose stool is not bloody is much less likely to have colonic ischemia. (Ch. 114; pg 2598)

90. a

Docusate salts are surfactants that soften the stool to permit easier defecation. Although laxatives composed of docusate sodium may be taken together with other laxatives, they can increase the absorption of certain laxatives, such as mineral oil, danthron and phenylophthalein. Docusate salts are not systemically absorbed and, unlike mineral oil, they do not cause malabsorption of the fat-soluble vitamins. Interestingly, placebo-controlled studies have failed to demonstrate changes in stool water content, stool weight, frequency of defecation, or colonic transit times. (Ch. 41, pg 921)

91. b

All of the following are stimulant laxatives except for magnesium sulfate which is a saline laxative. (Ch. 41; pg 921)

92. d

Foreign bodies are usually placed into the rectum for purposes of eroticism. Even if the object is palpable, abdominal radiography is appropriate, not only to document the position and the number of foreign bodies, but also to visualize possible free air, which is suggestive of a perforation. Transanal removal is possible even with glass objects. Proctosigmoidoscopy should be performed after the object is successfully removed to document the absence of other objects and to rule out traumatic damage to the rectosigmoid colon. (Ch. 91; pg 2099)

93. a

Colon cancer itself is not a risk factor for anal carcinoma. (Ch. 91; pg 2100)

94. d

Only 25% of patients are symptom-free; however, it is not unusual for the lesion to be discovered incidentally at routine examination. Although large or infiltrating lesions may require an abdominoperineal resection, most lesions can be treated for cure with a combination of radiotherapy and chemotherapy. The five-year survival rate is approximately 70%. (Ch. 91; pg 2100)

95. a

Although a solitary rectal ulcer may occur with internal prolapse and may be associated with straining during defecation and hematochezia, it is not necessarily associated with a long history of laxative abuse, chronic diarrhea, and narrow stools. The same is true of anal fissure. This patient is unlikely to have rectal carcinoma at her young age and her symptoms are not consistent with rectal prolapse. Anal stenosis is the most likely diagnosis. (Ch. 91; pg 2093)

96. c

For diminutive polyps, cold snaring and cold biopsy are safe and hemorrhage is rare, in comparison with hot cautery techniques. Hot biopsy forceps are five times more likely to produce a complication in the right than in the left colon. Snare cautery effectively removes the entire polyp, even if the polyp is smaller than 5 mm. Cold biopsy may be used to completely remove small polyps. (Ch. 130; pg 2893)

97. d

Only saline injection into the submucosa would raise an effective mound. This technique has not been associated with a risk of tumor seeding or peritonitis. Lesions smaller than 1.5 cm should be removed in a single piece if possible. The incidence of residual cancer and even of metastasis from sessile malignant polyps is clearly greater than that associated with pedunculated malignant polyps. (Ch. 130; pg 2894)

98. d

Finger palpation and transillumination in the right lower quadrant are sometimes effective in confirming passage of the endoscope tip to the cecum; however, they can on occasion be misleading. Using the length of endoscope inserted as a gauge is unreliable. Fluoroscopic confirmation may be helpful, but it is not practical and exposes the patient to unnecessary radiation. The ideal way to identify passage of the scope to the cecum is by using cecal landmarks. (Ch. 122; pg 2704)

99. a

Antibiotics are completely unnecessary even if a biopsy or polypectomy is performed, unless the patient has certain unusual risk factors for endocarditis. Routine avoidance of aspirin is unnecessary prior to colonoscopy. If aspirin is discontinued because of a planned polypectomy, discontinuation 1 week prior is sufficient. Oral sodium phosphate is not a balanced electrolyte solution. It is reasonable to avoid iron preparations for several days prior to colonoscopy, because they can produce a black, sticky residue in the colon, which makes the procedure difficult. (Ch. 122; pg 2705)

100. a

Chronic abdominal pain and long-standing functional symptoms, such as constipation or bleeding, are very low-yield indications for colonoscopy. A barium enema will usually suffice in these cases. The evaluation of any condition with blood loss possibly due to colonic disease or chronic diarrhea, which may require mucosal biopsy, is an appropriate indication for colonoscopy. (Ch. 122; pg 2713)

101. a.

The colonic wall lacks villi. (Ch. 80; pg 1762)

102. b

The cecum, transverse colon, and sigmoid colon are all intraperitoneal structures and are prone to volvulus because of their location and relative lack of fixation. (Ch. 80; pg 1765)

103. d

All have a strong association with adenomas, with the exception of cholecystectomy. (Ch. 88; pg 1967)

104. d

Tubular adenomas are most common, comprising 80% to 85% of all adenomas, followed by tubulovillous adenomas (10%) and villous adenomas (5%). (Ch. 88; pg 1968)

105. c

Based on percentages, 5% of colorectal adenomas are in the rectum, 45% in the sigmoid colon, 30% in the descending colon, 10% in the transverse colon, and 10% in the ascending colon. (Ch. 88; 1967)

106. d

Microsatellite instability due to DNA mismatch repair is the hallmark defect in hereditary nonpolyposis colorectal cancer syndrome. (Ch. 88; pg 1972)

107. b

Tubular adenomas are relatively common; therefore, a first-degree relative with only an adenoma is not an indication for colonoscopy (except in certain hereditary syndromes with multiple polyps). (Ch. 88; pg 1981)

108. d

All are poor prognostic factors except pedunculated malignant polyps. Some studies suggest that the outcome for patients with pedunculated malignant polyps is improved. (Ch. 88; pg 1984)

109. c

Once the polyp penetrates the submucosa, metastatic spread is possible because the lymphatics are located in the submucosa. (Ch. 88; pg 1985)

110. b

This mutation occurs in approximately half of colorectal adenomas larger than 1 cm. (Ch. 88; pg 1972)

111. a.

All are inherited in an autosomal dominant fashion, except hyperplastic polyposis, which is not an inherited syndrome. However, up to one-third of newly diagnosed cases of familial adenomatous polyposis appear to represent de novo mutations. (Ch. 89; pg 1996)

112. c.

In vitro protein synthesis (IVPS) would be the most reasonable initial genetic test. Linkage testing requires blood from two or more known affected persons in a family to identify DNA markers that associate with the mutant gene. Mutation identification uses direct DNA sequencing at gene sites to determine the precise gene mutation; however, it is primarily limited to research laboratories, and it is not commercially available at present. IVPS testing requires that only a single individual be tested. It has been shown to identify a protein truncation successfully in 80% of families with familial adenomatous polyposis tested. (Ch. 89; pg 1997)

113. c.

The majority of polyps are tubular adenomas, 90% of which are smaller than 0.5 cm. (Ch. 89; pg 1998)

114. a.

All of the extracolonic lesions listed are seen in Gardner syndrome except ovarian carcinoma. (Ch. 89; pg 2004)

115. b.

The APC gene (located on the long arm of chromosome 5) is mutated in familial adenomatous polyposis. The resultant mutation almost always causes a truncation of the APC protein, which is thought to function as a tumor suppressor gene. (Ch. 89; pg 1996)

116. d.

Juvenile polyposis is characterized by ten or more juvenile polyps. Juvenile polyps are considered non-neoplastic hamartomatous polyps, usually occurring in the colons of children between ages of 4 and 14 years. (Ch. 89; pg 2009)

117. e.

Other than defining associated diseases (e.g., human immunodeficiency virus, Gardner syndrome, and common variable immunodeficiency syndrome) so that they may be treated, no other specific therapy is needed. (Ch. 89; pg 2014)

118. a

Tobacco use has been associated with a 2- to 3-fold increase in adenoma prevalence, but not in colorectal cancer. Regular consumption of beer has been associated with a 2- to 3-fold increased risk. The ingestion of animal fat has been associated with a modest but statistically significant increased risk. Women who have received radiation therapy for gynecologic cancer have a 2- to 3.6-fold increased risk of colorectal cancer. (Ch. 90; pg 2026)

119. c

Patients with familial adenomatous polyposis experience a regression of their adenomas after treatment with sulindac. (Ch. 90; pg 2031)

120. c

The mode of transmission in hereditary nonpolyposis colorectal cancer is autosomal dominant. (Ch. 90; pg 2039)

121. b

The best clinical predictor of outcome in colorectal cancer is the pathologic stage, which is principally a reflection of depth of invasion. (Ch. 90; pg 2063) Most colorectal cancers are moderately or well-differentiated tumors. Only 20% are poorly or undifferentiated tumors, which are associated with a poorer outcome. (Ch. 90; pg 2046)

122. b

Levamisole plus 5-fluorouracil in Dukes stage C tumors has been shown in several studies to improve survival and the recurrence-free interval. There was no benefit found for stage B tumors. (Ch. 90; pg 2066)

123. d

All are components of the Amsterdam criteria except d. (Ch. 90; pg 2041)

124. c

Patients with acromegaly have a 3-fold higher incidence of colon cancer. Several studies and one meta-analysis have demonstrated no excess risk for adenomas or carcinomas after cholecystectomy. The effect of dietary fiber consumption on the prevalence of colorectal cancer remains controversial; however, the weight of available evidence suggests a protective effect. (Ch. 90; pgs 2029, 2045)

125. d

Indications for an ileal pouch–anal canal anastomosis include chronic ulcerative colitis, multiple colorectal malignancies, familial adenomatous polyposis, and younger age. It is contraindicated in persons with Crohn's disease, those with poor anal sphincter function, and those older than 65. (Ch. 82; pg 1842)

126. c

This woman may have functional bowel disease or microscopic colitis. Considering her age, the best choice is a colonoscopy. This procedure will exclude the presence of incidental colonic polyps and, with a biopsy, collagenous and lymphocytic colitis. A barium enema does not allow for a biopsy, and there is no clear-cut indication for computed tomography or ultrasonography. The yield of a stool culture for ova and parasites is very low in this situation. (Ch. 84; pg 1894)

127. e

Fatty liver, cholesterol gallstones, pericholangitis, and chronic active hepatitis have all been associated with inflammatory bowel disease (IBD). Hepatic hemangioma has not been associated with IBD. (Ch. 81; pg 1788)

128. c

Arthritis associated with inflammatory bowel disease (IBD) is usually migratory and affects large joints. The treatment of IBD with steroids often results in dramatic improvement of the associated arthritis. Unlike with ankylosing spondylitis, there is no association of IBD and arthritis with haplotype B27. Deformity with radiologic changes occurs in fewer than 25% of cases. (Ch. 81; pg 1787)

129. b

Crohn's disease is more common in people who smoke cigarettes. Growth failure and delayed sexual maturation occur in about 30% of children with Crohn's disease. Hypoalbuminemia is an accurate indicator of disease severity. Crohn's disease recurs at the anastomosis even when wide margins of normal intestine are resected. Increasing the length of microscopically normal intestine resected does not reduce the likelihood of recurrence. The incidence of recurrence after ileal resection for ileitis or ileocolic resection for ileocolic disease is at least 50% after 10 years and 75% after 15 years, as assessed by rates of reoperation. (Ch. 81; pgs 1776, 1784, 1821, 1830)

130. d

The terminal ileum, cecum, and rectosigmoid are segments involved in radiation enterocolitis because they are fixed in the pelvis and receive the greatest radiation exposure. A histologic examination would reveal ischemia with endarteritis, occasional partial villous atrophy, fibrosis, and strictures. Diarrhea may be caused by bile acid malabsorption if the terminal ileum is involved, and by bacterial overgrowth if small intestine strictures occur. Antidiarrheals may be used to control stool frequency and consistency; however, antiinflammatory drugs are of little benefit. (Ch. 40; pg 883)

131. c

Pregnancy can be safely completed in most patients with Crohn's disease. A cesarean section is not necessary in the absence of significant perianal disease. Metronidazole is contraindicated during pregnancy, particularly during the first trimester. Mesalamine and steroids can be used safely during pregnancy. (Ch. 81; pg 1830)

132. b

Sulfasalazine has been successfully used to treat mild to moderate ulcerative colitis. The usual dose is between 2 to 4 g/day. In some patients, the incidence of side effects is dose-dependent; in others, side effects are due to hypersensitivity. The dose-related toxic effects, which include headache, nausea and vomiting, and abdominal pain, are associated with serum sulfapyridine levels higher than 50 mcg/mL. Sulfapyridine is metabolized by acetylation; therefore, persons who are slow metabolizers have high levels of serum sulfapyridine and low levels of acetylated sulfapyridine. Dose-related side effects are more common in persons who are slow acetylators. Hypersensitivity reactions are not dependent on sulfapyridine levels. (Ch. 81; pg 1806)

133. d

134. c

The clinical presentation suggests pneumatosis cystoides intestinalis. Pneumatosis is most commonly associated with chronic obstructive pulmonary disease, intestinal obstruction, collagen vascular diseases, systemic amyloidosis, and iatrogenic conditions (e.g., after surgery or endoscopy). It has also been reported in patients with Crohn's disease, especially those taking steroids. Complications include volvulus, intussusception, intestinal perforation, obstruction, and tension pneumoperitoneum. (Ch. 83; pg 1877)

135. a

The major diagnostic challenge is to differentiate recurrent Crohn's disease from diversion colitis. Advanced diversion colitis has focal ulceration and a nodular appearance that mimics Crohn's disease. Endoscopic appearance and histologic features may help distinguish the two. A computed tomographic scan may detect abnormalities in the bowel wall thickness. Hydrocortisone enemas are usually not beneficial in the management of diversion colitis. Short-chain fatty acid enemas may induce a remission of diversion colitis in some patients. (Ch. 83; pg 1862)

136. b

The activity of ankylosing spondylitis in patients with inflammatory bowel disease does not follow that of the bowel disease, and the treatment of the bowel disease does not affect the spondylitis. Nonsteroidal antiinflammatory drugs reduce inflammation and pain but do not halt disease progression. Medical treatment of the colitis and colectomy are not helpful in managing ankylosing spondylitis. (Ch. 81; pg 1787)

137. c

The upper limit of normal colonic transit in healthy adults is approximately 70 hours. The mean transit time is approximately 36 hours. (Ch. 41; pg 916)

138. b

139. b

Of patients with significant diverticulosis, 70% remain asymptomatic and never develop complications. However, with long-term follow-up, 15% to 25% will develop acute diverticulitis and 5% to 15% may exhibit diverticular bleeding. (Ch. 86; pg 1928)

140. a

Careful follow-up of localized outbreaks of shigellosis indicate that 1% to 2% of infected people subsequently develop Reiter syndrome. (Ch. 87; pg 1949)

141. d

This patient demonstrates several of the typical features of the CREST syndrome, namely calcinosis. Raynaud phenomenon, esophageal hypomotility, sclerodactyly, and telangiectasia. (Ch. 113; pg 2573)

142. c

Carbohydrate malabsorption is a prominent cause of gas and bloating. Complex carbohydrates as found in pasta may be incompletely absorbed and may contribute to these symptoms. Although sorbitol in chewing gum can produce gas and bloating due to its incomplete absorption, gum chewing itself can evoke symptoms by causing aerophagia. In addition to being a component of fruits, fructose also is used to sweeten carbonated soft drinks, which may induce gas in susceptible individuals. Relationships between subtle malabsorption of lactose and symptoms may be difficult to ascertain based on the history alone; in some patients, hydrogen breath testing may be indicated to characterize the role of lactase deficiency in symptom development. (Ch. 37; pg 818)

143. d

Most patients with complaints of excess gas actually have normal volumes of intestinal gas as measured by argon washout techniques. Trapping of air in the colonic flexures may result from spastic activity of the colon. Hypothyroidism may produce constipation with bloating. Breath tests are commonly used to assist in the diagnosis of lactase deficiency and small bowel bacterial overgrowth. Although the discovery of increased hydrogen excretion after lactose ingestion is strongly suggestive of lactase deficiency, this finding does not prove that the disaccharidase deficiency is the cause of this patient's symptoms. Complex carbohydrates such as flour made from wheat, oats, and potatoes may be partially malabsorbed and thus may produce falsely abnormal results on a breath test; therefore, avoidance of complex carbohydrates as found in pasta is recommended prior to hydrogen breath testing. Methane is produced by 33% to 41% of healthy adults and thus is not the best gas for breath testing. (Ch. 37; pg 816)

144. b

The role of carbohydrate malabsorption in producing symptoms in patients with functional bowel disorders is uncertain. Some patients may be hypersensitive to bacterial fermentation of certain sugars; however, gas and bloating are prominent symptoms in irritable bowel syndrome and may not respond to dietary restriction. Simethicone alters the elasticity of bubbles in the gastrointestinal tract. The mechanism of fiber-induced bloating does not stem from increased gas production as a result of the inefficient conversion of fiber to gas. The administration of bacterial β-galactosidase may enhance the digestion of beans and other legumes rich in stachyose and raffinose. (Ch. 37; pg 818)

145. e

Aberrant gut motor patterns are commonly seen in patients with irritable bowel syndrome (IBS), but the pathogenic importance of these patterns is uncertain. Many of the abnormal contractile patterns can be induced by stressful events or by inducing somatic pain in healthy individuals. Other patterns such as discrete clustered contractions and prolonged propagated contractions can be related to painful episodes in patients with IBS. However, these patterns occur in healthy volunteers and do not evoke symptoms, suggesting that the perceptual responses to these patterns rather than the patterns themselves are the relevant abnormalities in IBS. Diarrhea-prone IBS patients exhibit an exaggerated gastrocolonic response relative to constipated patients, whereas small intestine motor patterns such as discrete clustered contractions and prolonged propagated contractions occur with equal frequency in diarrhea- and constipation-predominant

IBS, again raising questions as to their pathogenic importance. (Ch. 84; pg 1887)

146. a

Abnormalities of visceral sensory function are believed to play a prominent role in the pathogenesis of the irritable bowel syndrome (IBS). Hypersensitivity to colonic balloon distention is seen in most patients with IBS. In those patients with normal sensation to initial balloon distention, hypersensitivity may be induced by noxious repetitive distention of the sigmoid colon. There is significant overlap of IBS with other functional conditions such as functional dyspepsia, and patients with different functional disorders may exhibit abnormalities of visceral perception diffusely throughout the gut. However, most IBS patients have normal sensitivity to cutaneous stimulation indicating that the defect is selective for visceral sensory pathways. Although abnormal gas reflux patterns are seen in some patients with IBS, the total volume of gas in these individuals is normal. Altered visceral elastic properties are observed in some cases of IBS. Patients with constipation-predominant IBS may exhibit increased compliance of the rectum while diarrhea-prone individuals may exhibit a stiff, noncompliant rectum that does not accommodate to accept a fecal bolus. (Ch. 84; pg 1888)

147. b

Diarrhea-predominant irritable bowel syndrome (IBS) may respond to a variety of therapies. Lactase deficiency is a common condition that mimics IBS; thus, either a trial of a lactose-free diet or performance of a lactose tolerance test may be indicated for patients with diarrhea-predominant illness. Most studies suggest that fiber supplements are no better than placebos in managing diarrhea-prone IBS; some forms of fiber such as bran may increase flatulence and distention. Opiate antidiarrheals reduce diarrhea by inducing segmenting contractions that slow transit and promote the absorption of fecal water. Antispasmodics may benefit patients with meal-induced diarrhea because they inhibit the gastrocolonic response. (Ch. 84; pg 1895)

148. b

A number of therapies are useful in the management of constipation-predominant irritable bowel syndrome. As an initial treatment, any drugs that delay colonic transit (e.g., calcium channel blockers) should be discontinued. Fiber supplements such as psyllium and calcium polycarbophil are the first therapies to be considered, because they provide bulk and hydrate the stools. In more severe cases, osmotic laxatives may play a role. Isoosmotic preparations containing polyethylene glycol provide benefit for some patients who do not respond to standard agents such as milk of magnesia or lactulose. Prokinetic agents can enhance stool emptying in some patients; however, their effects are generally weak. Stimulant laxatives may cause catharctic colon and should not be used chronically. (Ch. 84; pgs 1895, 1900)

149. d

Common symptoms in irritable bowel syndrome (IBS) include persistent postprandial lower abdominal pain (possibly due to prolongation of the gastrocolonic response), increased fecal mucus, a sensation of incomplete fecal evacuation, and upper gastrointestinal symptoms such as heartburn, nausea, early satiety, and dyspepsia. Some patients with IBS do experience sleep disruption and thus may have pain at night. However, the presence of nocturnal symptoms is an indication to more aggressively exclude organic diseases of the gut. (Ch. 84; pg 1885)

150. d

Hirschsprung disease results from aganglionosis extending proximally from the anus. The rectoanal inhibitory reflex is absent in most persons with Hirschsprung disease; however, it may also be impaired in premature or low birth weight infants. Proctosigmoidoscopy usually reveals a normal, empty rectum, although stercoral ulcers may be seen in some patients. For accurate diagnosis, a deep rectal biopsy should be obtained at least 3 cm proximal to the pectinate line. Diarrhea may develop in 20% of patients as a result of pseudomembranous enterocolitis induced by the functional obstruction. Overflow incontinence can also be a feature of this condition. (Ch. 85; pg 1918)

151. a

Slow transit constipation typically produces hard, dry, pellet-like stools. Using bony landmarks, plain radiographs can be used to detect regional delays in transit of radiopaque markers. Patients with pelvic floor dysfunction as a cause for constipation may respond to biofeedback techniques. In contrast, surgical resection in these individuals may produce little benefit or may lead to uncontrolled diarrhea. (Ch. 85; pg 1914)

True/False

152. false

153. true

154. true

155. false

Pruritus ani may be caused by pinworms in children, but this is rarely the case in adults. Idiopathic pruritus ani is much more common. Pruritus ani may occur as a consequence of a variety of conditions, including fistulas, anal carcinoma, hemorrhoids, fecal incontinence, and psoriasis, and therefore it may respond to treatment of the underlying condition. Pruritus ani does not respond to local massage and vigorous mechanical cleansing measures, which instead often produce further irritation and excoriation of the anal mucosa. (Ch. 91; pg 2098)

156. false

157. false

158. true

159. true

160. true

161. true

External skin tags probably arise from thrombosis of an external hemorrhoid with redundancy of the overlying skin and previous resolution of the clot. External hemorrhoids are vascular structures arising from below the dentate line and are covered by squamous epithelium. Anorectal varices and hemorrhoids are unrelated. Hemorrhoids have no connection to the portal system, and the incidence of hemorrhoids is the same regardless of the presence of portal hypertension. Thrombosis of an external hemorrhoid may be a painful event. Simple surgical excision of the clot may offer immediate relief, although frequently patients respond to conservative medical therapy. Internal hemorrhoids are classified according to the degree of prolapse. Most third-degree and fourth-degree hemorrhoids require surgery because of the high risk of strangulation. Rubber-band ligation and infrared therapy are both standard treatment modalities for internal hemorrhoids not large enough to require a formal hemorrhoidectomy. Treatment of external hemorrhoids with these modalities would result in severe pain. (Ch. 91; pg 2085)

162. false

The internal anal sphincter is a distal continuation of the circular, not the longitudinal, muscle layer of the rectum. (Ch. 91; pg 2094)

163. true

The right colon receives its blood supply from the superior mesenteric artery and the left colon from the inferior mesenteric artery, with a watershed area located in the region of the splenic flexure. (Ch. 80; pg 1766)

164. true

Clostridium septicum is a causative organism of typhlitis. (Ch. 48; pg 1042)

165. true

Antiperistaltic contractions are prevalent in the right colon, whereas peristaltic contractions are prevalent in the left colon. (Ch. 11; pg 225)

166. true

Studies in both dogs and humans suggest that giant migrating contractions are the manometric correlates of mass movements of intracolonic contents observed radiographically prior to defecation. (Ch. 11; pg 226)

167. false

The presence of skin tags (acrochordons) does not warrant a change from the usual screening procedures for colonic neoplasm. Skin tags are associated with colonic adenomas in patients with acromegaly but not in the general population. (Ch. 90; pg 2044)

168. true

Approximately 50% of individuals with fecal occult blood have an adenoma or carcinoma on colonoscopy. (Ch. 90; pg 2056)

169. false

Insertion of a 60-cm sigmoidoscope will routinely examine the distal 50 cm of the colon and will detect about 50% to 60% of colonic neoplasms when used to screen unselected populations. (Ch. 88; pg 1980)

170. true

The sensitivity and specificity of carcinoembryonic antigen (CEA) testing for the purposes of colorectal neoplasia screening are low. The clinical use of CEA is limited to selected patients with previously diagnosed colorectal carcinoma to detect early recurrence of disease. (Ch. 90; pg 2068)

171. false

Carcinoma in situ, also referred to as high-grade dysplasia, is routinely treated and cured by polypectomy. When cancer cells penetrate the muscularis mucosae, evaluation of the margin of the polyp with serial sections is warranted, as is evaluation for lymphatic and capillary invasion. Poor prognostic features that indicate the need for surgery include large size, poor differentiation, lymphatic or capillary invasion, invasion into the stalk margin, and a short stalk or no stalk. (Ch. 88; pg 1983)

172. false

Although bleeding and diverticulitis are the two major complications of diverticulosis, it is very unusual for the two to present simultaneously. (Ch. 86; pg 1928)

173. false

174. false

175. true

Ischemic colitis commonly occurs as an iatrogenic consequence of inferior mesenteric artery interruption during aortic surgery. At colonoscopy, abnormal mucosa is usually seen extending proximally from the distal sigmoid colon. Most patients respond to supportive medical management. (Ch. 114; pg 2596)

176. true

Barium trapped proximal to a colonic obstruction is of concern because continued dehydration can lead to inspissation and impaction. In the small intestine, inspissation of barium is not a concern, because it remains in suspension, probably as a result of net fluid secretion in the small intestine. (Ch. 39; pg 853)

177. false

Acute colonic obstruction results in severe pain and distention. Pressure in the colon may rise rapidly and possibly cause rupture of the colon. Emergent decompression of the colon is required in this circumstance to decrease wall tension, improve mucosal blood flow, and decrease the risk of perforation. (Ch. 39; pg 846)

178. false

The volume of intestinal gas as determined by the washout technique is normal in patients complaining of excess gas. Patients with excess gas tend to reflux more gas from the intestine to the stomach. (Ch. 37; pg 817)

179. true

Bran ingestion accelerates colonic transit in individuals with a transit time longer than 3 days. Bran prolongs the transit time in subjects with a transit time of 1 day or less. (Ch. 84; pg 1895)

180. false

The rectoanal inhibitory reflex is absent in persons with Hirschsprung disease because of loss of ganglia in the rectum. However, in some patients with megarectum, the reflex may be absent with preservation of normal rectal ganglia. The definitive diagnosis of Hirschsprung disease requires appropriate biopsy findings. (Ch. 80; pg 1769)

181. false

182. true

183. false

184. true

Compliance with fecal occult blood testing is usually in the range of 30% to 60%. Controlled trials have demonstrated a reduction in colorectal cancer mortality with fecal occult blood testing. At very high concentrations, ethanol may induce hemorrhagic gastritis, but small to moderate amounts do not appear to induce bleeding. Cecal cancers do have a tendency to bleed more than other cancers in the colon. (Ch. 33; pgs 747, 753, 755)

185. true

The colon progressively diminishes in lumenal diameter when moving from the cecum to the sigmoid colon. (Ch. 80; pg 1765)

186. false

All three modalities are contraindicated if perforation and peritonitis are suspected. (Ch. 80; pg 1772)

187. false

A 43% recurrence rate after nonoperative reduction can be expected. (Ch. 80; pg 1772)

188. true

Once removed endoscopically, no further therapy is needed, only close surveillance. (Ch. 88; pg 1985)

189. false

Familial adenomatous polyposis, Gardner syndrome, and attenuated adenomatous polyposis coli are inherited in an autosomal dominant pattern. (Ch. 89; pg 1995)

190. false

Colorectal cancers in hereditary nonpolyposis colorectal cancer have a better outcome than sporadic tumors matched for stage. (Ch. 90; pg 2035)

191. false

Most polyps and cancers in hereditary nonpolyposis colorectal cancer are above the reach of the sigmoidoscope—65% to 88% occur in the proximal colon. Therefore, colonoscopy is recommended at about age 25, or 5 years before the earliest colorectal cancer developed in the family. It should be repeated every 2 years if polyps or tumors are found. (Ch. 90; pg 2060)

192. true

A study of 302 consecutive autopsies in patients with early metastatic cancer from an unknown primary lesion revealed that only 3.6% originated in the colon or rectum. (Ch. 90; pg 2065)

193. false

Radiation therapy as adjunctive treatment for colon cancer outside the rectum has not proven to be beneficial. (Ch. 90; pg 2068)

194. false

195. false

196. true

197. true

198. false

Fecal continence is preserved in ileal pouch–anal canal anastomosis and continent ileostomy (Kock). Diarrhea, which occurs over the long term in about one-third of patients with a Kock pouch, probably results from pouchitis caused by bacterial overgrowth. Pregnancy and spontaneous vaginal delivery are well tolerated in patients with an ileal pouch–anal anastomosis. (Ch. 82; pg 1844)

199. true

200. true

Older patients are more likely to experience long periods without relapse than are younger patients. The severity of the first attack and the degree of colonic involvement do not predict the likelihood of recurrence. However, these factors are predictive of the severity of recurrence and likelihood of subsequent colectomy. (Ch. 81; pg 1784)

201. true

202. false

203. true

204. false

205. true

Collagenous and lymphocytic colitis have been associated with thyroid disorders, asthma, diabetes, celiac disease, Sjögren's syndrome, vitiligo and pernicious anemia. Though idiopathic, these disorders appear to be caused by immunologic events. They have been associated with antigens HLA-A1 (lymphocytic) and HLA-A2 (collagenous) but not with HLA-B8 and -DR3. Perinuclear antineutrophil cytoplasmic antibody (p-ANCA) positivity is found in 20% of cases. (Ch. 83; pg 1859)

206. false

Several investigators have reported severe ischemic colitis in patients using large amounts of cocaine. The putative mechanism is catecholamine-induced mesenteric vasospasm. Colitis in previously asymptomatic individuals has been associated with numerous nonsteroidal antiinflammatory drugs, including diclofenac, but not with the new selective COX-2 inhibitors. (Ch. 83; pg 1869)

207. true

Perforating stercoral ulcers are usually located on the antimesenteric border of the sigmoid or rectosigmoid colon (77% of the time). (Ch. 83, pg 1873)

208. true

Melanosis can be detected in a biopsy specimen stained with hematoxylin and eosin even if it is not visible on endoscopy. (Ch. 83; pg 1867)

209. false

Motor activity in the colon of healthy volunteers is significantly greater during waking hours, and especially postprandially. (Ch. 11; pg 230)

210. false

Colonic scintigraphic studies demonstrate regional differences in the emptying efficiency of the marker: 20% of the marker is evacuated from the right colon, 32% from the left colon, and 66% from the rectum (approximations, thus total ≠ 100%). (Ch. 11; pg 235)

211. false

Approximately 50% of patients with diarrhea whose cytotoxin and culture tests are positive for *Clostridium difficile* have pseudomembranes. (Ch. 87; pg 1954)

Matching

212. b

213. e

214. a

Given the difference in cost, it is appropriate to begin treatment with sulfasalazine and reserve 5-aminosalicylic acid (5-ASA) enemas for those who cannot tolerate sulfasalazine. Oral 5-ASA preparations are an additional option. Metronidazole has documented efficacy in patients with colonic and perianal Crohn's disease. Indications for immunosuppressive therapy include an inability to taper steroids and unacceptable adverse effects from steroids. The risks of immunosuppressive therapy must be weighed against its benefits. Furthermore, at least 3 months of treatment are required before a significant therapeutic benefit can be expected from immunosuppressive therapy. (Ch. 81; pgs 1814, 1816)

215. b

216. d

217. a

The severity of disease in ulcerative colitis patients is based on stool frequency, bleeding, and systemic signs, including fever, pulse, anemia, and sedimentation rate. (Ch. 81; pg 1782)

218. c

219. b

220. a

221. c

222. d

Colonoscopic polypectomy may cause bleeding immediately or up to 12 days after the procedure (secondary hemorrhage). The transmural burn syndrome is characterized by a full-thickness burn of the colonic wall that manifests clinically 6 to 24 hours after polypectomy with localized pain, fever, and leukocytosis. Oversedation occurs only in the immediate time frame of the examination because of the short-acting nature of the sedatives and analgesics used. Colonic perforation may present immediately or up to 1 day after the examination. Colonic obstruction is not a complication of colonoscopy. (Ch. 122; pg 2714)

223. b

224. d

225. e

226. a

A loss of 5 to 10 mL of blood from the colon causes a fecal hemoglobin concentration of approximately 5 to 10 mg/g stool and results in a positive Hemoccult II test in 50% of stool samples. Positive tests are more likely with more distal sources of blood loss. More than 100 mL of blood loss is required to produce melena. Thus, 20 mL of blood lost from the cecum will almost always give a positive fecal occult blood test (FOBT) but will not produce melena. A loss of 5 mL of blood from the anorectum would be expected to give a positive FOBT result and cause a streak of bright red blood. A loss of 150 mL of blood from the cecum will produce melena and could easily produce hematochezia, depending upon colonic transit. A 4 mL loss of blood from the duodenum will undergo such degradation during its transit through the gut that it will not produce a positive result when standard tests for fecal occult blood are used. (Ch. 33; pg 747)

227. a

228. c

229. b

Reticulocyte counts are maximal within 7 to 10 days of initiating iron therapy. Normalization of the hemoglobin may occur within 2 months, whereas repletion of bone marrow stores may take up to 6 months. (Ch. 33; pg 756)

230. b

231. c

232. a

233. b

234. a

235. d

236. e

One of the major advantages of the immunochemical test is that dietary restrictions are unnecessary. The quantitative heme porphyrin assay is the most sensitive for upper gastrointestinal blood loss, requiring only slightly greater than 2 mL/day. All of the tests can detect as little as 3 mL/day of colonic blood loss (Ch. 33; pg 749, Table 33.5). Only uncooked vegetables as listed in the question need to be excluded for guaiac-based tests. (Ch. 33; pg 748)

237. c

238. d

239. b

Unlike hyperplastic and adenomatous polyps, lipomas are submucosal lesions. Villous adenomas are occasionally associated with watery diarrhea. Patients with chronic colitis can sometimes develop benign inflammatory pseudopolyps. (Ch. 88; pgs 1974, 1977, 1980)

240. a

Desmoid tumors are benign fibrous growths that occur in 3% to 20% of patients with familial adenomatous polyposis, and rarely in the general population. (Ch. 89; pg 2005)

241. e

Turcot syndrome resembles typical familial adenomatous polyposis, but with an associated brain cancer. (Ch. 89; pg 2006)

242. f

Mucocutaneous pigmentation in a patient with Peutz-Jeghers syndrome is characterized by melanin spots, especially in the perioral area and on the lips. (Ch. 89; pg 2007)

243. h

In vitro protein synthesis testing involves determining the presence of a relevant DNA mutation by the in vitro detection of protein truncation. (Ch. 89; pg 1997)

244. b

Gardner syndrome is the same as familial adenomatous polyposis, but with associated extracolonic lesions, such as osteomas and fibromas. (Ch. 89; pg 2004)

245. j

The most common extracolonic malignancy associated with familial adenomatous polyposis is duodenal carcinoma, most commonly in the periampullary area. (Ch. 89; pg 2001)

246. n

Cowden's disease is characterized by multiple facial trichilemmomas; hamartomatous gastrointestinal polyps occur in 35% of patients with this disease. (Ch. 89; pg 2011)

247. o

Cronkhite-Canada syndrome is characterized by polyposis throughout the gastrointestinal tract except the esophagus. (Ch. 89; pg 2013)

248. c

The average number of polyps in patients with familial adenomatous polyposis is approximately 1000 when the phenotype is fully expressed, although 100 or more is considered diagnostic. (Ch. 89; pg 1998)

249. d

Linkage testing uses DNA markers near or in the gene in question to identify mutant gene carriers in a kindred. (Ch. 89; pg 1997)

250. f

251. i

252. k

253. a

254. d

255. c

Cancers proximal to the transverse colon are treated with a right hemicolectomy, and tumors from the splenic flexure are treated with a left hemicolectomy. Lesions in the sigmoid colon are treated with segmental resection and an end-to-end primary colonic anastomosis. Cancers that extend into the submucosa but no further are stage A, cancers that extend through the muscularis propria and into the serosa or fat are considered stage B, and those that are associated with lymph node metastasis are considered stage C. Carcinoma in situ refers to a cancer not invading the muscularis mucosae. Stage D colon cancer is defined by the presence of distant metastasis. (Ch. 90; pgs 2033, 2048, 2065, 2067)

256. d

257. c

258. b

259. a

260. e

Bismuth may rarely cause encephalopathy when used in high doses or if given to patients with renal failure. Diphenoxylate may precipitate toxic megacolon and may prolong the excretion of pathogens. Psyllium may precipitate intestinal obstruction proximal to pre-existing strictures. The serotonin antagonist methysergide sometimes used to treat secretory diarrheas may cause tardive dyskinesia. Clonidine, an α_2-adrenergic antagonist, may cause postural hypotension. (Ch. 40; pg 897)

261. d

262. a

263. e

264. b

265. c

The α_2-adrenergic agonist clonidine is sometimes used to treat diarrhea accompanying opiate withdrawal. Indomethacin inhibits prostaglandin synthesis and secretion and may be used to treat AIDS enteropathy. Methysergide (a serotonin antagonist) may be useful to treat diarrhea of carcinoid syndrome. Promethazine, an H_1 antagonist, may be useful for systemic mastocytosis. Lansoprazole, a proton pump inhibitor, may be useful for the treatment of the hyperacidity of Zollinger-Ellison syndrome. (Ch. 40; pg 897)

CHAPTER 5

Multiple Choice

1. c

   Studies have suggested that biliary pancreatitis is triggered by the passage of stones through the ampulla of Vater into the duodenum. Although it is a common cause for acute pancreatitis, it does not result in chronic pancreatitis. Thus, chronic functional or morphologic abnormalities of the pancreas do not occur as a result of gallstone disease. Gallstone pancreatitis occurs more frequently in patients with multiple small stones. Gallstones are recovered from the feces of 30% to 85% of patients with hyperbilirubinemia and pancreatitis. Although the timing of acute cholecystectomy remains controversial, definitive treatment of underlying biliary obstruction should be performed prior to discharging the patient from the hospital. (Ch. 93; pg 2125)

2. e

   The most common form of nonalcoholic chronic pancreatitis in North America and Europe is the idiopathic type (10% to 40%). (Ch. 94; pg 2156)

3. c

   Under experimental conditions, alcohol has been shown to exert a direct toxic effect on pancreatic tissue. In general, patients with ethanol-related pancreatitis consume large quantities of alcohol for a prolonged period prior to the onset of symptoms. Thus, the pancreas is usually morphologically or functionally abnormal prior to the first attack of acute pancreatitis. Epidemiologic studies suggest that individuals who abuse ethanol and consume high-protein diets are more likely to develop acute pancreatitis. (Ch. 93; pg 2127)

4. d

   Postoperative pancreatitis can complicate a wide variety of surgical procedures. It occurs most commonly after manipulation of the pancreas or periampullary region or when a procedure is complicated by the development of hypotension. No evidence has been found to directly implicate halogenated anesthetic agents in the pathogenesis of postoperative pancreatitis. (Ch. 93; pg 2131)

5. c

   Tropical pancreatitis is more common in Afroasiatic countries and typically occurs in the setting of malnutrition. The ingestion of dietary toxins has also been suggested to play a role. This disorder is characterized by recurrent episodes of abdominal pain in childhood, the onset of diabetes mellitus around the time of puberty, and extensive pancreatic calcifications. (Ch. 94; pg 2154)

6. d

   Cytomegalovirus, *Mycobacterium avium*, *Cryptococcus* species, *Toxoplasma gondii*, *Mycobacterium tuberculosis*, and *Candida* species have been linked to the development of pancreatitis in patients infected with the human immunodeficiency virus (HIV). *Pneumocystis carinii* has not been reported to cause HIV-related pancreatitis. (Ch. 93; pg 2129)

7. b

   Both aerosolized and intravenous pentamidine have been associated with acute pancreatitis. Treatment with didanosine is complicated by the development of clinical pancreatitis in up to 20% of patients. Asymptomatic elevations of serum amylase are seen in 40% of patients taking didanosine. Trimethoprim-sulfamethoxazole is a less common cause of drug-induced pancreatic injury. Zidovudine has not been associated with acute pancreatitis. (Ch. 93; pg 2128)

8. b

   A diet high in fat and protein predisposes a person to alcohol-induced pancreatic injury. (Ch. 94; pg 2153)

9. d

   Immunohistologic studies of patients with chronic pancreatitis have shown that certain neurotransmitters associated with the development of pain, such as substance P, are quantitatively increased in afferent pancreatic nerves. (Ch. 94; pg 2157)

10. d

   In animals, chronic alcoholism causes a baseline hypersecretion of digestive enzymes, in part explained by increased cholinergic tone. In addition, in chronically alcoholic dogs and humans, the pancreas is more responsive to cholecystokinin stimulation. (Ch. 94; pg 2152)

11. b

   The serum half-life of amylase is approximately 2 hours. Thus, the measurement of lipase levels may be a more sensitive means of assessing patients with acute pancreatitis after the first day of symptoms. Amylase elevations in hypertriglyceridemia-induced acute pancreatitis may be underestimated by standard laboratory techniques. Dilution of the lactescent sera may eliminate this effect. Macroamylase has a much greater molecular weight than amylase (200 kd versus 45 kd) and is not cleared by the kidney. In patients with macroamylasemia and no pancreatic disease, lipase levels are normal. (Ch. 93; pg 2133)

12. a

   Hunger is the most reliable marker for initiating refeeding in the patient with acute pancreatitis. Nasogastric suction is clearly indicated in cases of severe pancreatitis with associated ileus. The routine use of antibiotics in patients with mild pancreatitis is unnecessary. However, there is emerging evidence suggesting that antibiotics are of benefit in the management of patients with pancreatic necrosis. Preoperative endoscopic retrograde cholangiopancreatography is indicated in patients with evidence of persistent common bile duct stones. (Ch. 93; pg 2139)

13. a

Ecchymosis of the flanks and periumbilical areas (Grey Turner and Cullen signs) result from retroperitoneal hemorrhage, which may occur with hemorrhagic pancreatitis. These signs often are indicative of a poor prognosis. Elevations of serum methemalbumin levels have been demonstrated to occur in this clinical setting. (Ch. 93; pg 2132)

14. c

Hypocalcemia with acute pancreatitis is a poor prognostic sign. Significant loss of albumin as a result of severe exudative inflammation in the peripancreatic region will cause a decline in total serum calcium. However, in severe pancreatitis, the fall in serum calcium exceeds that predicted for the level of hypoalbuminemia. Although hypocalcemia was initially felt to be secondary to fat necrosis with calcium sequestration, more recent studies suggest the decline is the result of diminished end-organ responsiveness to parathyroid hormone. There is no evidence suggesting that hypocalcemia observed in acute pancreatitis is due to hyperglucagonemia. (Ch. 93; pg 2139)

15. a

The onset of pancreatic insufficiency in patients with chronic pancreatitis has been associated with the resolution of abdominal pain in studies of patients with alcohol-induced pancreatitis. (Ch. 94; pg 2157)

16. a

Pseudocysts result from disruption of the pancreatic duct, resulting in a collection of pancreatic fluid encased in a simple fibrous membrane. Pseudocysts are capable of expanding and may erode into vascular structures in 5% of cases, resulting in massive hemorrhage with a resultant mortality of 40%. Although pseudocysts larger than 5 cm in size and lasting longer than 6 months seldom resolve spontaneously, in the absence of immediate complications, surgery is usually deferred until the fibrous membrane matures, a process that generally requires approximately 6 weeks. (Ch. 93; pg 2143)

17. c

Most pancreatic abscesses are polymicrobial, and although there have been a few reports of successful management with large percutaneous drains, prompt surgical debridement of necrosis remains the standard of care. (Ch. 93; pg 2143)

18. d

Given the presentation with high fevers, the low-attenuation region may represent infected necrotic tissue or a pancreatic abscess. To confirm the diagnosis, needle aspiration of the suspicious pancreatic region should be performed. Emergent surgery is not indicated unless the patient is unstable or the diagnosis of infected necrotic tissue or abscess is confirmed. (Ch. 93; pg 2143)

19. d

Acute pancreatitis may produce hypoxemia by several mechanisms. Most commonly, patients develop atelectasis as a result of poor respiratory effort and splinting in the setting of abdominal pain. Pleural effusions may result from diaphragmatic inflammation, transdiaphragmatic spread of pancreatic ascites, or extension of a pancreatic pseudocyst. The most serious complication is the development of adult respiratory distress syndrome, which results in an extended clinical course and frequently death. Pulmonary hemorrhage does not commonly result from acute pancreatitis. (Ch. 93; pg 2145)

20. c

Pancreatic pseudocysts are most frequently encountered after pancreatic inflammation resulting from alcohol- or gallstone-induced injury. Those pseudocysts that are larger than 6 cm and persist for more than 6 weeks should be considered for drainage. If the pancreatic duct is intact and does not communicate with the pseudocyst, percutaneous drainage may be attempted. However, if the pseudocyst is in continuity with the pancreatic duct, percutaneous drainage may result in the development of a pancreatic fistula. Recent advances in endoscopic methods have afforded the ability to endoscopically drain appropriately located pseudocysts into the stomach or small intestine. (Ch. 94; pg 2164)

21. c

As a rule, the degree of fecal weight increase due to pancreatic malabsorption is less than in other conditions with comparable steatorrhea. This relatively low weight reflects a lesser quantity of fecal water. Patients may pass bulky formed stool as opposed to the frank watery diarrhea observed in other conditions. (Ch. 94; pg. 2156)

22. d

The failure of enzyme replacements to correct pancreatic steatorrhea in chronic pancreatitis may be caused by an inadequate delivery of lipase to the small intestine. Inadequate dosing, peptic acid inactivation of lipase, and delayed entry of coated tablets into the duodenum in relation to the meal all may cause insufficient enzyme activity. In addition, a concomitant malabsorptive condition such as bacterial overgrowth may result in lipid maldigestion independent of pancreatic insufficiency. The use of an H$_2$-receptor antagonist can reduce the likelihood of acid-induced degradation of lipase and may enhance the response to a given dose of enzyme supplementation. (Ch. 94; pg 2171)

23. c

A 72-hour fecal collection is the gold standard for the detection of lipid maldigestion. The presence of 15 g/day of fecal fat (normal, 7 g/day) confirms lipid maldigestion as a cause for this patient's diarrhea. This test is not specific for pancreatic insufficiency and cannot provide a diagnosis in the absence of additional studies. Because of a significant reserve in the production of lipase by the normal pancreas, lipid digestion remains intact until more than 90% of pancreatic exocrine function is lost. A repeat 72-hour fecal collection taken while the patient consumes pancreatic enzyme supplements can be used to assess the adequacy of the enzyme replacement. (Ch. 132; pg 2932)

24. b

Pancreatic enzymes are synthesized within acinar cells, not ductal cells. (Ch. 16; pg 357)

25. b

Fat in the intestine stimulates pancreatic secretion by way of cholecystokinin (CCK) release. The potency of a given lipid to induce CCK release varies according to the chain length, the degree of saturation, and the concentration of bile salts relative to fatty acids in the intestinal lumen. Gastric acid is not required for lipid-evoked CCK release and pancreatic enzyme secretion. (Ch. 16; pg 372)

26. a

Both essential amino acids and fatty acids are potent stimuli of pancreatic enzyme secretion. Antral distention also leads to pancreatic enzyme secretion. In contrast, glucose causes little or no pancreatic secretion in humans. (Ch. 16; pg 372)

27. c

The presence of an intraduodenal pH of less than or equal to 4.5 stimulates secretin release and pancreatic bicarbonate secretion. The action of secretin to stimulate bicarbonate release is potentiated by cholecystokinin. Duodenal pH is the major regulator of secretin release. (Ch. 16; pg 359)

28. d

Cholecystokinin (CCK) is a potent stimulant of pancreatic secretion. CCK is released by the hydrolytic products of digestion, including the amino acids and fatty acids. Carbohydrates are not a potent stimulus of CCK release. (Ch. 16; pg 360)

29. c

The body of the pancreas lies across and is pushed anteriorly by the first and second lumbar vertebrae. This position, coupled with the fixed nature of the gland in this region, make the body portion of the pancreatic duct more susceptible to disruption from blunt abdominal injury. (Ch. 92; pg 2109)

30. d

Visceral pain from the pancreas usually is sensed as a severe constant discomfort in the epigastrium. Because the pancreas does not contact the parietal peritoneum (owing to its retroperitoneal location), sharply localized pain usually does not occur. (Ch. 92; pg 2114)

31. c

Patients with pancreas divisum and otherwise unexplained recurrent acute pancreatitis are most likely to respond to endoscopic therapy. Patients with chronic pancreatitis respond poorly to both surgical and endoscopic therapies. Only about 30% of patients with pancreas divisum and chronic pancreatitis experience symptomatic improvement following minor sphincterotomy. (Ch. 92; pg 2117) (Ch. 93; pg 2127)

32. b

The patients with pancreas divisum most likely to respond to therapy are those without evidence of chronic pancreatitis and without symptoms of chronic persistent pain. (Ch. 92; pg 2117)

33. e

Surgical division of the annulus is not recommended because of the high incidence of pancreatitis and pancreatic fistulas complicating this procedure. Bypass of the obstructed intestinal segment is preferred for the treatment of annular pancreas. (Ch. 92; pg 2116)

34. a

Seventy-five percent of pancreatic rests are located in the submucosa of the stomach or small intestine. They appear as firm yellow nodules, 2 to 4 cm in diameter, often with a central mucosal depression. (Ch. 92; pg 2116)

35. b

Gallstones occur in 12% of patients with cystic fibrosis; however, most of these patients never develop biliary symptoms. (Ch. 97; pg 2233)

36. d

Meconium ileus occurs in 15% of infants with cystic fibrosis. This condition is thought to result from reduced water content in the meconium, causing it to become impacted within the bowel. Complications such as volvulus and small bowel atresia may lead to peritonitis. In uncomplicated cases, it may be possible to relieve the obstruction with *N*-acetylcysteine, Hypaque, or Gastrografin enemas. In cases involving volvulus, small bowel atresia or peritonitis, surgery is necessary, and mortality rates may be as high as 30%. (Ch. 97; pg 2233)

37. a

Ninety percent of human pancreatic cancers originate from ductular cells, and 75% of all tumors are ductal cell mucin-producing adenocarcinomas. Acinar cell carcinomas are uncommon and are associated with elevated serum lipase levels, nonsuppurative panniculitis of the extremities, polyarthritis, and subcutaneous nodules. Islet cell tumors, including insulinomas, glucagonomas, and somatostatinomas cause a number of endocrine syndromes. Giant cell tumors can be divided into four histologic categories: giant cell, spindle cell, pleomorphic, and anaplastic. The prognosis for these tumors is generally worse than that for ductular cell tumors, although rarely patients will enjoy long-term survival. (Ch. 95; pg 2180)

38. c

Around the world, the risk factor most strongly associated with pancreatic cancer is cigarette smoking, which approximately doubles one's chance of developing the disease. (Ch. 95; pg 2179)

39. b

Two-thirds of pancreatic ductal adenocarcinomas occur in the head of the gland. Because of their proximity to the intrapancreatic portion of the common bile duct, tumors in the head usually compress and obstruct the bile duct as they grow, producing jaundice. (Ch. 95; pg 2180)

40. b

The most frequent genetic alteration in pancreatic adenocarcinoma is activation of the K-*ras* oncogene, which occurs in at least 85% of cases. (Ch. 95; pg 2179)

41. b

A variety of tumor-associated antigens have been studied; however, all are of limited value in detecting lesions smaller than 1 cm. Although the CA 19-9 tumor marker is the most sensitive (80%) and most specific (90%), levels in patients with small lesions are almost never significantly elevated. (Ch. 95; pg 2181)

42. c

Combination therapy using 5-fluorouracil (5-FU) and supervoltage radiation appears to improve survival in patients with both locally advanced and surgically resectable pancreatic cancer. In a study of patients with unresectable disease, 5-FU plus radiation resulted in a median survival of 10.4 months, compared to 6.3 months for patients receiving radiation alone. Gemcitabine is a newer chemotherapeutic agent with radiosensitizing properties. In several studies, only a small subpopulation of patients received a slight survival benefit with gemcitabine therapy compared to treatment with 5-FU alone. However, for about 25% of patients, gemcitabine reduced pain, increased weight, and improved the quality of life. Wire mesh stents should never be placed in potential candidates for pancreatic resection. These stents incite a severe inflammatory reaction and eventually may be incorporated into the bile duct wall, potentially complicating or even preventing surgical intervention. (Ch. 95; pg 2189)

43. c

The definitive diagnosis of VIPoma requires the establishment of a secretory diarrhea, an elevated serum level of vasoactive intestinal polypeptide (VIP), and the identification of a tumor. Diarrhea persists during fasting and is both iso-osmotic and high output; the volume of diarrhea was quantitated in one study as more than 1 L/day in 100% of patients and more than 3 L/day in 70% to 80% of patients. Because of the iso-osmotic nature of the diarrhea, a hydrogen breath test would not be indicated. A number of diseases may cause chronic secretory diarrhea with this volume, and therefore differentiation from VIPoma is required: midgut carcinoid, medullary thyroid carcinoma, Zollinger-Ellison syndrome, diffuse islet-cell hyperplasia, and surreptitious use of laxatives. Laxative abuse can be assessed using a number of tests, including the evaluation of stool or urine for phenolphthalein. (Ch. 96; pg 2198)

44. d

VIPoma is an endocrine tumor, usually located in the pancreas, that produces excessive amounts of vasoactive intestinal peptide (VIP). Patients with the VIPoma syndrome present with a number of characteristic abnormalities: large volume diarrhea despite fasting, hypokalemia, dehydration, hypochlorhydria, hyperglycemia, hypercalcemia, and flushing. Fasting hypoglycemia would suggest other conditions, such as insulinoma, inadvertent or deliberate insulin administration, ingestion of oral sulfonylurea, alcoholism with severe liver disease, and malnutrition. (Ch. 96; pg 2198)

45. c

Multiple endocrine neoplasia (MEN) syndrome type I is inherited in an autosomal dominant fashion and is associated with a defect on chromosome 11. The most common clinical abnormality in MEN I is hypercalcemia resulting from hyperparathyroidism. The most common pancreatic endocrine neoplasm in MEN I is gastrinoma, which frequently presents with multiple tumor foci in the pancreas. (Ch. 96; pg 2196)

46. b

In cases of glucagonoma, plasma glucagon levels exceed 1000 pg/mL in 48% to 90% and exceed 500 pg/mL in 86% to 97% of patients. Other conditions associated with increased plasma glucagon concentrations include renal insufficiency, acute pancreatitis, hyperadrenocorticism, hepatic insufficiency, severe stress, prolonged fasting and familial hyperglucagonemia. With the exception of cirrhosis, plasma glucagon usually is not elevated higher than 500 pg/mL in these conditions. (Ch. 96; pg 2201)

47. a

48. d

This patient has the classic findings of insulinoma. She is a woman between age 40 and 50, and her symptoms are associated with fasting. Symptoms suggest catecholamine-excess with diaphoresis as well as neuroglycopenia as evidenced by emotional irritability, headache, and confusion. The most reliable test to document hypoglycemia is a 72-hour fast done during an inpatient stay. During this exercise, patients are allowed free access to water. Most patients with insulinoma become symptomatic within 24 hours. During fasting, the diagnosis of insulinoma is suspected if serial insulin levels remain stable or increase in the face of serial glucose levels less than 50 mg/dL or if the insulin-glucose ratio is greater than 0.3. The differential diagnosis of fasting hypoglycemia includes insulinoma, B-cell hyperplasia, surreptitious administration of insulin or oral hypoglycemic agents, and autoantibodies to insulin or the insulin receptor. In patients with insulinomas, the proinsulin and C-peptide levels are usually elevated, no autoantibodies to insulin or the insulin receptor are detected, and there are no oral hypoglycemic agents in the blood. Adrenal insufficiency would not cause the test results described. (Ch. 96; pg 2197)

49. a

In general, the histologic classification of pancreatic endocrine tumors does not predict the growth pattern of the tumor nor determine whether it is malignant. Further, there is no definite correlation between the histologic pattern and the clinical syndrome with which the tumor is associated. In addition to producing multiple peptides, pancreatic endocrine tumors frequently express the α-chain and less frequently the β-chain of human chorionic gonadotropin or chromogranin A, and it has been proposed that their expression correlates with the development of malignancy. Malignancy, however, can be unequivocally established only in those patients who have metastatic tumor spread to lymph nodes or the liver, gross invasion or infiltration into adjacent organs, or clear blood vessel invasion. Because of this, it is not completely established what percentage of pancreatic endocrine tumors are malignant. The benign nature of the tumors can be established only by long-term follow-up. The size of the tumor usually is not related to the severity of hormonally induced symptoms; in general, however, there is a correlation between size and the occurrence of malignancy. (Ch. 96; pg 2195)

50. e

Endoscopic ultrasonography (EUS) is a sensitive imaging technique for evaluating patients with suspected pancreatic disease. EUS is the most sensitive technique for diagnosing endocrine tumors, and it is also useful for staging pancreatic adenocarcinoma, although the presence of enlarged peripancreatic lymph nodes does not confirm the presence of either malignancy or unresectability of a pancreatic mass. EUS has potential use in the diagnosis of chronic pancreatitis, although some localized areas of chronic pancreatitis may have an ultrasonographic appearance that is similar to adenocarcinoma. EUS reliably identifies neoplastic involvement of the portal and splenic veins; however, it is less reliable in detecting encasement of the major arterial structures. (Ch. 136; pg 3011)

51. d

In general, insulinomas are less responsive to octreotide than are glucagonomas, VIPomas, gastrinomas, and GRFomas. Some insulinomas may lack somatostatin receptors, explaining their poor clinical response to octreotide. There have been reports of patients with insulinoma deteriorating when treated with octreotide; thus, it is recommended that octreotide therapy for insulinomas be initiated only in the hospital. In one study, octreotide improved diarrhea and reduced plasma VIP concentrations in 86% of patients with VIPoma. For patients with glucagonoma, octreotide has been shown to improve necrolytic migratory erythema and reduce plasma glucagon concentrations. Octreotide reduces weight loss, pain, and diarrhea; however, it has little effect on diabetes mellitus or tumor size in patients with glucagonoma. Octreotide effectively reduces symptoms of growth hormone excess and the plasma concentration of GRF in patients with GRFomas. (Ch. 96; pg 2213)

52. b

Trypsinogen is normally secreted into pancreatic juice and is converted to trypsin upon reaching the duodenum, where it is exposed to enterokinase. However, small amounts of trypsinogen undergo autoactivation within the pancreas even under normal conditions. Pancreatic trypsin inhibitor produced by pancreatic acinar cells prevents intrapancreatic trypsin from damaging the host tissues. Alteration in this balance in favor of the activation of intrapancreatic trypsinogen has remained a central hypothesis for the development of acute pancreatitis. The identification of a mutation in the cationic trypsinogen gene in hereditary pancreatitis suggests that intrapancreatic trypsin activation likely plays a pathophysiologic role in this disease and possibly in other forms of acute pancreatitis. (Ch. 97; pg 2235)

53. d

Patients with insulin- or noninsulin-requiring diabetes resulting from pancreatic cancer have elevated levels of islet amyloid polypeptide (IAPP). The diabetes and high IAPP levels disappear in some patients after surgical resection of pancreatic cancer. (Ch. 95; pg 2181)

54. d

Solid and papillary epithelial neoplasms have a favorable prognosis, and most patients are cured by resection. However, some tumors may recur locally or metastasize to the liver. (Ch. 95; pg 2190)

55. b

Cholinergic stimuli acting through vagal efferents primarily modulate the action of gut peptides on pancreatic secretion. Acetylcholine has no physiologically relevant effect on the release of peptides that stimulate the pancreas—neither CCK nor secretin. (Ch. 16; pg 361)

56. c

The vein closest in proximity and with the widest exposure to the pancreatic tail and body is the splenic vein. It courses along the posterior extent of the tail and body. The invasion of tumors of the pancreatic head into the superior mesenteric vein (a more common clinical scenario) excludes their surgical resection. Tumors in the body and tail do not always invade by that route and must be staged and evaluated for surgical resection using other criteria. (Ch. 92; pg 2112)

True/False

57. false

Most patients with senile idiopathic chronic pancreatitis present with pancreatic insufficiency, diabetes, and a calcified pancreas with no attacks of abdominal pain. (Ch. 94; pg 2156)

58. true

Deficiencies of fat-soluble vitamins seldom occur in pancreatic insufficiency because lipolysis is relatively unimportant to their absorption. (Ch. 94; pg 2156)

59. true

The demonstration of diffuse, speckled calcification of the pancreas on plain abdominal radiography is diagnostic of chronic pancreatitis. Although the sensitivity of this finding is limited (30% to 40%), visible

evidence as such obviates the need for additional testing. (Ch. 94; pg 2161)

60. false

The finding of abdominal distention and ascites in an alcoholic patient with cirrhosis is often erroneously attributed to decompensated cirrhosis. Paracentesis in these patients commonly reveals elevated pancreatic enzymes and a high albumin level. (Ch. 94; pg 2165)

61. true

Obstruction of the distal common bile duct is frequently a complication of fibrosis of the pancreatic head. Clinically, this condition presents as an elevation of alkaline phosphatase and may progress to jaundice in cases of high-grade obstruction. (Ch. 94; pg 2159)

62. true

Splenic vein thrombosis with extrahepatic portal hypertension is a well-known complication of chronic pancreatitis. Varices involving the esophagus, stomach, duodenum, and colon with resultant hemorrhage have been described and can be cured with simple splenectomy. (Ch. 94; pg 2165)

63. false

The observation of diffuse calcification of the pancreas on plain radiography of the abdomen is diagnostic of chronic pancreatitis; unfortunately, it is seen in only 30% to 40% of patients. Pancreatic calcifications are most commonly seen in alcohol-induced chronic pancreatitis. Although computed tomography (CT) is 10% to 20% more sensitive than ultrasonography in the diagnosis of chronic pancreatitis, the specificities of the two imaging modalities are equivalent. Because of the expense and radiation exposure, some have suggested that CT be reserved for patients with negative or inadequate results on ultrasonographic examination. (Ch. 94; pg 2161)

64. false

Pancreatic pseudocysts occur in approximately 25% of patients with chronic pancreatitis. In contrast to pseudocysts complicating acute pancreatitis, pseudocysts that occur in patients with chronic pancreatitis seldom resolve spontaneously, particularly when larger than 6 cm. (Ch. 94; pg 2164)

65. true

66. true

When evaluating a pancreatic duct leak in the setting of an external pancreatic fistula, it is important to exclude any lesions that might impair drainage of the duct into the duodenum. In most patients, endoscopic retrograde cholangiopancreatography or fistulography performed after the tract has matured will provide this information. (Ch. 94; pgs 2161, 2165)

67. true

68. false

69. true

70. false

Postprandial pancreatic secretion represents the net result of stimulation and inhibition by intralumenal and postabsorptive effects of nutrients. Hyperglycemia and hyperaminoacidemia induced by intravenous nutrient administration inhibit pancreatic enzyme secretion. Nutrients such as lipids in the colon inhibit cholecystokinin-stimulated pancreatic enzyme and bicarbonate secretion in humans. Duodenal distention has been shown to stimulate pancreatic secretion by activation of a vagal cholinergic pathway. Acid entering the duodenum stimulates the release of secretin and pancreatic bicarbonate secretion. (Ch. 16; pg 371)

71. true

The importance of pancreatic divisum as a cause of pancreatitis remains controversial. A number of studies have suggested that the risk of pancreatitis in individuals with pancreas divisum is no higher than in those with normal ductal anatomy. (Ch. 92; pg 2117)

72. false

Patients with cystic fibrosis are characteristically hypersecretors of gastric acid, which exacerbates difficulties associated with acid degradation of orally administered enzymes. (Ch. 97; pg 2234)

73. true

74. true

75. true

Hereditary chronic pancreatitis characteristically presents with recurring episodes of abdominal pain at age 10 to 12 years. It follows a clinical course similar to that of nonhereditary pancreatitis, with the development of pancreatic insufficiency and overt diabetes 10 years after the first episode of pain in approximately 15% to 20% of patients. The inheritance pattern is autosomal dominant, with no evidence of linkage to a specific HLA haplotype. (Ch. 94; pg 2154)

76. true

77. true

78. true

Patients with pancreatic adenocarcinoma exhibit abnormal glucose tolerance testing in approximately 80% of cases. Diabetes mellitus is diagnosed in 50% of patients, although most patients with pancreatic cancer do not present with symptoms of diabetes. It has been postulated that pancreatic tumors may release a substance that stimulates the secretion of islet amyloid polypeptide (IAPP). IAPP then causes insulin resistance. The normalization of IAPP levels, with the

disappearance of diabetes, has been reported after resection of the tumor. Diabetes mellitus is associated with a 2- to 3-fold increased risk of pancreatic cancer. (Ch. 95; pg 2181)

79. false

80. true

81. true

Chemotherapy has not increased the survival rates of patients with pancreatic cancer. Surgical resection is the only chance for cure. Unfortunately, only 10% of patients have resectable lesions. For tumors of the pancreatic head, the Whipple procedure is the surgical treatment of choice. Neurolytic celiac plexus block provides some relief of pain in up to 90% of patients. (Ch. 95; pgs 2186, 2189)

82. false

Approximately 50% to 75% of patients with glucagonomas have metastasis at the time of diagnosis. (Ch. 96; pg 2216)

83. true

Less than 10% of insulinomas are malignant, and 75% to 95% of patients are curable with surgical resection of the primary tumor. (Ch. 96; pg 2216)

84. false

Abnormal cystic fibrosis transmembrane conductance regulator (CFTR) genotypes can lead to endocrine diseases without associated cystic fibrosis–related lung disease. CFTR genotypes were recently shown to be associated with idiopathic chronic pancreatitis in patients presenting without overt lung disease. (Ch. 97; pg 2235)

Matching

85. c

86. b

87. d

88. a

89. b

Both cystic fibrosis and hereditary pancreatitis in children can lead to clinical manifestations suggestive of pancreatic disease. More than 80% of patients with cystic fibrosis have clinically apparent pancreatic insufficiency by age 2 years. The mean age for the diagnosis of hereditary pancreatitis is 10 years. Hereditary pancreatitis is due to a G:A transition mutation in the cationic trypsinogen gene that renders the activated trypsin less susceptible to proteolytic degradation. Uninhibited trypsin initiates a cascade of events including the activation of pancreatic zymogens with resultant autodigestion and pancreatitis. Approximately 5% of patients with cystic fibrosis develop clinically apparent liver disease including neonatal jaundice, hypersplenism, esophageal varices, and bleeding. (Ch. 97; pgs 2229, 2235)

90. d

91. c

92. a

93. b

Endocrine tumors of the pancreas are classified according to the type of clinical syndrome they produce. *Gastrinomas* typically cause extensive, recurrent ulcerations throughout the gastrointestinal tract as a result of a continuous overstimulation of H^+,K^+-ATPase in the stomach by tumor-secreted gastrin. Cholelithiasis is reported in 65% to 95% of patients with *somatostatinomas* and is probably caused by impaired gallbladder emptying. Necrolytic migratory erythema, the characteristic skin rash of the *glucagonoma* syndrome, is a raised erythematous lesion often with a central bulla that is hyperpigmented on healing. GRFomas cause clinical symptoms that are indistinguishable from those of classic acromegaly. (Ch. 96; pg 2199) (Ch. 65; pg 1447)

94. b

95. c

96. d

97. a

The first patient most likely has sarcoidosis, which is associated with acute pancreatitis in 10% of cases as a result of secondary hypercalcemia. The second patient has acute pancreatitis, which may be the result of biliary microlithiasis caused by prolonged starvation. The third case provides a clinical picture consistent with systemic lupus erythematosus, which can rarely present with acute pancreatitis caused by vasculitis. In the final case, the patient has acute pancreatitis but a normal serum amylase level. Hyperlipidemia is known to erroneously reduce serum amylase measurements; thus, hyperlipidemia-induced pancreatitis should be considered in this patient. (Ch. 93; pg 2125)

98. d

99. a

100. b

The first patient most likely has pancreatic adenocarcinoma. The diagnosis can be reliably established by performing fine-needle aspiration of the pancreatic head mass. CA 19-9 lacks the sensitivity and specificity to be useful in this setting. The second patient has a clinical history consistent with chronic pancreatitis. The presence of a pseudocyst should be suspected in this individual with worsening of previously stable pain. This possibility is best evaluated by abdominal ultrasonography. The final case involves a woman with suspected biliary pancreatitis. Her clinical deterioration after admission is an indication for urgent endoscopic retrograde cholangiopancreatography to evaluate for and treat choledocholithiasis. (Ch. 93; pg 2134)

CHAPTER 6

Multiple Choice

1. b

   This patient has symptomatic gallstone disease. Bile acid therapy is more successful for cholesterol stones that are small (i.e., <1.5 cm diameter) and buoyant. Extracorporeal shock-wave lithotripsy can be successful with single, small stones; however, it is less effective with multiple, larger stones. Contact dissolution (therapy that involves infusion of the gallbladder with methyl-*tert*-butyl ether [MTBE]) can be performed within a few hours of the patient's attack and is successful in up to 90% of selected cases (i.e., if cholesterol stones are small, without calcified rims). Elective cholecystectomy remains the standard care for the majority of eligible patients, because recurrence rates are high after nonsurgical therapy. (Ch. 99; pgs 2265, 2270)

2. c

   Gallstones recur in approximately 50% of patients who show evidence of gallstone dissolution with chenodeoxycholic acid or ursodeoxycholic acid. The risk of recurrence is highest in the first year after dissolution and may be related to incomplete dissolution. Gallstones do not seem to recur if the patient remains free of stones for 5 years. (Ch. 99; pg 2273)

3. a

   Although 85% of all stones contain cholesterol, only 20% are relatively pure cholesterol stones. (Ch. 99; pg 2258)

4. e

   Bile acid malabsorption from ileal resection results in relative bile salt hyposecretion. Clofibrate leads to a decreased conversion of cholesterol to cholesterol esters. Estrogens are associated with an increased hepatic uptake of cholesterol. The underlying mechanisms for cholesterol hypersecretion during marked weight reduction are not well understood. The use of nonsteroidal antiinflammatory drugs are not a risk factor for the formation of cholesterol stones. (Ch. 99; pg 2259)

5. c

6. a

   This patient has gallstone ileus. Inflammation and necrosis of the gallbladder resulted in a fistula between the bowel and the gallbladder. After the stone passed into the bowel, the patient's symptoms subsided and the acute cholecystitis resolved. However, the stone caused bowel obstruction, which can occur with stones larger than 2.5 cm in diameter. The most common site of obstruction is the distal ileum (65% to 85% of cases) followed by the jejunum. Surgery is required to relieve the obstruction. (Ch. 99; pg 2269)

7. e

   There is no evidence to suggest that a prior performance of endoscopic retrograde cholangiopancreatography increases the risk of common bile duct stone formation. Bacterial glucuronidase with biliary infection deconjugates bilirubin, which binds to calcium, creating a nidus for stone formation. Foreign bodies, such as some adsorbable sutures used in cholecystectomy, have been shown to increase the risk for common bile duct stones. Patients with juxtapapillary diverticula have a higher incidence of choledocholithiasis as well. (Ch. 100; pg 2282)

8. d

   Choledochal cysts may be complicated by pancreatitis, cholangitis, cholecystitis, cyst rupture, biliary cirrhosis, portal hypertension, and cholangiocarcinoma. (Ch. 98; pg 2256)

9. a

   Abdominal radiographs are rarely helpful in identifying gallstones as the cause of abdominal pain, because only 13% to 17% of gallstones contain enough calcium to be radiopaque. (Ch. 99; pg 2267)

10. b

    Black pigment stones are found in western as well as Asian populations, whereas brown pigment stones are found mostly in Asian populations. Bile cultures usually are sterile in patients with black pigment stones, whereas brown pigment stones are associated with *Escherichia coli*, *Bacteroides* species, and parasitic infections. Black pigment stones are generally not recurrent, and up to 70% are radiopaque. In contrast, brown pigment stones frequently recur, and they are usually radiolucent. (Ch. 99; pg 2264)

11. c

    The intraduodenal segment of the common bile duct and the ampulla is surrounded by a sheath of smooth muscle fibers called the sphincter of Oddi. These muscle fibers act independently of the surrounding duodenal musculature. The resting pressure exerted by the sphincter is approximately 13 mm Hg above duodenal pressure, and the regulation of bile flow is primarily controlled by the sphincter. Relaxation of the sphincter occurs with cholecystokinin stimulation and is facilitated by parasympathetic stimulation. Sympathetic stimulation induces increased sphincter tone. (Ch. 98; pg 2250)

12. b

    The cholangiogram of a patient with sclerosing cholangitis generally reveals multiple strictures involving both the intrahepatic and extrahepatic ducts. A similar pattern may be seen with cholangiocarcinoma and with cytomegalovirus infection, and after radiotherapy or intraarterial chemotherapy directed at the liver. Trauma to the biliary tree typically is characterized by either a localized area of stricture or a leak in the extrahepatic duct system. (Ch. 100; pg 2305)

13. b

The most likely diagnosis is pancreatic carcinoma. Stent placement into the common bile duct is as effective as surgery for achieving biliary drainage; however, for palliation of nausea and pain it has not been compared in a controlled fashion with no intervention. (Ch. 123; pg 2735)

14. a

Seventy percent to 90% of reported choledochal cysts are type I, characterized by fusiform or saccular dilation of the common bile duct, without hepatic duct involvement. Type II choledochal cysts, true diverticula of the common bile duct, comprise less than 3% of all cases. Type III choledochal cysts, also known as choledochoceles, are located in the distal intraduodenal segment of the common bile duct and represent 2% to 20% of all cases. Type IV is the classification for multiple extrahepatic or mixed intra- and extrahepatic cysts, whereas type V represents intrahepatic cysts only—the condition known as Caroli disease. (Ch. 98; pg 2255)

15. d

Choledochal cysts are an anomaly characterized by saccular dilation of the extrahepatic biliary tract. They are more common in Asians than in whites, and four times more common among women than among men. There are five types of cysts (types I–V). The risk for adenocarcinoma is about 10%; therefore, the treatment of choice is complete excision rather than drainage. The etiology is unclear, but most accepted theories suggest that pancreatic reflux from an abnormal pancreatic-biliary duct junction is causative. (Ch. 100; pg 2292)

16. c

The best management plan in this situation is to remove the stones through the existing T tube when the tract is mature, usually 4 to 6 weeks postoperatively. If this fails, endoscopic retrograde cholangiopancreatography with sphincterotomy and stone extraction is indicated. Repeat laparotomy usually is unnecessary; however, if the other options fail it should be performed because common bile duct stones should not be left in situ. (Ch. 100; pg 2288)

17. a

A moderate rise in serum amylase is observed following 40% to 75% of pancreatograms. Typically, the hyperamylasemia is not accompanied by clinical symptoms and subsides in 1 to 2 days. Although overfilling of the pancreatic duct is claimed to be the main

causative factor in the development of acute pancreatitis, acute pancreatitis has been observed in some patients after unsuccessful cannulation of the pancreatic duct. This may in part be the result of repeated trauma and subsequent development of edema of the papilla. The addition of sphincter of Oddi manometry increases the risk of procedure-related pancreatitis, and patients should be advised of this risk. Infection of a pseudocyst and subsequent abscess formation can occur if the pseudocyst communicates with the pancreatic duct; therefore, endoscopic retrograde cholangiopancreatography should not be performed unless drainage of the pseudocyst is anticipated. (Ch. 123; pg 2719)

18. b

There is no evidence that proctocolectomy has any beneficial effect on the course of primary sclerosing cholangitis (PSC) nor that it will prevent the development of cholangiocarcinoma in patients with chronic ulcerative colitis. PSC may obscure the diagnosis of cholangiocarcinoma. The incidence of cholangiocarcinoma ranges from 7% to 15% in patients with PSC. About 10% of patients undergoing liver transplantation for PSC are found to have cholangiocarcinoma. Secondary biliary cirrhosis is found in 30% of patients at the time of diagnosis of PSC; therefore, liver transplantation should be considered for those with deterioration of hepatic synthetic function. (Ch. 100; pg 2306)

19. b

Acute pancreatitis is the most common complication of diagnostic endoscopic retrograde cholangiopancreatography (ERCP). An attack of clinically apparent acute pancreatitis after ERCP occurs in 0.7% to 7.4% of patients. (Ch. 123; pg 2720)

20. e

Overfilling of the pancreatic duct, which can result in instillation of contrast media into the pancreatic parenchyma (i.e., acinarization) is thought to be the main causative factor in the development of acute pancreatitis after endoscopic retrograde cholangiopancreatography (ERCP). Repeated attempts at cannulation or repeated pancreatic duct injections are risk factors for the development of acute pancreatitis. The addition of sphincter of Oddi manometry to diagnostic ERCP increases the incidence of postprocedural pancreatitis. A history of ERCP-induced pancreatitis does not increase the risk of pancreatitis after repeated diagnostic ERCP. (Ch. 123; pg 2720)

21. a

Most benign bile duct strictures are caused by a previous surgical injury. (Ch. 123; pg 2728)

22. c

An elevated basal pressure in the sphincter of Oddi is a better predictor of pain relief after endoscopic sphincterotomy than are cholangiographic findings of a dilated common bile duct or delayed drainage of contrast from the bile duct. (Ch. 102; pg 2350)

23. c

Delayed drainage of injected contrast material (i.e., >45 minutes) has been documented in many patients with sphincter of Oddi dysfunction. (Ch. 102; pg 2346)

24. d

Primary biliary cirrhosis may be associated with other autoimmune disorders, such as Sjögren syndrome and thyroiditis. An association between primary biliary cirrhosis and diabetes mellitus has not been reported. (Ch. 100; pg 2302)

25. b

This patient has painless jaundice and a palpable gallbladder (i.e., the Courvoisier sign). A tumor of pancreatic or bile duct origin is the most likely cause. Chronic pancreatitis may result in a stricture in the distal common bile duct, but this patient has no history of pancreatitis and his current symptoms are of short duration. (Ch. 43; pg 949)

26. d

Ultrasonography is the best imaging technique for the detection of cholelithiasis; conversely, in the typical patient with painless jaundice, a computed tomography (CT) scan may be the best initial investigative tool. If a pancreatic mass is noted without evidence of metastatic spread on the CT scan, further investigation is not needed before proceeding to surgery. If there is no mass visible on the CT scan, diagnostic endoscopic retrograde cholangiopancreatography may be performed to determine the site and type of obstruction. (Ch. 101; pg 2330)

27. d

Rotor syndrome is a familial condition caused by the markedly reduced storage capacity of the hepatocyte for conjugated bilirubin. Patients with Rotor syndrome have conjugated, rather than unconjugated, hyperbilirubinemia. (Ch. 42; pg 934)

28. c

The proper selection of patients is a key factor affecting the success of bile acid dissolution therapy. Favorable criteria include the following characteristics: gallstones composed chiefly of cholesterol, small stones (<1.5 cm diameter), stones with a large surface area in relation to mass, and stones that are mobile within the gallbladder. Pigment stones or calcified stones cannot be dissolved with bile acids. (Ch. 99; pg 2273)

29. a

Eighty-six percent of patients present before age 50 and the two sexes are equally affected. Malnutrition and lower socioeconomic levels are associated with a higher incidence of this syndrome. Only 15% to 33% of cases are associated with cholelithiasis. Typically, the cure rate after the first operation is low; attacks recur and reoperation is necessary. (Ch. 100; pg 2289)

30. d

Primary sclerosing cholangitis (PSC) may be associated with many disorders. The most common is ulcerative colitis, which occurs in 50% to 75% of patients with PSC. Other associated disorders include AIDS, pancreatitis, Riedel thyroiditis, celiac disease, and sarcoidosis. Hepatitis A and B do not cause PSC. (Ch. 100; pg 2302)

31. e

The prognosis for oriental cholangiohepatitis is poor despite aggressive initial management. Stone recurrences, cholangitis, the need for repeated operation, and secondary biliary cirrhosis are common. (Ch. 100; pg 2290)

32. a

Liver flukes such as *Clonorchis sinensis* can infect persons in Japan, China, Indochina, South Korea, and Taiwan who eat uncooked fish. The major pathologic changes induced by chronic infection occur in the bile ducts. (Ch. 109; pg 2455)

33. a

Adult liver flukes (e.g., *Clonorchis sinensis, Opisthorchis viverrini*, and *Fasciola hepatica*) live in the distal portion of the biliary tract. (Ch. 109; pg 2455)

34. d

The most common cause of acute cholecystitis is obstruction of the cystic duct by gallstones, resulting in acute inflammation of the gallbladder. Approximately 90% of cases are associated with cholelithiasis. (Ch. 99; pg 2265)

35. e

Hepatobiliary imaging using ^{99m}Tc-labeled iminodiacetic acid (IDA) compounds may be useful when evaluating parenchymal liver function and the structural integrity and patency of the hepatobiliary tree. Specific applications include studies of infants suspected of having biliary atresia, patients with primary biliary cirrhosis, and patients who have had a liver transplantation. Hepatobiliary scintigraphy is used most frequently to evaluate for the presence of acute cholecystitis. Quantitative measurement of the gallbladder response to stimulation to calculate the gallbladder ejection fraction has been advocated to evaluate patients with abdominal symptoms thought to be related to acalculous biliary disease. (Ch. 140; pg 3083)

36. e

Pregnancy, hypercholesterolemia, vagotomy, diabetes, sprue, and total parenteral nutrition have all been associated with gallbladder stasis. (Ch. 99; pg 2263)

37. b

Retrospective comparative studies have shown that laparoscopic cholecystectomy results in fewer complications, shorter hospital stays, more rapid returns to normal activities, and minimal use of postoperative analgesia. The estimated incidence of bile duct injury associated with laparoscopic cholecystectomy varies from 0.3% to 2.7%, compared to the incidence associated with open cholecystectomy, which ranges from 0.25% to 0.5%. (Ch. 99; pg 2270)

38. c

Alcohol abuse is not a risk factor for gallbladder carcinoma. (Ch. 101; pg 2336)

39. a

Papillary stenosis, sclerosing cholangitis, combined papillary stenosis with intrahepatic and extrahepatic sclerosing cholangitis, and long extrahepatic biliary strictures may be found in association with AIDS. The most common abnormalities are papillary stenosis with or without intrahepatic and extrahepatic sclerosing cholangitis. Pancreatic duct abnormalities, specifically strictures in the juxtaampullary pancreatic duct, have also been reported. (Ch. 100; pg 2315)

40. c

Clinically, patients with AIDS-associated cholangiopathy present with right upper quadrant or epigastric abdominal pain (64% to 88%), fever (20% to 65%), and cholestasis (75% to 80%). The serum bilirubin level is usually normal or minimally elevated, whereas the alkaline phosphatase level is typically elevated to a value in the range of 700 U/L. (Ch. 100; pg 2315)

41. d

Jaundice is a poor prognostic sign in gallbladder cancer; more than 85% of these patients having unresectable tumors. (Ch. 101; pg 2337)

42. d

Hepatobiliary diseases associated with AIDS include diffuse hepatocellular injury, granulomatous hepatitis, and sclerosing cholangitis. Fatty infiltration of the liver is common in patients with AIDS who have abnormal liver chemistries. A primary biliary cirrhosis–like syndrome has also been reported. Nodular regenerative hyperplasia is not reported to be associated with AIDS. (Ch. 107; pg 2413)

43. e

Although the pathogenesis of AIDS-associated cholangiopathy is unclear, most investigators favor infec-

tious causes with opportunistic agents including cytomegalovirus, *Cryptosporidium*, Microsporida, or even human immunodeficiency virus itself. (Ch. 100; pg 2316)

44. d

Cirrhosis has not been shown to be independently associated with a higher incidence of bile duct cancer. (Ch. 101; pg 2326)

45. d

No role for preoperative biliary drainage has been established in the management of bile duct cancer. Treatment should be targeted at resection, because this can clearly improve survival in selected patients. Unfortunately, only a very small percentage of patients with bile duct cancer are truly resectable for cure at the time of laparotomy; thus, overall survival rates have not significantly improved. Chemotherapy currently offers little additional benefit in terms of survival. (Ch. 101; pg 2334)

46. d

Gram-negative organisms are common pathogens in patients with cholangitis. Anaerobes account for 15% of the pathogenic organisms. The presence of gram-positive organisms other than enterococci is unusual. (Ch. 99; pg 2266)

47. d

The technique of percutaneous transhepatic cholangiography (PTC) involves a blind infusion of contrast media into the liver until the biliary tree is visualized. Iodinated contrast agent will enter the systemic circulation; thus, susceptible patients require prophylaxis against allergic reactions. The success of performing either a diagnostic or therapeutic PTC is improved if the intrahepatic biliary system is dilated. PTC is as effective as surgery for establishing drainage of the biliary system in obstructive jaundice. Several studies have shown endoscopic retrograde cholangiopancreatography and PTC to be equally effective in relieving obstructive jaundice. Endoscopic retrograde cholangiopancreatography is preferred in some settings because there is no external drain, whereas PTC may be preferred for relief of jaundice caused by lesions in the porta hepatis or in the liver. (Ch. 142; pg 3128)

48. a

In primary sclerosing cholangitis, the alkaline phosphatase level is elevated in more than 90% of cases; increased circulating immune complexes are measurable in 80% of cases, and the test for perinuclear antineutrophilic cytoplasmic antibody is positive in 80% to 85% of cases. Antimitochondrial antibody, rheumatoid factor, and smooth muscle antibody are absent in more than 90% of cases. (Ch. 100; pg 2304)

49. a

Only 10% of ductal injuries, such as a bile leak, are recognized in the first postoperative week. Patients with bile leaks usually present with acute bile peritonitis. Two-thirds of patients with ductal injury present with strictures as late as 1 year after the operation. The outcome is better if the repair of the ductal injury is immediate, either by endoscopic stent placement or by open laparotomy, than if the repair is delayed for several days. Most patients have virtually no symptoms after laparoscopic cholecystectomy. Therefore, the presence of any symptoms, such as nausea or pain, on the first postoperative day, even if vague, is justification for emergent biliary scintigraphy. Development of an ileus on the second postoperative day is an indication of a complication that must be evaluated. (Ch. 143; pg 3160) (Ch. 99; pg 2271)

50. e

This child presented with the triad of right upper quadrant pain, jaundice, and a palpable abdominal mass, which is consistent with a diagnosis of a choledochal cyst. Presentation features may also include pancreatitis, duodenal obstruction, or cholangitis. Ultrasonography is the best screening method for type I, II, IV, and V cysts. Hepatobiliary scintigraphy is a sensitive, noninvasive tool to diagnose these same cyst types. Endoscopic retrograde cholangiopancreatography may be helpful in the diagnosis of type III cysts, i.e., choledochoceles. Computed tomography has been advocated by some to be superior to ultrasonography. Oral cholecystography is of no use in the diagnosis of choledochal cysts. (Ch. 100; pg 2298)

51. b

Biliary cyst treatment is surgical. Medical therapy has been associated with a 97% mortality rate; death results from cyst rupture with secondary peritonitis, cholangitis, or liver cirrhosis with secondary complications. External drainage alone has been shown to be associated with a 65% mortality rate; moreover, it does not correct the underlying defect. (Ch. 100; pg 2299)

52. c

Several studies have illustrated that the majority of patients' gallstones remain asymptomatic. Although the rate of new-onset biliary colic may be 2% per year for the first 5 years, this rate plateaus, and the rate of new-onset biliary colic after 10 years ranges from 15% to 25%. Cohort studies following patients with gallstones who are symptomatic indicate that 58% to 72% of patients have ongoing symptoms. More than 90% of complications (e.g., cholecystitis, cholangitis, gallstone pancreatitis) are associated with antecedent attacks of pain. Complications of gangrene and perforation occur in 10% of cases of acute cholecystitis. (Ch. 99; pg 2269)

53. d

Ursodeoxycholic acid improves biochemical abnormalities in patients with primary sclerosing cholangitis (PSC), but survival results are conflicting. Patients with ulcerative colitis and PSC do not improve with proctocolectomy. Colchicine may have shown promise in early studies, but subsequent trials have not shown survival improvement. Liver transplantation improves the survival of patients with PSC. (Ch. 100; pg 2307)

True/False

54. true

In a prospective study of patients receiving long-term total parenteral nutrition (TPN), 50% developed biliary sludge after 4 to 6 weeks of TPN, and after 6 weeks of TPN, its appearance was universal. (Ch. 99; pg 2263)

55. false

Impaired Na^+,K^+-ATPase activity, the driving force for bile acid uptake, rather than an abnormality of the sinusoidal bile acid transport protein, appears to underlie the elevation of serum bile acids in cirrhosis. (Ch. 17; pg 385, Fig. 17.5)

56. true

In celiac sprue, the dynamics of the enterohepatic circulation are altered by a neuroendocrine mechanism. Reduced cholecystokinin release from the intestinal mucosa and impaired gallbladder emptying, which are reversed by a gluten-free diet, lead to infrequent cycling of the bile acid pool and stagnation of bile within the biliary tree. (Ch. 17; pg 395)

57. true

Serum alkaline phosphatase levels may be low in patients with hypothyroidism, pernicious anemia, zinc deficiency, and congenital hypophosphatasia. In addition, a decreased serum alkaline phosphatase level has been associated with the acute hemolytic anemia that complicates Wilson disease. (Ch. 43; pg 952)

58. true

High incidences of obesity and regular alcohol use have been demonstrated in patients with asymptomatic aminotransferase elevations. Consequently, fatty infiltration is the most common finding on liver biopsy specimens. However, the histologic confirmation of chronic persistent or active hepatitis in 20% of patients in one study has lent support to the use of percutaneous liver biopsy in the diagnostic approach to patients with persistently elevated levels of serum aminotransferases. (Ch. 43; pg 959)

59. true

Prolongation of the prothrombin time, often disproportionate to other signs of liver dysfunction, is the most common abnormality in patients with congestive heart failure, although elevations in serum bilirubin, primarily unconjugated, occur and are rarely greater than 3 mg/dL. Elevations in serum aminotransferases can also occur. (Ch. 43; pg 948)

60. true

Hepatocellular injury can be differentiated from cholestatic causes of prothrombin time prolongation by the parenteral administration of vitamin K. Intact hepatic function is established by a greater than 30% improvement in the prothrombin time within 24 hours of administration. A prolonged prothrombin time may occur in the absence of liver disease, such as with a dietary deficiency of vitamin K, consumption coagulopathies, anticoagulant and antibiotic use, and steatorrhea. Parenteral administration of vitamin K corrects the abnormal prothrombin time that occurs in these conditions. (Ch. 43; pg 950)

61. true

Even accounting for other risk factors, Mexican Americans and Native Americans have an especially high incidence of gallstone disease, which suggests that genetic factors contribute to the pathophysiology of cholelithiasis in these populations. (Ch. 99; pg 2258)

62. true

Concomitant choledocholithiasis is confirmed in at least 12% to 15% of patients undergoing cholecystectomy. Despite advances in biliary tract surgery, 3% to 5% of patients who have had exploration of the common bile duct are found to have a retained common bile duct stone in the immediate postoperative period. (Ch. 100; pg 2281)

63. true

Spontaneous biliary-enteric fistulas are caused by gallstones (90%), peptic ulcer disease (6%), malignancy or trauma (4%). (Ch. 100; pg 2314)

64. false

Primary common bile duct stones consist mostly of calcium bilirubinate with a cholesterol content of less than 25%; a very different chemical composition compared to that of the predominant type of gallbladder stones and of secondary bile duct stones. (Ch. 100; pg 2282)

65. false

In western populations, 70% to 80% of gallbladder stones are cholesterol stones, and 20% to 30% are pigment stones. Fifty-five percent to 70% of common duct stones, which are predominantly secondary duct stones, are cholesterol stones. (Ch. 100; pg 2282)

66. false

Trauma is the most common cause of hemobilia in young men; gallstone disease is the more common cause in elderly women. (Ch. 100; pg 2313)

67. false

Biliary colic is usually constant, lasting anywhere between 30 minutes to several hours. Typically, the pain is felt in the right upper quadrant or epigastrium, with frequent radiation to the interscapular area. (Ch. 38; pg 835)

68. true

In patients with acute bile duct obstruction, aspartate aminotransferase and alanine aminotransferase elevations are typically less than fivefold higher than normal; occasionally they are as high as those seen in patients with hepatitis. Alkaline phosphatase levels are also often elevated, but usually not more than five times above normal values. The serum bilirubin level is elevated in 50% to 72% of symptomatic patients with choledocholithiasis. (Ch. 100; pg 2285)

69. true

The rates of complications (e.g., bleeding, pancreatitis, cholangitis, and perforation) associated with endoscopic retrograde cholangiopancreatography are generally less than 10%. The exception is when endoscopic retrograde cholangiopancreatography is performed to evaluate for possible sphincter of Oddi dysfunction— the complication rate may be 20%. (Ch. 100; pg 2287)

70. true

The breakdown of senescent red blood cells in reticuloendothelial cells located in spleen, liver, and bone marrow contributes approximately 80% of the total daily bilirubin. (Ch. 42; pg 927)

71. false

Nonionic and lower osmolality contrast media, which are more expensive, offer no safety advantage. (Ch. 123; pg 2720)

72. false

Several studies conclude that there is no difference in outcomes for patients with mild pancreatitis treated conservatively or treated with endoscopic retrograde cholangiopancreatography. One large study illustrated a lack of benefit in using endoscopic retrograde cholangiopancreatography to treat patients with gallstone pancreatitis who had no evidence of severe biliary obstruction (i.e., bilirubin >5 mg/dL). (Ch. 123; pg 2725)

Matching

73. c

74. a

75. b

76. e

77. d

The left lobe is more dependent in the prone position and fills preferentially during endoscopic retrograde cholangiopancreatography. Right lobe filling may require tilting the patient's head down 15 to 20 degrees on the fluoroscopy table, or turning the patient to the supine position. Contrast media mix slowly with gallbladder bile, and final films are best taken with the patient in the supine position after endoscope withdrawal. Standard contrast media (e.g., meglumine diatriazoate) at a 50% to 60% concentration (full-strength) are used for pancreatography, whereas a 25% to 30% (half-strength) concentration is recommended for cholangiography. (Ch. 123; pg 2720)

78. b

79. a

80. d

81. c

In pregnancy, a substantial fraction of serum alkaline phosphatase may be derived from the placenta. Alcohol, presumably by enzyme induction, elicits elevated serum γ-glutamyltransferase levels. This finding has been invoked as a sensitive marker of chronic alcoholism that occurs independently of any liver damage. Falsely low aspartate aminotransferase levels, corrected by dialysis, have been reported in patients with uremia. Hypoceruloplasminemia may result from the diminution in hepatic synthetic function observed in non-Wilsonian fulminant hepatic injury, in chronic hepatitis, and less commonly, in severe malnutrition and other protein-losing states. (Ch. 43; pg 952)

82. a

83. a

84. b

85. a

Primary duct stones are associated with the following characteristics: a high frequency of bacterial bile infection, stone composition mostly consisting of calcium bilirubinate, and the presence of benign or malignant bile duct strictures. Common bile duct stones that are found within 2 years of cholecystectomy are generally thought to be secondary stones. (Ch. 100; pg 2282)

86. d

87. a

88. b

89. c

Isolated elevation of the serum alkaline phosphatase level is strongly suggestive of a systemic granulomatous disease such as brucellosis. The highest serum elevations of aspartate aminotransferase and alanine aminotransferase are seen in patients with viral, toxin-induced, and ischemic hepatitis. Hypoceruloplasminemia is an important diagnostic finding in Wilson disease. Similarly, hyperferritinemia is a significant diagnostic finding in hemochromatosis. (Ch. 43; pgs 954, 958)

90. b

91. a

92. c

93. a

Endoscopically placed stents can be used to treat biliary strictures caused by chronic pancreatitis, although some patients may eventually require surgery (Ch. 123; pg 2729). Patients with abdominal pain and documented AIDS-related papillary stenosis should undergo endoscopic sphincterotomy (Ch. 100; pg 2316). Biliary fistulas secondary to cholecystectomy injury may be endoscopically treated with biliary sphincterotomy, stenting, or nasobiliary tube drainage (Ch. 123; pg 2732). Cholangitis, pain, or pancreatitis caused by food or stones blocking the bypassed segment of a side-to-side choledochoduodenostomy (a condition known as sump syndrome) may be successfully managed with an endoscopic sphincterotomy. (Ch. 123; pg 2736)

94. d

95. e

96. a

97. c

98. b

Sphincter of Oddi dysfunction is defined as impedance to transsphincteric flow caused by either stenosis or a motility disorder. Sphincter of Oddi dysfunction is an uncommon cause of postcholecystectomy syndrome, which is characterized by biliary-type pain. Patients most likely to respond to sphincterotomy include those with elevated aminotransferases, a dilated common bile duct, or delayed drainage of the contrast agent during endoscopic retrograde cholangiopancreatography. Sphincter of Oddi manometry may be helpful in predicting the response to sphincterotomy, although its role remains controversial. Sphincter dysfunction presumably can occur in patients with intact gallbladders, although the diagnosis may overlap with gallbladder microlithiasis or dyskinesia. (Ch. 102; pg 2343)

99. a

100. b

101. c

102. b

Brown pigment stones are prevalent in Asia, and occur in the clinical settings of cholangitis, parasitic infections, and after surgery of the biliary tree. Recurrence of brown stones is common. Black pigment stones are found in both Asian and western populations and are associated with cirrhosis and hemolytic anemia. Cultures of bile from patients with black pigment stones are usually sterile. (Ch. 99; pg 2264)

CHAPTER 7

Multiple Choice

1. c

   Most diarrheal illnesses in patients infected with HIV-1 are caused by infectious agents, and using the current improved diagnostic techniques, a specific pathogen is identified in 50% to 85% of cases. Patients with low CD4 counts and systemic symptoms such as weight loss are more likely to be diagnosed with a specific causative pathogen. Some physicians advocate a three-phase work-up for these patients, beginning with stool cultures for routine bacterial pathogens, *Clostridium difficile*, and ova and parasites. Phase 2 involves esophagogastroduodenoscopy and colonoscopy to obtain biopsy specimens that are then stained specifically for mycobacteria, viruses, and fungi. Step 3 includes electron microscopy for Microsporida and adenovirus. *Cryptosporidium* species and *Isospora belli* are more commonly found in patients in developing countries. (Ch. 107; pg 2401)

2. b

   The aspartate aminotransferase–alanine aminotransferase ratio in serum is a useful indicator of alcoholic liver disease; a ratio greater than 2 is highly suggestive of alcohol-induced liver injury. Lesser elevations in serum aminotransferases (an aspartate aminotransferase level of 300 U/L) are usually observed in alcoholic hepatitis, whereas higher elevations (often 1000 U/L) occur with viral, toxin-induced, or ischemic hepatitis. (Ch. 43; pg 951)

3. d

   Chronic graft-versus-host disease occurs 80 to 400 days after bone marrow transplantation. The esophageal manifestations involve the upper and mid esophagus while the distal esophagus is usually spared, in contrast to the esophageal involvement in peptic esophagitis. Histology specimens usually show clusters of individual necrotic cells with apoptotic bodies. In contrast to scleroderma, fibrosis involves the mucosa, and sometimes the submucosa. The treatment of chronic graft-versus-host disease with immunosuppressives is often satisfactory. Esophageal dilation may be required for webs or strictures. (Ch. 112; pg 2560)

4. a

   High-output fistulas, when they involve the duodenum or proximal small bowel, are associated with metabolic acidosis as a result of alkaline fluid loss and can produce significant dehydration in rare cases. Gastric fistulas typically produce an alkalosis. Low-output fistulas (<500 mL/day) are associated with a high incidence of spontaneous closure; however, high-output fistulas rarely resolve without intervention. (Ch. 104; pg 2371)

5. c

   Only 10% to 12% of patients with peritonitis complicated by peritoneal dialysis require removal of their dialysis catheters. Refractory and recurrent infections are indications for removal. Most patients are infected with cutaneous organisms such as *Staphylococcus* species; gram-negative rod bacterial infections occur less often. Antibiotic therapy should cover these organisms. Patients usually present with abdominal pain and a cloudy dialysate. (Ch. 106; pg 2388)

6. d

   Spider angioma are increased by exposure to sunlight and may therefore not be prominent in all cirrhotics. The clinical diagnosis is ascites, which is the presenting complaint and the only major physical sign. Diagnostic paracentesis is indicated to confirm this impression and to better understand the etiology of the ascites. Determination of the serum-ascites albumin gradient can help in this regard. There is little merit in measuring lactate dehydrogenase or bilirubin levels in the ascitic fluid. (Ch. 44; pg 972)

7. c

   Psoriasis is not associated with gastrointestinal disease. Methotrexate, a therapy for refractory psoriasis, is associated with gastrointestinal complications such as nausea and vomiting, fatty liver, hepatic fibrosis, cirrhosis, and rarely, colitis. (Ch. 111; pg 2504)

8. c

   Down syndrome is associated with a variety of gastrointestinal manifestations, including esophageal stenosis, tracheoesophageal fistula, gastroesophageal reflux, duodenal stenosis, duodenal atresia, imperforate anus, Hirschsprung disease, and hepatitis B. There is no increase in the incidence of Crohn's disease with Down syndrome. (Ch. 111; pg 2507)

9. c

   Acute intermittent porphyria is an autosomal dominant disease associated with recurrent attacks of abdominal pain, nausea, vomiting, constipation, seizures, and peripheral neuropathy. Attacks may be precipitated by the administration of certain drugs (e.g., barbiturates, steroids, sulfa drugs, alcohol), by surgery, and by pregnancy. Variegate porphyria, hereditary coproporphyria, porphyria cutanea tarda, and protoporphyria are often associated with skin lesions; however, acute intermittent porphyria is not. (Ch. 111; pg 2508)

10. c

   Patients with acute arsenic poisoning have hepatomegaly and jaundice as part of the characteristic clinical presentation; however, liver biopsy specimens from these patients do not reveal granulomas. (Ch. 111; pg 2516)

11. e

This patient's symptoms are compatible with the HELLP syndrome. Nevertheless, this diagnosis should be distinguished from the other possibilities. The HELLP syndrome is a variant of toxemia in pregnancy. Its features suggest a thrombotic micro-angiopathic disease, and delivery of the fetus is the therapy of choice when possible. (Ch. 111; pg 2531)

12. d

Infiltration of the liver and spleen with amyloid proteins causes hepatosplenomegaly in patients with systemic amyloidosis, but portal hypertension and liver failure are rare. Fulminant liver failure does not occur. (Ch. 111; pg 2520)

13. a

Several studies have suggested that drug metabolites generated within the enterocyte may reenter the gut lumen, never to be reabsorbed. This may result from the trapping of metabolites within enterocytes that are subsequently shed from the villus tip, or from energy-dependent pumps such as p-glycoprotein. (Ch. 26; pg 618)

14. d

Chylous ascites is more suggestive of lymphatic obstruction (e.g., lymphoma) and is not usually associated with fulminant hepatic failure. (Ch. 44; pg 968)

15. a

Although peritoneal carcinomatosis is the leading cause of malignant ascites, not all malignancy-related ascites are caused by this condition. Ascites associated with malignancy may result from massive liver metastases, tumor-induced portal hypertension, or tumor-induced chylous ascites. (Ch. 44; pg 967)

16. d

The utility of the serum-ascites albumin concentration gradient is based on the concept of oncotic-hydrostatic balance. A high oncotic gradient will match a high portal pressure, and, of the serum proteins, albumin has the most effect on the oncotic pressure of serum. In patients with portal hypertension, there are large differences between serum and ascitic fluid albumin concentrations. The albumin gradient is approximately 97% accurate in grouping patients with ascites into those with and those without portal hypertension. Those with a low albumin gradient (<1.1 g/dL) include patients with peritoneal carcinomatosis, tuberculosis, pancreatic ascites, or nephrotic syndrome. A high albumin gradient (≥1.1 g/dL) is seen in patients with portal hypertension, including those with cirrhosis, alcoholic hepatitis, cardiac ascites, Budd-Chiari syndrome, or portal vein thrombosis. (Ch. 44; pg 972)

17. b

Spontaneous bacterial peritonitis (SBP) usually occurs in patients with severe liver disease and low-protein ascites. SBP rarely occurs in patients with ascites caused by heart failure or in patients with peritoneal carcinomatosis, both of whom have high-protein ascites. SBP is believed to result from the seeding of ascites after transient bacteremia. As a result, most cases of SBP result from contamination with a single organism. (Ch. 44; pg 978)

18. b

A serum-ascites albumin gradient of greater than or equal to 1.1 g/dL indicates the presence of portal hypertension with greater than 90% reliability. Conversely, a gradient of less than 1.1 g/dL indicates the absence of portal hypertension with more than 90% reliability. This patient has a serum-ascites albumin gradient of 1.8 g/dL, as would occur with cirrhosis, constrictive pericarditis, or portal vein thrombosis. Peritoneal carcinomatosis invariably exhibits a low serum-ascites albumin gradient. (Ch. 44; pg 972)

19. b

Salt restriction is a cornerstone of effective diuresis in patients with cirrhosis and ascites, and it alone is adequate for the control of ascites in some patients. In those patients requiring diuretic treatment, spironolactone is the agent of choice for single-drug therapy, being effective in 95% of patients compared with furosemide, which is effective in 58% of patients. (Ch. 44; pg 984)

20. c

Spontaneous bacterial peritonitis (SBP) must be considered in the differential diagnosis of any patient with stable cirrhosis who has a sudden worsening in clinical status. Many patients do not present with fever, abdominal pain, and leukocytosis. Studies have shown that 10% to 27% of patients with ascites admitted to the hospital have SBP, even in the absence of any clinical suspicion. The most accurate and sensitive parameters to check for SBP are the total leukocyte count, absolute neutrophil count, and ascites culture. There is no need to perform a therapeutic paracentesis in this patient, because he is described as having only moderate ascites. (Ch. 44; pg 978)

21. b

Although ampicillin and gentamicin were recommended as therapy for spontaneous bacterial peritonitis (SBP) in the past, aminoglycosides are associated with a high incidence of nephrotoxicity in patients with cirrhosis and should be avoided. Third-generation cephalosporins have been shown to be more efficacious than ampicillin and gentamicin, and they do not induce renal toxicity. Norfloxacin is indicated for SBP prophylaxis, not for treatment of the active infection. Patients with SBP should not have a Denver shunt placed until after the infection has resolved. There is no clinical information provided to suggest that the patient is resistant to diuretics and will require repeated paracentesis. (Ch. 44; pg 980)

22. d

The correct diagnosis is tylosis, which is an uncommon autosomal dominant disorder associated with a 90% probability of developing esophageal carcinoma by the age of 65. The phenotypic manifestation is hyperkeratosis of the palms of the hands and the soles of the feet. (Ch. 111; pg 2513)

23. b

Spontaneous bacterial peritonitis is more common in adults than in children, and the incidence is equal in men and women. Gram-negative organisms are most common in patients with spontaneous bacterial peritonitis, but they are also found in a significant subset of individuals with peritonitis associated with peritoneal dialysis. (Ch. 104; pg 2367)

24. b

Although the total leukocyte count may rise during clinically significant diuresis, neutrophil counts remain stable, presumably because of the short half-life of neutrophils. The usual cutoff value for the diagnosis of spontaneous bacterial peritonitis is a neutrophil concentration in ascitic fluid of 250/mm^3, even with rapid diuresis. (Ch. 44; pg 972)

25. a

Hermansky-Pudlak syndrome is an autosomal-recessive disease occurring most frequently in persons from Puerto Rico, where the prevalence is one in every 2000 individuals. Thus, it is a genetic disease as common among the Puerto Rican population as cystic fibrosis is among the white population in the United States. Hermansky-Pudlak syndrome is a storage disorder characterized by the accumulation of a ceroid-like substance. Clinical features include partial albinism, restrictive lung disease, and platelet abnormalities. Inflammatory bowel disease is also common in Puerto Rico, and the combination of inflammatory bowel disease and defective platelets can contribute to recurrent gastrointestinal bleeding in these patients. (Ch. 110; pg 2482)

26. b

Retractile mesenteritis is an inflammatory disease of unknown etiology. The pathologic process involves the degeneration of fat, leading to fibrosis, which results in a thickened fibrotic mesentery with plaques. The disease affects adults, and its clinical symptoms include abdominal pain and fever. Mesenteric biopsy specimens confirm the diagnosis. Resection is usually not possible, and moreover, should not be attempted because the fibrous and fatty mesenteric masses always recur after resection. (Ch. 105; pg 2376)

27. b

Familial Mediterranean fever almost exclusively affects persons of Armenian, Arabic, or Jewish origin. Up to one-half of the patients with this syndrome are Sephardic Jews, so the diagnosis should be particularly considered in this patient population. (Ch. 110; pgs 2487, 2490)

28. a

The child is infected with *Trichuris trichiura*, a helminth that is prevalent in the tropics. Infection with this whipworm can be asymptomatic. Rectal prolapse is a rare but serious complication of a large parasitic burden. The infection is contracted by the ingestion of worm ova, and is particularly common in areas without latrines or where human feces is used as a fertilizer. (Ch. 109; pg 2442)

29. a

Although granulomas are seen in patients with Crohn's disease, granulomatous peritonitis is not a complication of Crohn's disease. Granulomatous peritonitis refers to a number of diseases with the common characteristic of granuloma formation, and it is associated with a high incidence of subsequent formation of adhesions. The disease processes most commonly associated with granulomatous peritonitis are tuberculosis and fungal and parasitic infections. The introduction of foreign bodies such as cellulose fibers or talc into the peritoneal cavity at laparotomy can induce iatrogenic granulomatous peritonitis. (Ch. 106; pg 2386)

30. a

Retroperitoneal fibrosis is a chronic inflammatory process that originates in the lower peritoneum and spreads bilaterally toward the renal hilus, encircling the vessels and ureters. In many cases, retroperitoneal fibrosis may be secondary to an allergic reaction to lipids. Serotonin produced by carcinoid tumors may produce the syndrome, as can the serotonin receptor agonist/antagonist methysergide. (Ch. 106; pg 2393)

31. g

A Dieulafoy lesion is a distinct vascular abnormality that is twice as common in men as in women, usually presenting in the sixth decade of life. Although quite rare, this lesion is the source of bleeding in 1% to 2% of patients with massive upper gastrointestinal hemorrhage. In over 80% of patients, the lesion is detected within 6 cm of the gastroesophageal junction and proximal to the lesser curvature. Angiography is only successful if the patient is actively bleeding, and even then the lesion can be missed. Repeat endoscopic evaluation is indicated for the patient with recurrent massive upper gastro-intestinal hemorrhage, especially if symptoms suggest a Dieulafoy lesion. (Ch. 113; pg 2576)

32. c

Mesenteric venous thrombosis is generally idiopathic but may be a result of trauma, hypercoagulability, peritoneal irritation, or portal hypertension. This patient has no clear risk factors for mesenteric arterial thrombosis, strangulation, or nonocclusive mesenteric ischemia. (Ch. 114; pg 2593)

33. c

Mesenteric arteriography should be perfomed promptly if small bowel ischemia is suspected. There are no laboratory tests that are sufficiently specific to be helpful in the initial diagnosis; therefore, the physician must persist with other diagnostic procedures to confirm or exclude ischemia. The patient should be stabilized prior to angiographic study. Computed tomography and ultrasonography are appropriate initial tests for patients with a history of deep vein thrombosis or a family history of coagulation disorders, who are likely to have mesenteric vein thrombosis. (Ch. 114; pg 2597)

34. b

Nonocclusive mesenteric ischemia occurs during low-flow states with systemic disease and does not result from mesenteric arterial narrowing. (Ch. 114, pg 2590)

35. e

Splenic artery aneurysms usually do not require surgical resection. Only when an aneurysm occurs in persons who are pregnant or who have pancreatitis is resection recommended because of an increased rate of splenic artery aneurysm rupture in these two groups. (Ch. 141; pg 3106) (Ch. 135; pg 2988)

36. b

Splenic vein occlusion is a common cause of the development of isolated gastric varices, which present a significant risk for spontaneous hemorrhage. This condition is best treated by surgical resection of the spleen. Esophageal varices are rare in patients with splenic vein occlusion. (Ch. 141; pg 3107) (Ch. 94; pg 2165)

37. b

This presentation is characteristic of hepatic vein occlusion, also known as Budd-Chiari syndrome. Hepatic venography is the diagnostic test of choice, because the results of ultrasonography with Doppler examination are associated with a high false-negative rate. The venous drainage of the caudate lobe is distinct from the other hepatic regions and thus may not be involved in Budd-Chiari syndrome. (Ch. 141; pg 3107)

38. b

This person is infected with *Taenia saginata*, a beef tapeworm renowned for its length, which can reach 6 meters. *Ascaris lumbricoides* is a large wormlike nematode. Infection with this roundworm can involve large numbers of worms. *Enterobius vermicularis* is a pinworm, most renowned for causing perianal itching. Infection with *Echinococcus granulosis* leads to the development of hydatid cysts in humans. (Ch. 109; pg 2443)

39. e

This patient has spontaneous bacterial peritonitis, confirmed by a polymorphonuclear leukocyte count of greater than $250/mm^3$ in the ascitic fluid. He should receive immediate empiric antibiotic therapy consisting of either a third-generation cephalosporin or a quinolone. Once a specific organism has been isolated, a more specific antimicrobial therapy may be administered. (Ch. 44; pg 978)

40. d

This patient has an aortoenteric fistula, which may not be visualized during aortography. Computed tomography almost never identifies the fistula but commonly reveals signs of inflammation (i.e., fluid or gas) in the perigraft region. It is this inflammation that leads to fistula formation. An alternative to performing computed tomography is to proceed directly to exploratory laparotomy in the potentially clinically unstable patient. (Ch. 32; pg 727)

41. d

This patient's lengthy history and the results of laboratory studies suggest tuberculous peritonitis. While other diagnoses need to be excluded, tuberculous peritonitis should be considered in high-risk patients. Because tuberculous peritonitis is difficult to diagnose, suspicion based on the clinical presentation, a non-exudative ascites, and a high-risk patient population should lead to an aggressive diagnostic approach, including laparoscopic peritoneal biopsy. Polymerase chain reaction tests for *Mycobacterium tuberculosis* facilitate a more rapid diagnosis, as cultures of ascitic fluid can take 4 to 6 weeks to incubate and the results of acid-fast staining are rarely positive unless large volumes (>1 L) of ascitic fluid are obtained and concentrated. Carcinoma should be included in the differential diagnosis of this patient. (Ch. 106; pg 2386)

42. d

Although computed tomography is critical in evaluating severe Crohn's disease of the small intestine and in excluding abscess formation, early disease is usually not detected by computed tomography; barium radiographic studies are preferable. (Ch. 137; pg 3024)

43. a

The probable lesion is telangiectasia or vascular ectasia of the small bowel. Turner syndrome is associated with a phenotype of a short heavy female with a webbed neck. Turner syndrome has been associated with telangiectasia of the gut; bleeding of these lesions can be recurrent. (Ch. 113; pg 2573)

44. c

Benign lymph nodes are usually hyperechoic with an irregular shape and poorly defined margins. Malignant nodes are more commonly hypoechoic and round with sharply defined borders. Endoscopic ultrasonography cannot distinguish between leiomyoma and leiomyosarcoma without needle aspiration. The normal gastrointestinal wall thickness is 3 to 5 mm. (Ch. 136; pg 3005)

45. d

Changes in the sonographic appearance of the intestinal wall do not reliably distinguish between Crohn's disease and ulcerative colitis. The other choices are well-defined clinical indications for the performance of endoscopic ultrasonography. (Ch. 136; pg 3016)

46. a

The timing of the onset of symptoms following the induction of radiation therapy suggests radiation-induced esophagitis. Endoscopic evaluation is the diagnostic test of choice, although radiologic and endoscopic findings can mimic opportunistic infections, in particular candidiasis, so biopsies may be helpful. The motility disorder induced by radiation therapy usually does not appear for 4 to 12 weeks after the induction of radiation therapy, and stricture formation may take 6 to 8 months. Opportunistic infections, such as candidiasis, herpes simplex, or cytomegalovirus infections, particularly if accompanied by severe ulcerative esophagitis, must be excluded. Following long-term radiation therapy, it is possible to see radiation-induced fibrosis and progressive nerve loss that can mimic diseases such as scleroderma or achalasia. (Ch. 115; pg 2607)

47. e

The splenic vein traverses the retroperitoneum immediately posterior to the pancreas. Pancreatic diseases, including malignancies and chronic or acute pancreatitis, are the major causes of isolated splenic vein thrombosis. (Ch. 93; pg 2145) (Ch. 92; pg 2112)

48. e

Of the vasculitis syndromes that affect the gastrointestinal tract, Henoch-Schönlein purpura is the condition most likely affecting this child. Henoch-Schönlein purpura is associated with a classic triad of symptoms: palpable purpuric rash, abdominal cramping, and hematuria. It is a small-vessel systemic vasculitis capable of affecting any part of the gastrointestinal tract. Usually the disease is self-limited without chronic sequelae. Radiographic findings include thickening of the small bowel folds, colonic wall edema, and possibly, intussusception of the bowel. (Ch. 111; pg 2536)

49. d

Common variable hypogammaglobulinemia is a heterogeneous group of disorders with an intrinsic B-cell defect. Alterations in T-cell functions have also been found in many patients. Patients present in the second or third decade of life with respiratory tract infections or diarrhea. Nodular lymphoid hyperplasia is thought to reflect the presence of B cells that are unable to undergo full differentiation to immunoglobulin-secreting plasma cells. A transient form of selective IgA deficiency exists after the administration of medications such as phenytoin and penicillamine; however, no drug-induced transient form of common variable hypogammaglobulinemia has been documented. (Ch. 112; pg 2548)

50. a

Familial Mediterranean fever is an autosomal recessive disorder. Since this patient does not know her family history as she is adopted, the diagnosis is somewhat difficult. It is important to remember that there is no family history of the disease in 50% of patients at the time of the presentation. Half of all affected people are of Sephardic Jewish descent, about 20% are Armenian, 20% are Turkish or Arabic, and the remainder are Italian, Greek, or Ashkenazi Jews. This disease is rare in people of northern Europe. The history of episodic febrile attacks and pain secondary to inflammation involving serosal surfaces suggests the diagnosis. Colchicine effectively prevents the acute febrile attacks associated with this disease. (Ch. 110; pgs 2487, 2490)

51. d

On ultrasonographic evaluation, a mesenteric desmoid tumor appears as a solid mass; on computed tomography, it is usually nonenhanced. (Ch. 105; pg 2377)

52. b

Umbilical hernias tend to heal and reduce spontaneously. They are more common in African American and male infants. Strangulation is reported in less than 5% of umbilical hernias and should not be surgically repaired before the patient is 3 years of age unless large defects, incarceration, or strangulation occur. (Ch. 103; pg 2358)

53. b

The most important laboratory test and the one least likely to mislead the physician in diagnosing spontaneous bacterial peritonitis is the polymorphonuclear leukocyte (PMN) count. The upper limit of a "normal" total white blood cell count in uncomplicated cirrhotic ascites is 500 cells/mm³. The upper limit cutoff of the absolute PMN count is 250 cells/mm³. The PMN count remains relatively constant during diuresis, likely because of the short half-life of PMNs. Cultures of ascitic fluid should be sent to the laboratory in blood culture bottles. This has been shown to enhance the detection of bacterial infection from 43% to 93%. (Ch. 44; pg 972)

54. b

Considering this patient's presentation, a 24-hour urine sample should be obtained for porphyrin determination. Endoscopy is unlikely to reveal any significant pathology in this patient and might exacerbate the patient's abdominal pain. *Yersinia* infection is associated with a variety of dermatologic manifestations and abdominal pain; however, recurring episodes are less common and are not associated with extensor surface blistering. The distribution of skin lesions and the character of the abdominal pain are atypical for serositis or pancreatitis occurring with systemic lupus erythematosus. Peripheral nerve conduction studies are unlikely to be revealing in a patient who does not complain of appendicular-skeletal pain. (Ch. 45; pg 1002)

55. d

Acute graft-versus-host disease is a common complication of bone marrow transplantation. Classically, patients develop watery diarrhea, mucositis, and hepatic abnormalities including hyperbilirubinemia beginning 3 weeks after bone marrow transplantation. Arthritis is not typically reported in acute disease. (Ch. 112; pg 2558)

56. a

Acute graft-versus-host disease develops in 20% to 50% of bone marrow transplant patients, typically occurring 20 to 80 days following transplantation, and may produce jaundice, diarrhea, and gastrointestinal blood loss. Other clinical manifestations commonly include dermatitis, protein-losing enteropathy, vomiting, abdominal pain, and ileus, but pancreatitis is rarely observed. (Ch. 112; pg 2558)

57. c

Chronic graft-versus-host disease (GVHD) commonly develops 3 to 9 months after bone marrow transplantion and may be associated with esophageal desquamation and stricture formation, small bowel bacterial overgrowth, and chronic cholestasis. Typhlitis (i.e., neutropenic enterocolitis) may occur with acute GVHD, but it is not a common manifestation of GVHD. (Ch. 112; pg 2559)

58. e

Clinical evidence of infection in patients with spontaneous bacterial peritonitis (SBP) can be subtle or absent. In one study, more than 10% of patients with SBP had no signs or symptoms. However, most patients present with fever, abdominal pain, or mental status change. There are very few contraindications to paracentesis. Even in the patient with coagulopathy, paracentesis causes minimal complications; and cirrhotics do not bleed seriously from needle sticks, unless conditions such as fibrinolysis or disseminated intravascular coagulation are concurrent. Ascitic fluid analysis from culture-negative neutrocytic ascites, secondary bacterial peritonitis, and SBP will show more than 250 polymorphonuclear leukocytes per mm³. Tuberculous peritonitis and peritoneal carcinomatosis cause an elevated white cell count, but the differential is primarily lymphocytic. (Ch. 44; pgs 971, 979)

59. b

The optimal duration of treatment for spontaneous bacterial peritonitis, both intravenous and oral, remains controversial. Treatment regimens cannot be stratified by the duration of infection because a variable number of patients will be asymptomatic. Others may be evaluated at different times after the onset of infection and will have different therapeutic needs. At present, cefotaxime, a third-generation cephalosporin, has been shown to be superior to ampicillin plus tobramycin in controlled trials, and is an excellent initial therapy for suspected spontaneous bacterial peritonitis. After susceptibility testing, a more narrow spectrum drug can be chosen. (Ch. 44; pg 980)

60. d

Chronic graft-versus-host disease typically presents with clinical features similar to scleroderma and includes the sicca complex among its manifestations. (Ch. 112; pg 2560)

61. a

The most likely diagnosis is Plummer-Vinson-Kelly syndrome. This syndrome is characterized by dysphagia, esophageal webs, and iron-deficiency anemia. Middle-aged women are most commonly affected, and symptoms can include glossitis, dyspepsia, atrophic gastritis, diarrhea, hoarseness, and paresthesias. The webs are usually thin fibrous tissue. Esophageal dysmotility has been reported as well. Therapy includes dilation of the webs and fibrous tissue, and treatment with iron and vitamin supplements to correct the iron deficiency. Note that careful endoscopic evaluation of the hypopharynx and upper esophagus should be performed to exclude malignancy. (Ch. 111; pg 2520)

62. c

Bipolar electrocoagulation is the only thermal contact method of tissue destruction mentioned in this list. The argon plasma coagulator and the Nd:YAG laser are noncontact methods of tissue destruction, and injection therapy has no thermal component. (Ch. 130; pg 2883)

True/False

63. true

64. false

65. true

66. false

Milky or opalescent ascitic fluid usually indicates a high triglyceride content in the fluid. This can be confirmed by measuring the triglyceride level or by observing for layering of the lipid after refrigeration of the ascitic fluid for 48 to 72 hours. Cholesterol and alkaline phosphatase measurements would not be helpful in this situation. (Ch. 44; pg 977)

67. true

The majority of patients with tuberculosis peritonitis do not have radiographic evidence of pulmonary or gastrointestinal tuberculosis; however, almost all affected individuals will have an identifiable focus at autopsy. (Ch. 106; pg 2386)

68. false

69. false

70. true

71. false

Visceral pain is usually perceived in the midline as a result of bilateral innervation patterns. Pain from the jejunum or ileum is usually perceived in the periumbilical region because of the midgut embryonic origins of these organs. Visceral pain may result from distention, forceful contractions, traction, torsion, or noxious chemicals. Pain from pancreatic disease usually radiates to the back. (Ch. 36; pg 797)

72. false

The visceral peritoneum receives afferent innervation from the autonomic nervous system and responds primarily to traction and pressure. Noxious stimuli are perceived as a poorly localized dull pain. The parietal peritoneum is innervated by somatic and visceral afferent nerves, resulting in the perception of noxious stimuli as sharp localized pain, as is observed with rebound tenderness. (Ch. 36; pgs 797, 806)

73. false

The onset of acute graft-versus-host disease usually occurs 3 to 4 weeks following bone marrow transplantation and may persist for up to 80 days. (Ch. 112; pg 2558)

74. false

75. true

76. true

77. true

No laboratory tests are pathognomonic for mesenteric ischemia. The timing of symptoms depends on the mechanism of injury. Mesenteric arterial emboli usually cause sudden pain, whereas pain from mesenteric thrombosis may be more insidious in onset. Iatrogenic ischemia may result from angiography-induced atheroma release or arterial dissection. Nonocclusive mesenteric ischemia is sometimes managed by administering intraarterial papaverine or intravenous glucagon. (Ch. 114; pg 2600)

78. false

79. true

80. false

81. true

Endoscopic surveillance is recommended for patients with Barrett esophagus and for individuals who have undergone endoscopic removal of adenomatous gastric polyps, because the incidence of adenocarcinoma in these patients is significantly greater than that in the population as a whole. The slight increases in the risk of developing malignancy with achalasia and pernicious anemia do not warrant endoscopic surveillance. (Ch. 120; pg 2689)

82. true

83. false

84. true

85. false

Intraabdominal abscesses frequently arise in the postoperative setting, with 50% to 75% occurring after abdominal surgery. The detection of an intraabdominal abscess in the postoperative period is often challenging because of incisional pain, the use of analgesics, and the difficulty of conducting a clinical examination in the presence of drains and bandages. Clinical signs of abscess manifest approximately 8 days postoperatively on average. Although most intraabdominal abscesses are polymicrobial, most commonly *Bacteroides fragilis* and *Escherichia coli,* only aerobes are cultured in more than half the cases. (Ch. 104; pg 2366)

Matching

86. h

87. c

88. e

89. f

90. d

91. i

92. a

93. g

94. b

Scleroderma is frequently associated with esophageal dysmotility. Behçet disease is classically associated with oral aphthous ulcers. Inflammatory bowel disease should be considered in patients with pyoderma gangrenosum. Acanthosis nigricans is found with recurrent abdominal adenocarcinoma. Tylosis, keratoderma of the palms and soles, is strongly associated with squamous cell carcinoma of the esophagus. Gastrointestinal involvement in pseudoxanthoma elasticum may present with recurrent upper and lower gastrointestinal bleeding. Hypertrichosis is associated with pancreatic or colonic carcinoma. Flushing is an important manifestation of the carcinoid syndrome. Necrolytic migratory erythema, typically affecting perioral, lower abdominal, and perineal sites, occurs with a glucagon-secreting islet cell tumor of the pancreas. (Ch. 45; pg 992)

95. b

96. a

97. d

98. c

Although few chemotherapeutic drug regimens cause significant mucosal injury, therapy with high-dose cytarabine can result in abdominal pain, diarrhea, peritoneal signs, gastrointestinal hemorrhage, and mucosal necrosis. Peliosis hepatis is a complication of therapy with hydroxyurea, azathioprine, 6-thioguanine, and androgens. Venoocclusive disease can complicate bone marrow transplantation and usually occurs within the first month posttransplantation. The cause of venoocclusive disease is related to the cumulative pretransplant total-body irradiation and chemotherapeutic treatments (particularly cyclophosphamide) received by the patient. Other chemotherapeutic agents that can cause venoocclusive disease include azathioprine, 6-thioguanine, and pyrolizidine alkaloids ("bush tea poisoning"). *Vinca* alkaloids are neurotoxic and can cause dysphagia or colonic pseudoobstruction. (Ch. 111; pg 2521)

99. a

100. a

101. c

102. b

A ruptured or dissecting abdominal aortic aneurysm classically presents with diffuse abdominal pain, hypotension, and a pulsatile abdominal mass. The pain may radiate to the back, flank, or groin. The diagnosis may be confirmed by emergent ultrasonography and treatment consists of emergent surgery. Acute cholecystitis presents with fever and right upper quadrant pain that radiates to the scapula and not the back. The diagnosis may be confirmed by ultrasonography or by biliary scintigraphy. The optimal management of cholecystitis is surgical excision of the gallbladder; however, this is rarely performed emergently. (Ch. 38; pgs 835, 837)

103. e

104. d

105. c

106. b

Familial Mediterranean fever is an autosomal recessive disorder characterized by brief episodic febrile attacks associated with inflammation and serositis. It is also known as recurrent familial polyserositis. Fabry disease, or diffuse angiokeratoma, is a lysosomal storage disorder caused by a deficiency of α-galactosidase. The deposition of lipoid material in tissues likely causes the attacks of pain in the abdomen or extremities, as well as vascular lesions in the ocular fundi and in the kidney, corneal opacities, hypertrophic cardiomyopathy, and skin lesions. Hereditary angioneurotic edema is an autosomal dominant disorder affecting the respiratory and gastrointestinal tracts. Deficiency of C1-esterase inhibitor is the underlying pathophysiologic defect, and gastrointestinal symptoms include abdominal pain, nausea, vomiting, and diarrhea. Hereditary pancreatitis is characterized by steatorrhea, recurrent attacks of severe abdominal pain, fever, and elevated serum amylase levels (which distinguish the disorder, clinically, from familial Mediterranean fever). Splenic or portal vein thrombosis can complicate recurrent episodes of pancreatitis. (Ch. 110; pg 2487)

CHAPTER 8

Multiple Choice

1. c

   The Na$^+$,K$^+$-ATPase pump, in the presence of Mg^{2+}, catalyzes the efflux of three Na$^+$ ions out of the cell and the uptake of two K$^+$ ions into the cell. This action is electrogenic and acts to maintain a high extracellular concentration of Na$^+$. The gradient established by this pump is then used to drive many Na$^+$-dependent transporters. The pump is located on the basolateral membrane and exists in all intestinal epithelial cells. (Ch. 15; pg 327)

2. b

   The intercellular regulatory mechanisms of electrolyte transport include endocrine (blood-borne hormones from distant sites), paracrine (local), nerve endings within the enteric nervous system, and resident and infiltrating immune and inflammatory cell types. The mediators released by these pathways generally are regulated by Ca^{++} or cAMP, which act as second messengers. (Ch. 15; pg 343)

3. d

   Although bicarbonate secretion is important in selected regions of the gut (e.g., bile and pancreatic ducts, duodenal mucosa), secretory mechanisms throughout the gastrointestinal tract largely center on the active transcellular secretion of chloride into the lumen. Sodium, potassium, and water follow passively through the tight junctions. (Ch. 15; pg 336)

4. a

   A lack of bile salts at effective micellar concentrations may occur as a result of low intralumenal levels of bile salts (e.g., cholestasis), bacterial deconjugation (e.g., bacterial overgrowth), or abnormal acidic conditions (e.g., Zollinger-Ellison syndrome). (Ch. 19; pg 433)

5. c

   Fatty acid-binding proteins (FABPs) are two cytosolic proteins that are independently regulated, with separate roles in the liver and the intestine. In the intestine, FABPs are essential in the directed intracellular trafficking of absorbed long-chain fatty acids, retinyl esters, and probably cholesterol. By so directing the movement of lipids intracellularly and assisting in their uptake from the lumen, FABPs are ultimately involved in the disposition of cellular lipids into secretable forms such as chylomicrons and very-low-density lipoprotein. FABPs are obligate intracellular peptides that are not exported out of the cell. (Ch. 19; pg 435)

6. a

   Monosaccharides are not readily absorbed by the colonic mucosa. Fermentation converts monosaccha-rides to short-chain fatty acids (i.e., acetate, propionate, and butyrate), which are readily absorbed. (Ch. 85; pg 1911)

7. a

   False-negative results from a hydrogen breath test may occur in a minority of individuals who have colonic flora that do not produce appreciable amounts of hydrogen during fermentation. In such cases, the measurement of breath methane excretion can be of benefit. The clinical setting in this case is highly suggestive of lactase deficiency, and the low level of fasting breath hydrogen suggests that the "normal" breath hydrogen value represents a false-negative result. (Ch. 75; pg 1690)

8. b

   Sorbitol and fructose are commonly used as sweeteners and may produce gas, bloating, and diarrhea resulting from their malabsorption if ingested in excess. Ingested starch from foods such as wheat, corn, oats, potatoes and beans, but not rice, can also be malabsorbed. (Ch. 37; pg 818)

9. b

   Brush border saccharidases are ectoenzymes that are anchored to the apical membrane of enterocytes. These enzymes are responsible for the further breakdown of lumenal hydrolysis products and ingested disaccharides, leading to the production of monosaccharides that can be transported across the apical membrane. Changes in diet can markedly affect the regulation of the saccharidases. Sucrose is the most potent inducer of the saccharidases, whereas starvation leads to their rapid decline. In diabetes mellitus there is a striking up-regulation of saccharidases, resulting in an increased uptake of sugars. Saccharidases are degraded by pancreatic protease; therefore, pancreatic exocrine insufficiency and bacterial overgrowth result in increased saccharidase activity. (Ch. 18; pg 410)

10. d

    Anticonvulsants, trimethoprim, pyrimethamine, and sulfasalazine interfere with intestinal folate deconjugase activity and enterocyte transport, which results in folate deficiency. Methotrexate impairs folate absorption by inhibiting dihydrofolate reductase, which regulates the intracellular production of tetrahydrofolic acid. In celiac disease, a reduced number of proximal bowel enterocytes, coupled with enhanced cell turnover and alkalization of lumenal pH, contribute to folate deficiency. In contrast, reduced bicarbonate output in pancreatic insufficiency increases lumenal acidification, which enhances folate absorption. (Ch. 21; pg 469)

11. b

    The decrease of intrinsic factor secretion in pernicious anemia, the impairment of R protein degradation in

Zollinger-Ellison syndrome, and the direct binding of cobalamin to organisms in bacterial overgrowth may all lead to cobalamin malabsorption. Specific ileal receptors are involved in the uptake of the intrinsic factor–B_{12} complex; therefore, ileal disease or resection of the terminal 100 cm of the ileum often produces vitamin B_{12} deficiency (e.g., Crohn's disease). Bile salt micelles do not play a role in cobalamin absorption; thus, cholestasis does not cause vitamin B_{12} deficiency. Vitamin B_{12} malabsorption is a rare occurrence in the setting of pancreatic insufficiency, resulting from the reduced release of proteolytic enzymes involved in the degradation of R proteins bound to dietary cobalamin. (Ch. 21; pg 471)

12. c

Following gastrectomy, there is a lack of intrinsic factor (IF), which is necessary for the absorption of cobalamin. Similarly, therapy with H_2-receptor antagonists can decrease IF production. Stage II of the Schilling test provides the IF necessary for cobalamin absorption and thus should normalize cobalamin absorption in conditions of reduced endogenous IF production. (Ch. 21; pg 471)

13. d

The two major sources of dietary iron are heme and nonheme iron. Meat, fish, and poultry provide heme iron. These sources offer high bioavailability because the iron is absorbed intact within the porphyrin ring of hemoglobin and myoglobin. Nonheme iron is present in vegetables, grains, and fruits. Absorption of nonheme iron is highly variable and is affected by other meal components. (Ch. 21; pg 476)

14. d

Sarcoidosis is associated with enhanced calcium absorption secondary to elevated levels of $1,25(OH)_2$ vitamin D_3. In contrast, calcium absorption is decreased in conditions with decreased absorptive surface area (e.g., celiac sprue), impaired micellar solubilization (e.g., chronic cholestasis), and suppression of parathyroid hormone secretion, which is a secondary effect of hyperthyroidism. (Ch. 21; pg 477)

15. b

Transthyretin (i.e., prealbumin) is a plasma transporter of vitamin A and does not hold any prognostic value in assessing postoperative morbidity and mortality. (Ch. 51; pg 1081)

16. a

Excessive caloric infusion results in an increased level of unoxidized glucose, which is diverted into the synthesis of glycogen and fat. The result is of no nutritional benefit. In fact, excessive caloric infusion can lead to hyperglycemia, hepatic steatosis, and excess carbon dioxide production. It does not, however, lead

to an increased susceptibility to infection. (Ch. 51; pg 1088)

17. c

The short-term prognosis for patients with anorexia nervosa is generally favorable. More than three-fourths of patients attain a body weight greater than 75% of their ideal body weight. Menses resumes in at least one-half of patients, but less than one-third of patients attain normal eating patterns. The long-term prognosis is variable, and relapses requiring hospitalization occur in about one-half of patients. The long-term mortality rate ranges from 4% to 13%, with the main causes of death being inanition, cardiac arrhythmias, and suicide. It appears that the degree of social integration (e.g., with parents, spouse, friends, coworkers) achieved by the patient is a stronger predictor of long-term outcome than medical treatment and psychotherapy. (Ch. 34; pg 767)

18. a

Enteral nutrition may provide nutrients not available from parenteral nutrition. The best example of this is the short-chain fatty acids that are formed by the bacterial degradation of dietary fiber or unabsorbed carbohydrates. Short-chain fatty acids provide an important source of energy for colonocytes that helps maintain colonic function. (Ch. 51; pg 1085)

19. d

There is no increased risk of hemolysis in patients receiving total parenteral nutrition. Elevated liver chemistries in patients receiving total parenteral nutrition are likely to be multifactorial, including hepatic steatosis and calculous as well as acalculous cholecystitis. (Ch. 51; pg 1089)

20. c

Hypermetabolism, negative nitrogen balance, insulin resistance leading to hyperglycemia, and increased mobilization of adipose tissue triglycerides characterize the metabolic response to illness and injury. (Ch. 22; pg 503)

21. b

Liver disease in obese patients is common. It is often, but not always, detected with elevations in levels of alanine aminotransferase, aspartate aminotransferase, and alkaline phosphatase—usually not more than 2 times the upper limit of normal. The android pattern confers a greater health risk, and obesity may be associated with some cancers, including breast, uterus, ovary, and colon. The risk of new gallstones is greater in patients ingesting 1 g of fat per day with a low-calorie diet. Ingesting adequate amounts of fat during dieting may be particularly important to stimulate regular gallbladder emptying. Mortality rates for obese men are higher than those for obese women. (Ch. 22; pg 509)

22. c

The goal of enteral or parenteral supplementation in the patient with anorexia nervosa is to slowly increase the patient's body weight out of the range of medical risk. Rapid refeeding produces excess water stores and edema, secondary metabolic disturbances, and possibly cardiac failure. Acute gastric or duodenal dilation, refeeding pancreatitis, and diarrhea may occur. The diarrhea may be caused by depletion of pancreatic and intestinal brush-border enzymes. Elevations occur in serum amylase of salivary and pancreatic origin, and ultrasonography has shown decreased echogenicity of the pancreas, possibly because of atrophy. Mesenteric ischemia has not been reported. (Ch. 34; pg 767)

23. b

This is a typical presentation of anorexia nervosa. In the majority of cases, the disease occurs within 7 years of menarche and exists for many years before it is recognized and diagnosed. These patients have very little insight into their disease and perceive themselves to be fat and ugly. They lose weight in an attempt to gain control of their environment, often having been raised in affluent families with unachievable expectations and poor emotional support. Amenorrhea results from a combination of pituitary dysfunction and reduced ovarian responsiveness to circulating gonadotropins. (Ch. 34; pg 765)

24. b

Bulimic patients have normal body weight and rarely report significant weight loss. A childhood history of being overweight is often noted, as is an association of food and meals with important social rituals. These patients undergo episodes of uncontrolled eating lasting up to several days, followed by feelings of guilt and depression leading to self-induced emesis and laxative abuse. These patients are usually very cognizant of their weight and will often use diuretics as well. Most patients will binge and purge in private and do not report symptoms to their physicians. Hypokalemia and hypochloremic metabolic alkalosis from chronic emesis are observed in more than 50% of bulimic patients. (Ch. 34; pg 769)

25. e

An initial medical interview and physical examination will readily point to an underlying cause of weight loss in the majority of patients. In the elderly, diagnoses of malignancy and adverse drug effects are commonly made. Gastrointestinal disorders account for 25% to 40% of the underlying causes of weight loss. Even with a defined underlying medical illness, reduced calorie consumption as documented by a food diary is the most common pathophysiologic reason for weight loss, not chronic inflammatory conditions as

was once believed. In approximately 25% of patients who undergo medical evaluation for weight loss, no clear-cut etiology is determined. Two-year follow-up in this group reveals a benign course without progressive weight loss or development of other disease. A large number of these patients are thought to have reduced food intake related to a psychological process. (Ch. 34; pg 761)

26. c

The loss of 100 cm of ileum results in bile acid malabsorption. Deconjugated bile acids, resulting from colonic bacterial fermentation, present an osmotic load and directly stimulate active anion secretion to produce a secretory diarrhea. (Ch. 77; pg 1705)

27. a

Vitamin K is passively absorbed in the small intestine, a process that requires bile-salt micelles and pancreatic enzymes. Unlike the other fat-soluble vitamins, there are no large adipose tissue stores of this vitamin. (Ch. 22; pg 497)

28. b

Glutamine and glutamic acid are major energy sources for enterocytes and are the only amino acids that are consistently taken up from the circulation by the small intestine mucosa. (Ch. 22; pg 504)

29. c

Malabsorption (leading to osmotic diarrhea), increased lumenal secretion, and fat malabsorption all occur in short bowel syndrome. Bacterial overgrowth is not commonly encountered in patients with short bowel syndrome. (Ch. 77; pg 1709)

30. b

The first phase of short bowel syndrome is characterized by severe diarrhea during oral nutrition, with the development of dehydration and electrolyte abnormalities. The diarrhea is caused by decreased transit time secondary to physical shortening of the small intestine and motility disturbances. Incomplete digestion and absorption of carbohydrates increases the osmotic load, drawing more water into the lumen. Gastric hypersecretion occurs, as does steatorrhea. Bacterial overgrowth can contribute to the diarrhea by increasing the osmotic load of the gut but is less likely to be a problem in the early postoperative period. Generally, at least 30 to 50 cm of healthy small intestine and an intact colon are necessary for the patient to be maintained without parenteral nutrition. Although functional pancreatic enzyme insufficiency can occur, pancreatic enzyme replacements are not needed in most patients. Oral nutrition should be encouraged to stimulate intestinal mucosal adaptation. Antidiarrheal agents may provide symptom relief. H_2-receptor antagonists may reduce diarrhea by decreasing the

gastric secretory component of the stool output.
(Ch. 77; pgs 1709, 1713)

31. d

This patient has signs of vitamin B_{12} and/or thiamine deficiency. Glucose administration prior to thiamine supplementation in deficient patients can lead to an acute clinical deterioration. Because the body has such large stores of vitamin B_{12}, it may take individuals consuming a diet deficient in vitamin B_{12} as long as 1 to 3 years to develop evidence of deficiency. Most patients with vitamin B_{12} deficiency will also be lacking in the other B vitamins. (Ch. 51; pgs 1096, 1098)

32. d

Short bowel syndrome predisposes the patient to hyperoxaluria and oxalate kidney stones. Normally, dietary oxalates are bound by dietary calcium to form insoluble calcium oxalate. In patients with steatorrhea, fatty acids compete for dietary calcium, preventing the formation of calcium oxalate, and free oxalate is available for absorption, especially in the colon. In addition, malabsorption of bile salts and free fatty acids alters the permeability of the colonic mucosa, which further increases the absorption of oxalate. For this sequence of events to occur, the colon must be intact. (Ch. 77; pg 1711)

33. d

Dietary nutrients are major stimuli of mucosal growth and adaptation after small intestine resection. Nonnutritive bulking agents do not have the same effect. Biliary and pancreatic secretions have been shown to induce mucosal hyperplasia in animal models. Hormones such as enteroglucagon and corticosteroids appear to induce mucosal hyperplasia, as do epidermal growth factor, prostaglandins, and growth hormone-releasing factor. Polyamines (e.g., putrescine, spermidine, and spermine) may play an important role in small bowel adaptive hyperplasia and are a topic of current investigation. (Ch. 77; pg 1707)

34. d

Percutaneous endoscopic gastrostomy tube placement is absolutely contraindicated in patients with uncorrectable coagulopathy, intestinal obstruction, peritonitis, peritoneal dialysis, or gastric varices. Paracentesis prior to gastrostomy tube placement may improve safety in patients with ascites. Tube placement is considered safe in patients with a ventriculoperitoneal shunt using a preprocedure radiograph to help avoid the catheter. A cut-down through skin and subcutaneous tissue under local anesthesia facilitates safe tube placement in obese patients. (Ch. 127; pg 2829)

35. a

In experimental models, the induction of oral tolerance depends on the type of antigen, the amount of antigen, the frequency of antigen sensitization, the type and genetic background of the animal being studied, the age of the animal, and the particular immune response being evaluated. Both T-cell suppression and clonal anergy have been suggested to play a role in the development of oral tolerance. (Ch. 6; pg 119)

36. c

At birth, pancreatic amylase activity is only 10% of adult levels, whereas the intestinal glucoamylase activity is nearly 70% to 100%. Salivary and mammary amylase also aid in the digestion of starch in the term infant. (Ch. 24; pg 558)

37. b

Carbohydrates account for approximately 50% of the total daily calories and serve as a fuel source for humans. Starches, which are complex polysaccharides, are the most common form of naturally occurring carbohydrate ingested and digested by humans. The monosaccharides include glucose, galactose, and maltose, as well as the five-carbon sugar fructose. Carbohydrates are only taken up by enterocytes in their monosaccharide form after undergoing cleavage from larger substrates by brush-border enzymes. Many plant sources of carbohydrate contain linkages that are not hydrolyzed by human intestinal enzymes and are therefore not absorbed. It is estimated that approximately 2% to 20% of ingested carbohydrates are malabsorbed and enter the colonic lumen for further fermentation by colonic bacteria. (Ch. 18; pg 405)

38. a

The actual composition of dietary fiber varies among plant sources, but in general, it contains large carbohydrate and noncarbohydrate polymers, which are not susceptible to amylase digestion. These carbohydrates can, however, be broken down anaerobically by colonic bacteria into short-chain fatty acids, hydrogen, methane, and sulfur gases. The short-chain fatty acids have been shown to be an excellent fuel source for the colonic epithelium and may be important in colonic cell turnover. (Ch. 18; pg 409)

39. b

Sucrase-isomaltase is the only enzyme capable of sucrose cleavage to glucose and fructose. The enzyme is down-regulated with infection and inflammation, which may contribute to symptoms of diarrhea. The enzyme is expressed between weeks 8 to 14 of gestation. The enzyme is anchored to the apical membrane of enterocytes. (Ch. 18; pg 410)

40. a

Although starvation in adults leads to a reduction of many saccharidases, lactase-phlorizin hydrolase activity is not reduced. Human immunodeficiency virus infection, corticosteroids, and inflammatory conditions are all associated with reduced enzyme activity. (Ch. 18; pg 414)

41. d

During fatty acid absorption, conjugated bile salts are passively absorbed by enterocytes in the upper small intestine. In addition, sodium-coupled active transport retrieves bile salts in the ileum. Together, these absorptive processes are very efficient, with a nearly 95% recovery of bile acids in the bloodstream. A small percentage of circulating bile salts enter the colon, where they are deconjugated and dehydroxylated by colonic bacteria and passed in the stool. Short-chain fatty acids are generated by the colonic metabolism of unabsorbed dietary carbohydrates. (Ch. 19; pg 434)

42. b

Pepsinogens are secreted by chief cells in response to gastrin, histamine, and vagal stimulation, the same factors that regulate acid secretion. Activation of pepsinogens to pepsins I and II is extremely pH-dependent and will not occur above a pH of 4.5. Patients who are achlorhydric or who have had a gastrectomy do not show evidence of protein maldigestion because of the extensive contribution of pancreatic proteases and intestinal brush-border enzymes to the digestion of protein, indicating that intestinal events are more significant than gastric factors for protein digestion. (Ch. 20; pg 457)

43. a

Intestinal epithelial cells can assimilate dipeptides and tripeptides as well as single amino acids. This has been shown in congenital diseases such as Hartnup disease and cystinuria, wherein defects in basic amino acid transporters occur in the small intestine and renal epithelium. In these conditions, measurable levels of the excluded amino acids are absorbed as a result of the intracellular processing of absorbed dipeptides and tripeptides. (Ch. 20; pg 460)

44. e

Pernicious anemia is an autoimmune disorder characterized by atrophic gastritis and the absence of intrinsic factor secretion. It is most common in older white persons of European descent. Pernicious anemia is diagnosed by the measurement of a low level of serum vitamin B_{12} and an abnormal result from a stage I Schilling test that normalizes with intrinsic factor administration (stage II). Treatment consists of intramuscular vitamin B_{12} injections (i.e., a loading dose of 1000 µg, then 100 µg every month). (Ch. 110; pg 2492)

45. a

Vitamin K is concentrated in the liver, albeit in small amounts. Dietary intake and colonic bacterial production are the principal sources of vitamin K in humans. Broad-spectrum antibiotic therapy for hospitalized patients of marginal nutritional status frequently leads to vitamin K deficiency as a consequence of the sterilization of the colon. Intravenous vitamin K administration may cause anaphylaxis; thus, vitamin K should only be given subcutaneously. (Ch. 21; pg 474)

46. e

The intestinal transport of calcium is primarily regulated by circulating levels of active vitamin D. Calcium salts in dairy products and foods require acid-mediated solubilization for absorption by the small intestine. Older persons with reduced vitamin D levels, patients with reduced acid production and poor micelle formation required for vitamin D absorption following gastric surgery, and long-term corticosteroid users who have reduced intestinal calcium transport should receive supplements of 1000 to 1500 mg of calcium per day. Patients with chronic cholestasis should receive supplements of parenteral vitamin D and calcium salts because of the risk of developing a negative calcium balance and resultant osteoporosis. Patients with hypophosphatemia have enhanced intestinal calcium absorption. Patients with idiopathic calcium stones may have inappropriately high levels of vitamin D_3, leading to enhanced intestinal calcium absorption. Calcium supplements are most commonly administered orally in the form of calcium carbonate, which has a much lower bioavailability than does calcium citrate. (Ch. 21; pg 477)

47. c

Although alcohol directly affects the acid microclimate of the intestine, alcoholics commonly become folate deficient because of decreased folate intake and malnutrition. Oral contraceptives inhibit folylpolyglutamate hydrolase, thereby causing malabsorption of folylpolyglutamate, a dietary form of folate. (Ch. 21; pg 468)

48. d

Iron absorption involves carrier-mediated translocation across the intestinal brush border. (Ch. 21; pg 476)

49. a

The recommended daily allowance is the level judged to be high enough to ensure an adequate intake for the majority of the normal population. (Ch. 22; pg 487)

50. c

Medium-chain triglycerides do not provide essential fatty acids. Animal studies have shown that a parenteral administration of 100% medium-chain triglyceride as the sole lipid source leads to essential fatty acid deficiency. (Ch. 22; pg 495)

51. d

A significant component of the hypokalemia that occurs with emesis is the result of increased renal losses of potassium. The metabolic alkalosis that occurs with gastric acid loss during emesis is compensated for by the kidney by increased H^+-K^+ exchange. Decreased intake or decreased absorption of sodium is rarely a cause of hyponatremia. Hypomagnesemia in alcoholic patients results from decreased dietary intake and increased renal losses. (Ch. 51; pgs 1090, 1092)

52. d

In severe liver disease, the liver cannot convert the various forms of vitamin D to the 25-hydroxy form. Thus, 25-hydroxycholecalciferol (calcifediol) must be provided for this patient. (Ch. 51; pg 1100)

53. a

Whenever possible, oral feeding should be used to meet the patient's nutritional requirements rather than total parenteral nutrition. Malnourished preoperative patients, those with severe Crohn's disease, and patients with pancreatic pseudocysts have been shown to benefit from total parenteral nutrition. Elderly patients who cannot swallow are better managed by enteral feedings provided through a feeding tube. (Ch. 51; pg 1085)

54. c

In general, the degree of obesity is directly correlated with comorbidity risk. The body mass index is a useful measure of obesity, but is calculated as the weight in kilograms divided by the square of the height in meters. Upper body fat is more of a risk factor for diabetes, hypertension, and ischemic heart disease than lower body fat. Men more commonly have upper body obesity compared to women. (Ch. 22; pg 506)

55. a

Only a minority of cases of "food allergy" are immune-mediated. Many are the result of food intolerance from a variety of nonimmunologically mediated causes. Most cases of immunologic food allergy are IgE-mediated, causing an immediate-type hypersensitivity as a result of the degranulation of mass cells. Most food allergens are small (<70 kd) and are heat- and acid-stable. Skin testing or food challenges in patients with severe anaphylactic reactions can be dangerous. In vitro tests for antigen-specific IgE (e.g., RAST) may be helpful in these cases. (Ch. 112; pg 2554)

True/False

56. false

Intravenous infusions of fats should be administered with caution to patients with sepsis, as fats may impair host defense mechanisms. (Ch. 51; pg 1088)

57. false

Crypt and villus cells are capable of both absorption and secretion. (Ch. 15; pg 320)

58. true

Without bile acids, micellarization is severely compromised. However, unless pancreatic secretion is inhibited, lipolysis proceeds normally, and subsequent triglyceride malabsorption is relatively mild in patients with total biliary obstruction. (Ch. 19; pg 449)

59. false

Cholesterol is absorbed across the brush border by passive diffusion. (Ch. 19; pg 437)

60. false

Patients without apolipoprotein B cannot assemble or secrete triglycerides from enterocytes or liver. Small bowel biopsy specimens reveal fat-filled enterocytes. (Ch. 19; pg 446)

61. true

Only 50% of dietary cholesterol is absorbed, and this rate of absorption appears to be unrelated to the hyperlipidemic phenotype or circulating low-density lipoprotein cholesterol levels. (Ch. 19; pg 437)

62. false

Human studies have demonstrated that lactase activity cannot be maintained or induced by a continued feeding of lactose. Treatment of lactase deficiency includes avoidance of dietary lactose or the administration of supplemental lactase with meals. (Ch. 75; pg 1688)

63. true

Although the intestinal transport of several essential amino acids can become defective in some disease states, the development of nutritional deficiencies is minimized by the capacity of the intestine to absorb amino acids in the form of dipeptides and tripeptides. (Ch. 20; pg 461)

64. true

The rate-limiting step in the assimilation of dietary sucrose and glucose is transport across the apical membrane of the enterocyte. This is in contrast to the assimilation of lactose, which is limited by the availability of hydrolase activity. (Ch. 18; pg 422)

65. false

In hypokalemia or starvation, serum magnesium levels may be normal in the presence of tissue depletion. The diagnosis of zinc deficiency is difficult, because plasma levels do not reflect total body stores. (Ch. 21; pg 478)

66. false

Dietary proteins are largely cleaved to oligopeptides by proteases secreted by the stomach and pancreas. Membrane-bound oligopeptidases on the intestinal brush border then cleave the oligopeptides further to free amino acids as well as dipeptides and tripeptides. (Ch. 20; pg 457)

67. false

Free amino acids, dipeptides, and tripeptides are transported across the brush border membrane into small bowel enterocytes. (Ch. 20; pg 460)

68. false

High proline contents in proteins such as gluten or casein reduce their digestibility. (Ch. 20; pg 460)

69. false

All of the pancreatic proteases are synthesized, stored in zymogen granules, and secreted as inactive precursors. (Ch. 20; pg 459)

70. true

Exocrine pancreatic insufficiency is by far the most common cause of defective intralumenal proteolysis. Chronic pancreatitis and malignancy are the most common causes of exocrine pancreatic insufficiency. (Ch. 20; pg 463)

71. false

A variety of neurotransmitters and hormones released both centrally and peripherally are responsible for the complex process of satiation. (Ch. 22; pg 506)

72. true

The resting energy expenditure does decrease with reduced caloric intake and may contribute to the difficulty of achieving and maintaining weight loss. (Ch. 22; pg 508)

73. true

Pharmacotherapy can be effective in helping patients achieve clinically important weight loss. Unfortunately, even with continued drug use, weight loss usually plateaus and weight gain may resume. (Ch. 22; pg 511)

74. false

Patients with trypsinogen deficiency present in early infancy with failure to thrive, hypoproteinemia, and edema. (Ch. 20; pg 463)

75. false

Only monosaccharides can be absorbed into enterocytes by a combination of passive diffusion, active transport, and facilitated diffusion. (Ch. 18; pg 416)

76. false

Protein digestion begins in the stomach with the release of gastric pepsinogen. (Ch. 20; pg 457)

77. true

Administration of a single preoperative dose of an intravenous cephalosporin minimizes the infectious complications associated with percutaneous endoscopic gastrostomy. (Ch. 127; pg 2830)

78. true

Although the duration of dependence on total parenteral nutrition (TPN) is variable, patients without residual colon require at least 60 cm of viable small intestine to avoid permanent TPN. With preservation of an intact colon, 30 to 50 cm of residual small intestine may be sufficient to allow weaning a patient from TPN. (Ch. 77; pg 1711)

79. false

Medium-chain triglycerides are directly absorbed into the portal circulation and are rapidly used as a fuel source. Because they can be absorbed in the absence of bile salts, medium-chain triglycerides can be used as a caloric supplement in patients with short bowel syndrome in whom there is malabsorption of long-chain fatty acids. (Ch. 77; pg 1713)

80. false

Severe metabolic bone disease developing during total parenteral nutrition is multifactorial and involves a negative calcium balance induced by organic acids contained in the total parenteral nutrition solution, as well as possible aluminum toxicity. (Ch. 51; pg 1089)

81. true

Salivary and gastric R proteins avidly bind dietary vitamin B_{12}. These R proteins must be degraded before intrinsic factor can bind the vitamin B_{12} and intestinal absorption can occur. This process is impaired if pancreatic proteolytic enzymes are not available to cleave the peptide bond linking the R protein to vitamin B_{12}. (Ch. 40; pg 892)

82. false

The only acceptable management of food allergy is avoidance of the offending food. (Ch. 112; pg 2557)

83. true

Lumenal bacteria, particularly anaerobic species, compete with the host for uptake of cobalamin–intrinsic factor complexes. The production of inactive, nonabsorbable cobalamin analogs by lumenal bacteria also impairs the intestinal absorption of cobalamin. In contrast, folate is produced by bacteria during fermentation and becomes available for intestinal absorption and use by the host. This produces the commonly observed pattern in bacterial overgrowth of vitamin B_{12} deficiency in the presence of folate excess. (Ch. 75; pg 1686)

84. false

Seventy-five percent to 95% of lumenal protein is absorbed by the small intestine despite the multiple steps required for processing. The lumenal proteins are initially acted upon by gastric factors and pancreatic enzymes, followed by brush-border enzymes. The majority of this protein is derived from dietary sources (70 to 100 g/day); endogenous secretions (20 to 30 g/day) and desquamated epithelium (20 to 30 g/day) constitute the remainder. Only about 1 to 3 g/day of protein enters the colon. (Ch. 20; pg 458)

85. false

Animal proteins are more readily digested and more efficiently absorbed than plant proteins. (Ch. 22; pg 492)

86. true

Dietary sources of vitamin B_{12} are ultimately derived from bacterial and protozoal sources. However, mammalian tissues concentrate vitamin B_{12}, and the consumption of meat and eggs provides an adequate dietary source of this vitamin. The body stores of vitamin B_{12}, (2 to 3 g) far exceed the daily requirement of 0.5 to 1.0 mg/day. (Ch. 21; pg 469)

87. true

Increases in γ-glutamyltransferase, lactate dehydrogenase, alanine aminotransferase, aspartate aminotransferase, and cholesterol levels often occur in patients with anorexia nervosa, as do decreases in serum proteins, albumin, globulins, and blood sugar. The liver chemistry abnormalities are secondary to steatosis or nonspecific periportal infiltrates and usually require no further evaluation. (Ch. 34; pg 767)

Matching

88. c

Zinc deficiency can occur as a result of diarrhea. (Ch. 51; pg 1095)

89. d

Thiamine deficiency can result from decreased oral intake and is common in chronic alcoholics. (Ch. 51; pg 1096)

90. a

Vitamin A is a fat-soluble vitamin and can be deficient in fat-malabsorptive diseases such as pancreatic insufficiency. (Ch. 51; pg 1100)

91. b

Vitamin K deficiency can occur with fat malabsorption. However, because bacteria in the intestine synthesize it, deficiencies can occur with broad-spectrum antibiotic use. (Ch. 51; pg 1101)

92. c

Chylomicrons are synthesized in the intestine and are the primary mode of transport for dietary triglycerides. (Ch. 19; pg 443)

93. d

Very-low-density lipoproteins are synthesized in the liver and are the primary transport vehicle for endogenously formed triglycerides. (Ch. 19; pg 443)

94. a

Low-density lipoproteins primarily consist of cholesterol esters and are the major transporters of cholesterol. (Ch. 19; pg 443)

95. b

Both the intestine and the liver synthesize high-density lipoproteins. (Ch. 19; pg 443)

96. a

97. b

98. a

99. b

100. a

101. b

Folate, vitamin K, and zinc are absorbed primarily in the proximal small intestine. Cobalamin, magnesium, and calcium are absorbed primarily in the more distal small intestine. (Ch. 21; pgs 468, 470, 474, 477, 479)

102. c

103. e

104. a

105. f

106. b

107. d

The classic symptoms of micronutrient deficiency are as listed. (Ch. 51; pg 1090)